THERAPY OF STUTTERING

THERAPY OF STUTTERING

Preschool through Adolescence

RICHARD E. HAM, Ph.D.

Professor, Speech/Language Pathology
Florida State University, Tallahassee, FL

Professor Emeritus, Hearing and Speech Sciences
Ohio University, Athens, OH

PRENTICE HALL, Englewood Cliffs, New Jersey 07632

Library of Congress Cataloging-in-Publication Data

Ham, Richard,
    Therapy of stuttering, preschool through adolescence / Richard
Ham.
        p.   cm.
    Bibliography: p.
    Includes index.
    ISBN 0-13-914748-9
    1. Stuttering in children--Treatment. 2. Speech therapy for
children.   I. Title.
RJ496.S8H34 1989
616.85'54--dc19   89-30330
                                                         CIP

Editorial/production supervision
  and interior design: **Mary Kathryn Leclercq**
Cover design: **Photo Plus Art**
Manufacturing buyer: **Peter Havens**

© 1990 by Prentice-Hall, Inc.
A Division of Simon & Schuster
Englewood Cliffs, New Jersey 07632

Printed in the United States of America
10 9 8 7 6 5 4 3 2 1

ISBN   0-13-914748-9

Prentice-Hall International (UK) Limited, *London*
Prentice-Hall of Australia Pty. Limited, *Sydney*
Prentice-Hall Canada Inc., *Toronto*
Prentice-Hall Hispanoamericana, S.A., *Mexico*
Prentice-Hall of India Private Limited, *New Delhi*
Prentice-Hall of Japan, Inc., *Tokyo*
Simon & Schuster Asia Pte. Ltd., *Singapore*
Editora Prentice-Hall do Brasil, Ltda., *Rio de Janeiro*

To dedicate in the literary sense is to recognize things, persons, or causes with affection and respect because of their significance. In 1952 I was assigned my first stutterer. A year later I was given my first assistant to train, beginning a long line of student clinicians that continues to this day. During this time, my introduction to stuttering came from Charles Elliot, followed by one Charles Van Riper—followed by many other mentors and colleagues who have influenced me over the years. Certainly, "affection and respect" describe my feelings toward the stutterers, the student clinicians, and the colleagues I have known. Also circa 1952 I met a young woman whom I married in 1953. For 35 years she has asked, "How was your day?" and listened to my answers. To all these sources, and particularly to Ann, my wife, this book is dedicated—with affection and respect.

CONTENTS

PREFACE

If stuttering has been one of the most perplexing of clinical problems in the field of communication disorders, stuttering among children has become a relatively recent addition to the dimensions of that perplexity. With approximately 35 years of experience in therapy of stuttering, the author has seen therapy with children occupy significant attention only during the latter half of that period. This book is an effort to present some of the approaches currently involved in therapy, approaches that we are still sorting among—much as we sort through the box of souvenirs collected over years of vacations. We are not sure what to retain, what to discard, what to combine, and exactly what to do with all that we keep. An effort is made in this book to provide information to help in making decisions, but in many instances the research data to suggest decisions is lacking and the decision making must be left to the perceptions and talents of individual clinicians.

Initial chapters of this book review concerns and information relative to our definitions of fluency and of stuttering, showing that we start off with some confusion, controversy, and information deficits. Theories of stuttering are reviewed, more in anticipation of "resolution someday" than in settlement, although the author expounds his biases. Evaluation is covered in some detail, but not in terms of recommending one outline or form that diagnosis and assessment should follow. Instead, multiple points or possibilities are covered, more than most clinicians will have the time or inclination to utilize. This organization allows the clinician to review possible measures and procedures, and then those applicable across different situations. Evaluation is followed by a short chapter discussing preparation for and planning of therapy. The chapter is deliberately short because it would otherwise overwhelm the book, causing other areas to lose coverage. The rest of the book, the bulk, is devoted to various procedures and methods of therapy. With few exceptions, total programs of therapy are avoided, since they are available from other sources. Research concerning various approaches is reviewed, but more for indicative trends than to resolve issues and draw conclusions. In most instances the research is too sparse to allow decisions, even if its adequacy were such as to encourage resolution. The reader will also find repetitive occurrences of the controversies between fluency reinforcement therapy and symptom modification therapy where belligerency and diplomacy often collide. In general, efforts are made here to provide enough information for the reader to understand what each method or procedure involves and to provide reference citations if greater depth is desired. Some portions of the text are written in how-to form, but many areas are limited to a range of descriptions for reader evaluation.

As much as possible, application sections are distributed across three age groups. These age groups comprise preschool children, early school children, and adolescent school children. This application, along with technique overlaps, results in a fair amount of redundancy at times. However, rather than constantly referring the reader back to chapter so-and-so, the author has committed the redundancies and hopes the reader will agree with that decision. It is assumed that readers are familiar with normal development and age stages, as well as having had typical courses in foundation areas of communication and disordered communication. In such a context, this text will serve as an orientation to therapy among stuttering children and as a continuing reference during future professional activity.

Finally, I wish to thank the reviewers of this book: Peter R. Ramig, University of Colorado; Robert L. Casteel, Portland State University; and Raymond Quist, Indiana State University.

Richard E. Ham

THERAPY OF STUTTERING

CHAPTER ONE
THE STUTTERING PROBLEM

SECTION INTRODUCTION

This first of three sections considers some of the information and the speculations concerning stuttering. The second section of this book discusses diagnosis and assessment of stuttering. The third, and longest, section deals with therapy of stuttering.

In order to discuss the information and procedures covered in the second and third sections, it will help here to survey basic information about stuttering, review definitional problems surrounding stuttering, and consider the differences between dysfluency and disfluency. In the process of this survey and consideration, the reader may feel that we "don't know a whole lot about much," and what we do know frequently seems to need revision or amendment. This is true! However, we have learned a great deal about the subject, and the information input from clinicians is constant. If we set retrospective points and look back, we are surprised at how much we have gained rather than frustrated over how much we have yet to find out.

OVERVIEW

Speech and language disorders often are what society declares them to be. The lisping quality of Castilian Spanish supposedly is the result of a royal lisp which became "normal," since it was easier for a whole population to lisp than for a king not to. Regional dialects, a disappearing factor today, were once inescapable classifications and part of insular attitudes. Today, and in more specific terms, the clinician often has to decide at what point a phoneme production is in error, a resonance is undesirable, or a vocal quality is unacceptable. A number of speech-rating scales have statements equivalent to "Production error that would not be obvious to a layperson." This problem of definition can be a vexing one, and so it will be discussed in the next section. It will also be reviewed further in the chapter on diagnosis and assessment.

Concomitant with problems in defining fluency and stuttering is the difficulty we have in accounting for stuttering. Theories of stuttering tend to be rather like disreputable relatives—they are inevitable and unavoidable, but it really isn't courteous to talk about them! Most clinicians function either in an atheoretic frame of reference or glibly state, "I'm an eclectic when it comes to theory" and change the subject. As a result, therapy tends to be applied pragmatically rather than with reference to a theory basis. In the next chapter, we will look at recent theory history and where we are (or seem to be) going in terms of stuttering theory.

After discussing incidence and prevalence in stuttering, this chapter considers the behaviors thought to be associated with stuttering on a typical developmental pattern. This leads to a discussion of efforts to establish "tracks" for the development of stuttering. This is followed by a summary of what has been said with reference to definition, behaviors, and tracks, and at this point the reader is prepared for the following chapter on theories.

DEFINITIONS

Fluency and Other Terms

Before discussing a definition of stuttering, it is useful to consider what we mean by *fluency* and what the two terms *disfluency* and *dysfluency* imply. By way of explanation before discussion, initial "use" definitions might be the following:

- **fluent**—the speech of people who do not stutter; the nonstuttered speech of stutterers.

- **disfluent**—the nonfluent speech of people who do not stutter; the nonstuttered, nonfluent speech of people who do stutter.
- **dysfluent**—the stuttered speech of stutterers; the stuttered speech of people who do not stutter usually.

Please note that the preceding were stipulated as "use" definitions. All of the applications can be found in various texts and references in our profession and are drawn from statements such as the following:

- Most stutterers are fluent most of the time.
- All speakers exhibit normal nonfluencies (disfluencies) on occasion.
- Most people report having stuttered at times.
- Stutterers (dysfluent) typically produce normal nonfluencies (disfluent) as they talk.

The point made here is that we have variable fluency in stutterers and in nonstutterers both, and our terminology tends to confuse further an already confusing situation.

The term *fluency* is derived from the Latin root *fluere*. It refers to many things but seems to relate, in communication, to the smooth and easy flow of utterance (Stein 1967). Unfortunately, we have not defined what "smooth and easy flow" really means. If it means to be without irregularity or perturbation, then no one is ever consistently fluent. Fluency, after all, is a perceptual judgment subject to the criteria of listener and speaker, the demands of the situation, and the requirements of the linguistic unit. Different listeners, and different speakers, can have different expectations for fluency as words are uttered. On another basis, one expects casual conversational speech to carry a different level of fluency than would a formal report. The same message delivered to different auditors can carry different fluency expectations, for instance, a clinician describing his or her workload to a colleague, to a supervisor, or to a meeting of the school board. Other factors may also affect fluency. We can define fluency strictly in terms of mechanical elements such as production accuracy, rhythm, timing, and stress. We can also define fluency in terms of the clarity of the information, the rapport between speaker and listener, and the response of listeners.

In considering stuttering, fluency has often been defined only in the "production accuracy" elements mentioned. However, problems occur when fluency disruptions are separated into disfluency and dysfluency. Adams (1984a) comments that our historical failure to achieve normal fluency in stutterers may be a result, at least partially, of our inexact and incomplete understanding of how speakers produce normally fluent output (and what normally fluent output is). Wingate (1984a, 1984b) has criticized careless and ambiguous use of the terms *fluency, disfluency,* and *dysfluency.* He states that fluency should be our basic referent so that *dis-* or *dys-* are definable in terms of how they depart from the suffix. This is a laudable desire, but one frequently disappointed. Most often it seems that we find fluency defined in terms of how it deviates from the prefixes, that is, what it is not rather than what it is. Wingate also criticized the misuse of *disfluency* where the prefix indicates speech features that are the opposite of fluency, and *dysfluency* in which the prefix should refer to an abnormal fluency condition. Wingate may be correct in that *normal dysfluencies* is contradictory, and *stuttering disfluencies* is at least confusing. Common use becomes muddied, since dysfluent stutterers will also have disfluent (nonstuttered) utterances and so-called fluent speakers can have moments of dysfluency. It is not clear how disfluency and dysfluency separate from each other, especially since some evaluations count all fluency failures without trying to differentiate between *dys-* and *dis-*.

Starkweather (1986, 1981) has made notable contributions to fluency and fluency disruption concepts. He has drawn together much of the relevant research on fluency development, normal disfluency parameters, and stuttering dysfluency to suggest parallels, observe incongruities, and raise pointed questions. Much of the material in the following paragraphs is a summary, rephrasing, reaction to, and extension of his thoughts expressed in *The Development of Fluency in Normal Children* (Starkweather 1986) in publication 20 of the Speech Foundation of America (SFA) (P.O. Box 11749, Memphis, Tennessee 38111).

To begin with, Starkweather suggests that there are three basics in speech fluency:

- RATE of utterance.
- CONTINUITY from moment to moment of utterance.
- EFFORT or ease, cognitively and physically, of production.

These three characteristics will be continuously and variably affected by ongoing and shifting factors such as information load, predictability of utterances, and situational factors.

Continuity reflects the smooth movement from phoneme to phoneme, between syllables, across words, and from phrase to phrase. Probably all of us know or have observed speakers who are distracting to listen to because their speech fails to flow smoothly. The significant disruptor of normal continuity is the hesitation. Pauses occur in two forms, *filled* or *unfilled.* An unfilled pause is a silent hesitation, while a filled pause is a vocalized hesitation. Hesitations also include false starts and retrials, repetitions of one's own or others' utterances, and parenthetical remarks or asides that delay the main utterance. Hesitations may occur for a variety of reasons:

- As a failure to hear or comprehend a statement or question.
- As a planned or practiced pause to create a dramatic effect or call attention to a stressed word or thought.
- As a listening device to encourage further utterance from the first speaker.
- As a tactic to allow time to formulate the cognitive and/or linguistic content and sequence of the next utterance.
- As a method of preplanning the neuromotor production sequence of speech sounds.
- As an avoidance device to delay the onset of utterance where problems in production, content acceptability, or auditor reaction are anticipated.

Everybody pauses, and does so frequently. Everybody, every day, pauses for all the reasons just cited. Starkweather points out that continuity and hesitation patterns show that from kindergarten through twelfth grade, the average frequency of "vocal hesitations" (filled pauses) decreases by about 2 percent only. However, when the type of vocal hesitation is plotted, there is a steady decrement of certain types and an increase in one type. In a summary of discontinuities (see Figure 1-1), he reported that from kindergarten (K) to twelfth grade (12) the following occurred:

FIGURE 1-1. Developmental fluency discontinuities of children, K–12. (Adapted from Starkweather, 1986.)

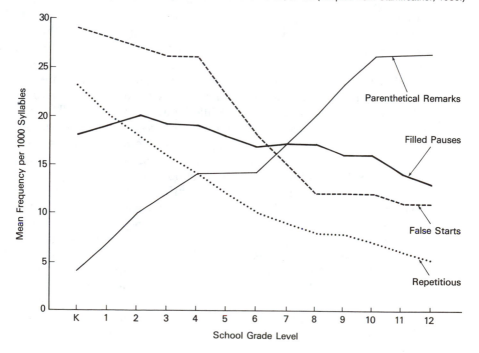

- Filled pauses dropped about 65 percent from their highest point.
- False starts dropped about 62 percent.
- Repetitions dropped about 78 percent.
- Parenthetical remarks increased by about 85 percent from their lowest level.

There is the suggestion that as we mature, our frequency of hesitation discontinuities decreases only slightly. However, we adroitly fill the time by more sophisticated forms of delay. Starkweather suggests that even though we do show some maturation in our planning resources and skills, the primary change is to a more sophisticated "filler" to allow for adequate response planning time.

Rate is typically measured in terms of words or syllables per minute. Overall rate will be affected by the length of words used, by word familiarity, message significance, situational concerns, and other factors. Sentence or phrase rate can differ significantly from overall rate as we slow down or speed up utterances. Other affecting factors include physiological considerations, the sound or sound sequence being produced, coarticulation effects within units, duration of utterance, and prosodic stress points. Starkweather notes that as children mature, their syllable rates increase while rate variability decreases. He suggests that pauses may help us in achieving faster intraphrase rates by creating brief planning intervals to prepare for rapid motor execution on the subsequent sequence. He questions a tendency to regard all or most pauses as disfluencies, since they actually may be very appropriate planning intervals, and he suggests that duration of pauses, rather than frequency, might be a disfluency criterion. This is reasonable, up to a point. Starkweather refers to Kowal, O'Connell, and Sabin (1975) who reported that by the second grade, unfilled (silent) pause durations decreased by about 60 percent, while the pause duration reduction from second through twelfth grades is only about 25 percent. The duration of unfilled pauses related well to the number of syllables that followed. Caution is necessary because we do not know to what degree pause duration represents language planning, motor-sequencing plans, other factors, or combinations. Also, Kowal, O'Connell, and Sabin warned that at early school ages the standard deviation is so wide that judgmental decisions are difficult to make accurately.

Rhythm, as an aspect of rate and continuity, is determined by the pattern of stress and unstress in syllable production. Stress points in utterances tend to follow predictable patterns based on "law and custom" of a particular language. Indeed, listeners' intuitive judgments of stress have been found to be related adequately to objective measures of stress (Wingate 1984c). Rate changes relate to stress points in that we tend to slow syllable rate prior to a stress point and then increase syllable rate following it. It is possible that the prestress rate reduction is an example of intraphrase planning activity. Most of our extra addition in the form of gestures, loudness, pitch variations, and so on, tend to occur at or around stress points in utterances.

Effort refers to the ease with which an act is performed. Although speech may require considerable attention in our formative years, the reverse is true at mature ages. "In normal speakers, very little thought is devoted to speech production. It runs mostly on automatic pilot" (Starkweather 1986, p. 94). This author would observe that the content of many responses also tends to follow an automatic course. Many speakers repeat or paraphrase utterances they have used before, learned from parents, or heard in use by peers and pundits. Some utterances are so prescribed that they are totally automatic and are delivered with minimal cognitive attention or awareness. Effort can, therefore, be neuromuscular in the timing and coordination of respiration, phonation, and articulation, using the formula of 14 phonemes per second multiplied by 100 muscles involved per sound production, multiplied by 100 motor units per muscle (Darley, Aronson & Brown 1975). Effort can also be mental in terms of formulating the content of a response and arranging content in an appropriate syntactic sequence. We know that cortical activity (evidenced by alpha wave alteration) occurs prior to utterance, and the extrapyramial unit (cerebellum, thalamus, basal ganglia) initiates impulses prior to the onset of cortical activity. Research suggests that planning and execution are different activities, and Starkweather stated that pauses can be related to fluency, as follows:

1. If pauses are prolonged unduly, but production meets the criteria—there is a planning disfluency.
2. If pauses are appropriate in place and duration, but the production is erroneous—there is an execution disfluency.
3. If pauses are inappropriate or prolonged unduly, and the production also is in error—there is a combined planning and execution disfluency.

Starkweather discusses effort and relates it to continuity, rate, rhythm, and stress. He notes that gestures may possibly reduce effort, on the idea that "entrained" movements reflect the stress characteristics of the primary movement sequence, or utterance. He refers to research where finger tapping in time with syllable production disclosed a more forceful finger tap when an uttered syllable was stressed (Kelso, Tuller & Harris 1983).

It is possible that fluency disorders typically are reflections of, or effects of, abnormal effort in planning and/or execution. "It is tempting to suggest that fluency is ease of speech, and that continuity and rate are observable results of it" (Starkweather 1986, p.70). On this basis, a fluency disorder could result from a problem in planning or execution, and the discontinuities we observe are, on the one side, overt symptoms of planning errors and, on the other side, the results of efforts to compensate for these errors. Starkweather has proposed the following as a tentative disfluency definition (p.98):

> Fluency is deviant when speech is produced with effort, when speech is more discontinuous than normal, or when the discontinuities are immature, when the rhythm of speech is atypical, or when it is not serving the speaker by making the speech production easier.

The writer would recast Starkweather's definition, as follows:

> Fluency is deviant when planning and/or execution effort is excessive, when discontinuities occur at a frequency and/or to a degree inappropriate for speaker age, or when speech rhythm is atypical or occurs in such a way as to impede or disrupt the speech production.

The preceding cannot be final definitions of fluency disruption, if for no other reason than that we still have so much more to find out about fluency itself. Also, as we will see in the section on definitions of stuttering, there is a problem as to when a fluency deviation can be called stuttering. Finally, the reader is urged to return to this section for review when the section "Linguistic Considerations" is reached in the Chapter 2 discussions on theory.

Incidence and Prevalence

Certain word pairs create problems for us, as we must know when to use which word. The pairs *lie/lay*, *lead/led*, *effect/affect* and *appraise/apprise* cause problems combining meaning and phonology. However, we also tend to confuse pairs such as *acute/severe* and *hereditary/acquired*. A similar confusion occurs with the words *incidence* and *prevalence*. Therefore, a brief definition is in order:

* **Incidence**—throughout the population considered, how frequently does the factor ever occur?
* **Prevalence**—throughout the population considered, how frequently does the factor continue?

The linkage between incidence and prevalence is duration. The incidence of stuttering is based on the question of whether or not a person has ever been diagnosed or labeled as being a stutterer. Prevalence of stuttering reflects the information as to how many persons continue to stutter, either over time in general or within a particular age range.

In general, population prevalence is usually pegged at about 1 percent. Enderby and Philipp (1986) reviewed various reports and estimated (in the United Kingdom) an incidence of approximately 3.5 percent and a prevalence of 1.07 percent. This excluded fluency problems accompanying mental handicap, diabetes, brain damage, and other primary disorders. In the so-called thousand families study (Andrews et al. 1964), data were collected from 1947 to 1962. The highest risk level for stuttering, about 50 percent, occurred between 3 and 4 years of age, and it had dropped to 25 percent by 5 to 6 years of age. In general, the prevalence figure was slightly over 1 percent. Porfert and Rosenfield (1978) used a questionnaire form with 2,107 subjects about 21 years of age. Subject to the serious factor of subjects' memories, they found that 2.1 percent considered themselves to be stutterers, 3.4 percent reported past stuttering, and 1.3 percent fell into the category of "doubtful stutterers." It was suggested that socioeconomic characteristics may have affected the results. A review of a number of studies on stuttering incidence, taking median of their ranges, places stuttering incidence near the 5 percent figure.

If we consider the total population, incidence estimates cluster around 5 percent, and prevalence estimates cluster around 1 percent. After next considering briefly the sex factor in stuttering, the section following introduces an added figure that confuses these tentative incidence and prevalence figures.

Sex

Estimates of the sex differential factor, where more males than females stutter, range around a 3 : 1 to 4 : 1 ratio (Andrews et al. 1983; Brady & Hall 1976; Gillespie & Cooper 1973). Explanations over the past 30 years have focused on learning theory compatibility explanations and suggested that female children were more sheltered, were subject to lower parental expectations, met less peer pressure, and so forth. It has also been pointed out that females at birth are more developed neurologically than are males and generally develop speech and language at earlier ages on the developmental continuum. Yairi (1983) used parents' reports and stated the sexes, at two to three years of age, were about the same in stuttering occurrences. It was suggested that spontaneous recovery (see later) in the females occurred at earlier ages and more quickly, which might explain the overall imbalance (but not the reason).

Spontaneous Recovery

Spontaneous recovery, from anything, refers to the achievement of or return to normalcy without the intervention of outside agents. Since stuttering incidence drops sharply after 9 to 11 years of age, we are interested in the recovery rate and its effect on statistics. Estimates of spontaneous recovery have ranged from below 40 percent to over 80 percent! Van Riper (1982) summarized the results of eight recovery studies. He reported they averaged 63.48 percent, with a range from 17.8 to 94 percent. Wingate (1976) devoted 53 pages of text to stuttering remission, covering early and more recent studies. He cited problems with data completeness, design adequacy, and other limiting factors. Overall, Wingate found a recovery occurrence of 42 percent to be typical. Ingham (1984), also, provides an extensive review of spontaneous recovery and is critical of methodological procedures. He is particularly critical of studies that identified stutterers (usually by questionnaire) without sampling or cross-checking the results. Ingham inserts an interesting point—the extent to which many of the recoveries truly were "spontaneous." His evaluations and interpretations of various studies led him to suspect that the corrective efforts of family members and others, and the self-corrective efforts of some stutterers, in many ways parallel the relaxation, rate control, breathing revision, easy-onset, and other procedures of established therapy. This is noteworthy in view of Wingate's (1976) conclusion that "professional therapy is by no means necessary or sufficient to recovery from stuttering" (p.107). Ingham's (1984) conclusion is that the "putative unassisted" (p.76) recovery rate probably falls in the range of 30 to 50 percent (p. 76).

Definitions of Stuttering

Definitions of stuttering (dysfluency) have also had a difficult time. Ingham (1984) has discussed the problem of defining stuttering, reviewing a number of different approaches. He concludes that broken words, prolongations, and part-word repetitions on first sounds "are the disfluency types that typify most stuttering" (p. 19). However, he notes that each occurrence of these behaviors is not necessarily stuttering, and that as measures the occurrences themselves are not as valid as judgments made by listeners. Research has demonstrated that even untrained listeners can identify stutterers, even if they cannot agree consistently in identifying different stuttering events. Curlee (1985) avoids any definition at all of stuttering and, instead, writes about "disorders of fluency." In this context he also sidesteps a definition but identifies common "disfluency" types that may occur in stuttering, cluttering, neurologic, and psychiatric disorders and, at times, in normal speech. Van Riper (1978) attempted to define stuttering, stating that

> stuttering occurs when the forward flow of speech is interrupted abnormally by repetitions of a sound, syllable, or articulatory posture or by avoidance and struggle behaviors. (p.257)

This definition, in its specificity, omits certain speech and behavioral considerations that others might feel are requirements. In contrast, Shames and Florance (1982) seem to veer too far in the opposite direction of generality:

> Perhaps stuttering is best characterized as a problem that involves a cluster of a particular kind of speech behaviors, feelings, beliefs, self-concepts, and social interactions. (p. 189)

Unfortunately, this definition would also apply to articulation and phonatory disorders, language disturbances, alaryngeal speech, dysphasia, and other behaviors such as fear of public speaking. Wall and Myers (1984) depend upon Wingate (1964a) for referents, noting that

> the essence of a definition of stuttering consists of anomalies in the flow or rate of speech that are minimally distinguished by repetitions and prolongations, particularly of units of utterance smaller than a word. (p. 6)

As in the Van Riper definition earlier, this application seems to suffer from a constriction of referents and to omit factors or behaviors others might regard as being integral to stuttering.

Quite a few writers refer to Wingate's summation of stuttering characteristics (1964a) and to a definition based on these characteristics. The definition or summary breaks into several parts, with the first section covering the core spasm:

> Disruptions are involuntary and mostly uncontrollable. They occur frequently or are noticeable, and usually are in the form of vocal or nonvocal repetitions or prolongations. Occurrence loci usually are monosyllabic words, syllables, and sounds. (p. 488)

The reader will recognize that, to some extent, the occurrences described may be present in their own speech or in the speech of others not regarded as being stutterers. Also, these characteristics may occur in neuromotor, neurosymbolic, and psychiatric syndromes where they are not often regarded as stuttering. The second segment of Wingate's standard definition refers to what some have called mannerisms, associated behaviors, secondaries, and so on:

> There usually will be struggle activities during stuttering spasms. These usually will involve parts of the speech production mechanism, body areas associated with the speech act (e.g., gesture movements), and/or body areas uninvolved in speech (e.g., posture changes, foot movements). Stereotyped sound or word productions also may be involved. (p. 488)

Again, the reader may know of persons who produce inappropriate grimaces, jerks, tics, gestures, sounds, words, and phrases as part of their communication, but they are not identified as stutterers. Further, these behaviors can be associated with the abnormal, but nonstuttering, syndromes identified in the prior discussion. Wingate's third segment approaches the emotional aspects of stuttering:

There will be emotional states. These can be on a continuum that extends from a generalized anxiety or tension about speaking, to particular emotional feelings. (p.488)

As before, anxiety and tension over speaking occur in nonstutterers also. Specific emotional reactions and attitudes can occur in nonstutterers, and all these can also be present and associated with the dysfluencies of persons with neuromotor or psychiatric problems.

Overall, then, Wingate (1964) has not supplied a definition of stuttering. His excellent summary and collective description is just that—a summary and description. Definitions must supply the criteria by which apparently similar items can be excluded or included on the basis of differentiation referenced to the characteristics of the definition. This does not obtain in any of the definitions discussed thus far.

Perkins (1984) questioned the use of disfluency categories to define the presence of stuttering. Instead, he suggested that the word *involuntary* as a modifier of *disfluencies* was required before the disfluencies of normal speech can be differentiated from stuttering dysfluencies. Wingate (1984b) objected to this characterization, arguing that nonstuttering disfluencies were involuntary also, and that Perkins's criterion was inappropriate. Perkins (1984) replied to Wingate, proposing that the two clinicians were on different points of the semantic differential; he stated that normal disfluencies usually occur as disruptions in voluntary efforts to control fluency. This differentiation has characteristics of linguistic hair splitting and raises the question of whether Perkins actually meant that all stuttering spasms occur during a speaker's overt efforts to control speech. In view of current therapy procedures aimed at raising stutterer awareness and trying to increase self-monitoring skills and willingness, this proposition is quite doubtful. However, these disagreements illustrate the degree to which we lack commonly accepted referents on which to base a definition of stuttering.

Although there is a general lack of agreement on definition, as has already been pointed out, listeners are fairly accurate in identifying stuttering, even when the listeners are untrained and uninstructed. And so it has been suggested that stuttering is best defined as whatever a "reliable observer" calls stuttering and is generally agreed with as being stuttering. This is a semantogenic definition (stuttering is in the ear of the listener) and more or less says, "I may not understand stuttering, but I know it when I see it or hear it."

While writing these paragraphs the author was teaching a graduate class in stuttering and wondered how the class would respond to a "new" definition of stuttering, particularly since they had just finished a ten-week project in learning how to pseudostutter. Accordingly, the definition that follows was constructed and presented to them as a final project:

Stuttering is a syndrome characterized by involuntary disruptions in the on-going flow of speech, tending to occur on syllables or sounds in the form of clonic and/or tonic productions. Disruptions often are accompanied by stereotyped utterances, physical struggle, and distortions in parts of the speech mechanism and/or other body areas. There may be emotional reactions and behavior related to specific moments of stuttering, and attitude and behavior characteristics related to the condition of stuttering.

The definition was reviewed by the twenty students with the following results: Two students approved of the "stereotyped" usage, three objected that all speakers have stereotyped behaviors, and two others objected on other grounds; two students objected to "ongoing flow," feeling that it suggested that stutterer fluency was indistinguishable from nonstutterer fluency, and several objected on the basis that it suggested that everything prior to emission of stuttering was normal and/or ignored covert behaviors and problems; five students approved of the "emotional reactions and behaviors" statement (although one criticized it for being a run-on sentence), two felt it was too vague or insufficient, and one objected because covert and overt feelings were not distinguished; five students specifically approved of "syndrome" and nine specifically objected because to them it suggested connotations of "disease states"; five students specifically agreed with the modifier "involuntary," while eight objected to it, arguing that nonstutterers also suffer from involuntary disruptions and/or that truly involuntary disruptions would not be so easily amenable to fluency-inducing methods. Finally, seven students submitted their own original definitions of stuttering to replace the one offered! At the moment, this all might suggest that the "reliable observer" definition may be the most functional one we have.

It is quite probable that spontaneous recovery affects significantly the prevalence of stuttering statistics. One can also question the appropriateness of many of the "stuttering" labels placed on young children. If this is correct, and the degree rather than the idea probably is the only aspect open to question, then spontaneous recovery figures would drop considerably. Young (1975a) reviewed onset, prevalence, and recovery figures from various studies and introduced an additional question based on the following points:

1. Prevalence in the school-age population is about 1 percent.
2. Prevalence in the young-adult population is about 1 percent.
3. Incidence of stuttering, after age nine, drops to a near-nothing level.

The question becomes then, if spontaneous recovery is in the 60 to 80 percent range, and new stutterers rarely develop after nine years of age, why is the young adult prevalence nearly the same as that for school-age children? The answer possibilities should tend to cluster around interaction between corrected recovery figures and improved identification statistics. Nevertheless, the question is valid.

DEVELOPMENT OF STUTTERING

Under most conditions behavior is not static, particularly at early ages. As we develop and mature, so do our various behaviors. So do our feelings, attitudes, signal reactions, and autonomic responses. Behavioral changes are a mix of programmed responses, trial-and-error experiments, and cognitive planning. As these changes occur, major variations or oscillations tend to reduce and we move toward a more stable persona that other people come to identify as "you." This also is true in stuttering. Dysfluencies (and disfluencies) usually change as a result of altered motor skills, self-awareness, reactions to the dysfluencies, and reactions to the responses of others.

Numerous efforts have been made to organize developmental behaviors and describe stuttering evolution. Bluemel (1932) is one example with his early concept of primary stuttering in children and secondary stuttering in adults. Others also worked with early concepts of stuttering stages (Van Riper 1982), and some of the modern learning theories have described developmental stages. Van Riper (1982) inserted a transitional stage between primary and secondary, and subsequently a fourth category was used to cover developmental stuttering that still would not "fit." Van Riper stated that he had become uncomfortable with his stages of development, and he concluded that they had been "sheer folly" (p. 92) and that classification and therapy should be based on observed characteristics rather than on the confining rigidities of unbending categories. After reviewing client folders, Van Riper reported that a little over 90 percent of 44 longitudinal cases and about 77 percent of 300 shorter-term observations distributed over four broad tracks of development. He divided the four tracks, arranging them into onset summaries and into patterns of subsequent development. The adaptations that follow are drawn from his discussion (1982) on pages 95 through 105 and the summary tables on pages 106 and 107 of his text.

Onset and Early Development Tracks

Track 1—onset development   Children in this track begin speech development with apparent fluency, normal articulation and prosody, and a well-integrated speech pattern. Stuttering appears between 2.5 and 4.0 years of age, developing gradually. Speech errors will be primarily in the form of easy, unforced syllable repetitions tending to localize on initial and function words. Disruption periods will be cyclic, and there likely will be long remission periods. The child will have little or no awareness, not show frustration, and will not have speech fears or a reluctance to talk.

Track 1—subsequent development   Syllable repetitions increase in rate and frequency and lose their rhythmic pattern. Prolongations start to appear at the end of repetitive patterns, and they will show increasing tension and struggle. There will be a general overflow of tension and struggle that will develop into facial contortions and other struggle signs. Speech output decreases; retrials and other behaviors occur. As this track progresses, awareness develops into concern, speech output reduces, frustration shows, and embarrassment occurs. Word fears and avoidances develop and may progress to phoneme fears and situation fears. The dysfluencies may turn into tonic stoppages with struggle. Eye contact deteriorates and disguise tricks may be observed.

Track 2—onset development   The track 2 child also has had a gradual onset of stuttering, but occurring later, often not until the stage of sentence utterance has been reached. Development is steady, without remissions. Overall, the child was never very fluent, articulation is poor, and rate tends to be irregular and rapid. Syllable and word repetitions will be mixed with extended hesitations and revisions, but there will be little or no tension and tremor. Dysfluencies will locate on initial words, longer words, general distribution across a sentence, and on content words. These children will show more variable speech patterns, but will resemble track 1 in lacking awareness, fears, and frustration and in being willing to talk.

Track 2—subsequent development   As time passes, children in this track show less change and development in dysfluencies and behaviors. Frequency and rate of dysfluency increase, and long syllabic repetition strings develop. Awareness increases slowly and there is little development of situation fears, avoidance behaviors, sound/word fears, or loss of eye contact. There may be occasional situation fears that show some increase over time. In general, this person develops into an overt, rather uncomplicated stutterer who is willing to try to communicate.

Track 3—onset development   The child in this track will have started with fluency and, after establishing connected speech, will have had an acute onset of dysfluency, often after some type of trauma. The development pattern tends to be steady with a few, brief remissions. Articulation is normal. Pauses will be significant and there will be extensive tension, articulator tremors, laryngospasms, and silent prolongations, and the rate will tend to be slow. The dysfluency pattern will tend to be consistent, even though nonstuttererd speech will sound quite fluent. The person will be very aware of the problem, develop word and situation fears, and show obvious frustration.

Track 3—subsequent development   Maturation tends to be accompanied by sharp changes in stuttering severity, increases in bizarre forms, and extensive development of avoidances. Speech output reduces drastically, eye contact drops off, and nonstuttered speech becomes irregular and unsure. All these behaviors occur developmentally and take individualized forms.

Track 4—onset development   In this track, stuttering typically occurs after four years of age. There will be no remissions, even though there may have been a previous history of fluency, and the development will be erratic. Articulation and rate factors are usually normal. Van Riper suggests that these children are very aware of their stuttering and overt in it. It seems as if the stuttering individual watches the listener during dysfluencies, does not seem to be concerned, and may even back up and stutter on a previously fluent phrase. Stuttering occurs mainly on initial words, on content words, and not often on function words. The pattern usually is stable, there are few or no fears, nonstuttered speech is very fluent, and the child is talkative.

Track 4—subsequent development   As this person develops, stuttering shows few changes except to increase in frequency. Avoidance and release behaviors are not common, loci are inconsistent, and there are few fears. These people are talkative, open in their stuttering, and have good eye contact. Van Riper notes that such persons talk about the suffering and consequences of stuttering but seem to display few of the behaviors that would substantiate such feelings or effects.

Discussion of Development

For some, the establishment of criterion points, stages, levels, or tracks in stuttering is logical and appropriate. Brutten and Shoemaker (1967) discuss three stages of development in which the child comes to associate negative emotions with dysfluency occurrences and then extends these reactions to a broader range of stimuli. Bloodstein (1974) argued that anticipation, with associated emotional reaction and struggle, results in the spread and intensification of struggle. While disagreeing with the prediction-anticipation factor, Perkins (1980a) cited beginning and advanced forms of stuttering. He stated that "an overall pattern of development can be discerned" (p.57) and that though fluctuating, stuttering would not remain in the same form.

The sureness of development is considered by Wingate (1976), and he discusses suggestions by Brutten and Shoemaker (1967) and by Bloodstein (1961a) and the general concept of stuttering progression. Wingate objected, stating that progression concepts present stuttering only as becoming worse and do not provide for conditions of no-change, of fluctuation, or of improvement. Also, he objected to the idea that progression concepts "always" link age and severity together, that is, as we get older, we get worse. "In fact, we have absolutely no grounds for predicting either course or destination for any case of stuttering" (p.67). Wingate suggests we abandon development labels or stages and just talk in terms of simple or complicated patterns, with appropriate descriptions.

Wingate's criticisms appear to be an overreaction to the excesses of those who have been too rigid and too inclusive in their categories, and too inadequate in their substantiating data. Wall and Myers (1984) reviewed the tracks suggested by Van Riper (1982) and others, in addition to the six subtypes suggested by Luchsinger and Arnold in 1965 (clutter stutter subtype, organic brain syndrome subtype, familial psychoneurosis subtype, physiological and learning subtype, traumatic subtype, hysterical subtype). Wingate's (1976) criticisms (discussed in the previous paragraph) are also reviewed. In terms of Wingate's rejection of the "stuttering gets worse" view, Wall and Myers counter that this has been verified in "a good many" (p.66) of their clients. Of course, this does not speak to those who are not clients, never having been enrolled. They also point out that Bloodstein and Van Riper both issued cautions and subgroup qualifications in guarding against overly rigid categorization by stages.

There is no question, or there should not be, that most stutterers develop in their stuttering. The value of descriptive categories is noted, and the dangers admitted. A compromise between Wingate's descriptive approach and the rigidities of firm categories or tracks is appropriate.

CHAPTER SUMMARY

In this first chapter, a number of topics have been considered as we have looked at the problem of stuttering. It was pointed out that we have no adequate definition of speech fluency against which we can compare disfluency or the effects of therapy. However, research and development and speculation are active, and interesting possibilities in describing and defining fluency were pointed out. Starkweather's (1986, 1981) research and synthesis efforts seem to hold particular promise. As with fluency, definition of stuttering is in disarray. Definitions vary from the encyclopedic and cumbersomely inefficient to streamlined phrases of succinct crispness that result in too many exceptions for broad use. Although observers show overall agreement on what is and is not stuttering, specific judgments can be quite variable, and guidelines or definition information may complicate identification (Martin & Haroldson 1981). Indeed, progress toward a definition of stuttering seems to be retrograde at present as we explore the dysfluency/disfluency controversies, disagree over what is a disfluency or dysfluency, and consider possible stuttering subgroups.

The incidence and prevalence of stuttering was discussed and we find incidence and prevalence also is somewhat shaky. In general, round figures of 5 percent incidence in early years and a population prevalence of about 1 percent seem acceptable. These figures are clouded by data on spontaneous remission. Unfortunately, these data are not too clean overall and raise questions about the incidence and prevalence ratios. Spontaneous recovery was discussed, and the interesting possibility or question was raised that some or perhaps many, child stutterers (particularly those with mild problems) recover because their parents or they themselves apply some of the remedial procedures currently used in organized therapy.

As a final section, the developmental course of stuttering was examined. That stuttering, unlike most behaviors, does not develop, was not accepted. However, appropriate questions were raised about the absolute certainty of the timing, progressive sequence, and ultimate outcomes of development.

Although the discussions in this chapter have not shown many illuminative answers, they have indicated many developments and progressions in our understanding. These lights will lead us to the better answers that we seek. In the following chapter we will move from the how, when, and where of stuttering to ask the fascinating and frustrating question, Why?

CHAPTER TWO
THEORETIC
APPROACHES
TO STUTTERING

Reviews and discussions of theory abound in literature on stuttering. Van Riper (1982) provides exhaustive coverage. Rieber and Wollock (1977) and Rieber (1977) look particularly at our roots in theory and therapy, and Froeschels (1962) has a fascinating survey of European writing on stuttering, from the sixteenth up through the early twentieth centuries. Wall and Myers (1984) provide a useful, condensed sampling of major theory areas and, of particular interest, discuss the presumed therapy implications of each theory area. Shames and Rubin (1986) have provided an extended coverage of significant theories from recent decades past, presenting the theories in then-and-now contexts for the reader. Wingate's chapter in this reference is particularly valuable in discussing how theory popularity can overweigh the scientific method and objectivity.

Theory has been a difficult area in stuttering, because none of the theories have ever satisfied criteria of adequacy. Wingate (1976) wrote that current theories "are little more than favored speculative notions supported by partial observations, preferred facts, and contrived explanations" (p. 3). Ten years later, Perkins (1986) noted that the multiple varia-

19

tions in stuttering therapy reflect the uncertainty of our theoretical positions. Theories have tended to run in waves or cycles of predominance, with nonfavored, emergent, or recurrent theories struggling against the dominant theory. Prior to World War II, pathophysiological theories were dominant, followed in the 1940–60 era by theories stressing the interactive effects of the speaker and the environment in learning paradigms (psychosocial). This wave, in the 1960s, was joined by a sharp increase in applications of operant orientations and some cognitive psychology applications. As learning theory applications began to wane in the early 1970s (Adams 1984a), a resurgence of interest in pathophysiology theories developed. At the same time, linguistic formulations concerning stuttering began to develop clearer delineation, and the concept of stuttering subgroups finally began to achieve wider acceptance. Today, we have no encompassing theory, and there is a question of whether failure to develop a stable, overall theory will result in separation of stutterers into X numbers of subgroups with an onset theory to explain each subgroup and a more common theory to explain development and maintenance of stuttering.

THEORY REVIEW

Theories have been arranged or categorized under a variety of labels. In general, they subdivide into onset theories explaining the cause or causes of stuttering onset and development theories that deal with the evolution of stuttering after it has occurred. Some theories encompass both aspects. Johnson (1959) suggested that all theories subdivide into two types: (1) speech theories, where the focus is on the speaker and the speech and (2) interaction theories, where focus is on the interaction effects between speakers and auditors. Within the divisions of onset and development and speech and interactive theories, different writers have summarized theories in a variety of ways, and these different compilations will not be reviewed. In our review here, three general categories will be established: psychological, linguistic, and pathophysiological. Where appropriate, subcategories will be set as the individual theories are reviewed. It should be noted that the linguistic category is tentative, since it may appropriately belong under one, the other, or both of the other two categories.

PSYCHOLOGICAL THEORIES

The category of psychological theories exemplifies the confusions we have in stuttering theory. Some of the theories in the other two categories do not deny psychological significance in the development of stuttering, and others accept psychological factors as part of the precipitating possibilities. However, these theories do not propose psychological factors as the only etiological source of stuttering. In this section, psychological theories are subdivided into psychoanalytic theories and psychosocial theories.

Psychoanalytic Theories

In the first 40 years of this century, psychoanalytic theories of stuttering were prevalent, but in more recent times, interest in and acceptance of such orientations has reduced sharply. However, there continue to be adherents to psychoanalytic concepts of stuttering. It also must be stated that some psychoneurotics stutter, and some stuttering may have its roots in neurosis. At this point, a definition of neurosis is appropriate. Hoerr and Osol (1956) provide us with a clear definition:

> A neurosis is a group of reactions characterized by anxiety, which may be directly felt and expressed or unconsciously controlled by means of a defence mechanism, the recognition of which becomes the basis for the specific diagnostic terms applied. Psychoneurotics usually present a history of unusual difficulties in development related to special stress or deprivations in early life, which influence the form of the disorder in terms of symptoms and susceptibilities. (p. 983)

Thus, stuttering would be a symptom of an underlying neurosis, rather than being a primary disorder.

Travis (1971) theorized that desires and repressions surrounding eating, elimination, sexual behavior, and feeding create a conflict that can paralyze behavior. "Out of this soil stuttering flowers. Thoughts must not be thought; feelings must not be felt; and words must not be spoken" (1971, p. 1022). Coriat (1943) is famous for identifying stuttering as a perseveration of pregenital drives to oral nursing. Oral gratification in nursing is disrupted by weaning, and the stuttering tongue, lip, and jaw movements are symbolic nursing movements. On a different basis, Fenichel (1945) felt that stuttering was a conversion neurosis, not an oral perseveration, in which unacceptable anal sadism is transformed to oral "messing" in dysfluencies. As toilet training and social demands constrain the young child's bowel elimination behavior, a conversion to verbal soiling provides a more acceptable social form of aggression. A third explanation of stuttering was expressed by Glauber (1958), who argued that stuttering is the result of an id-ego-superego conflict. The presumably unspeakable feelings and thoughts of the id are suppressed or rechanneled by the superego, under normal conditions. However, when the control balance breaks down (superego over id), the conflict may be expressed in the ego-based function of speech. Id efforts to break through, and superego efforts to suppress, result in the jerking, interrupted patterns of stuttering.

A more subdued view has been expressed by Barbara (1965a, 1965b, 1962, 1954) in his extensive writings on stuttering. In his neoanalytic approach, the stuttering child typically is the result of inconsistent, perfectionistic, rigid, demanding parents. The resultant conflicts in the child's feelings are expressed in speech behavior. Other psychoanalytic theories exist and can be explored in some of the sources cited in the overview, of the theory section.

As noted earlier, current support for and interest in the neurosis theories is low. Curlee (1985) rejects psychogenesis as a cause in most stuttering, and Wall and Myers (1984) do not accept the idea that emotional disturbance is a valid stuttering etiology. Perkins (1983a) began with a personal psychoanalytic orientation but noted that about 90 percent of his clients improved in their self-feelings but not in their speech. Van Riper (1982) provides an extensive review of research relative to neurosis theories but fails to find general support, a view also shared by Shames and Florance (1982). Perkins (1980a) states that the results of research "leave considerable doubt about the validity of the psychoanalytic concept of stuttering" (p. 464). Beech and Fransella (1968) agree that, overall, studies do not support the concept of a "stuttering personality."

The reader should not conclude that no stutterers are neurotic, or vice versa. Similarly, it would be inappropriate to conclude that many stutterers do not have conflicts, anxiety levels, and behavior patterns associated with their communication difficulties. Andrews and others (1983) note that stutterers generally have more social adjustment problems than do nonstutterers, but they suggest that this is a result of stuttering, not a cause. Bloodstein (1969), reviewing many studies, concluded that stutterers seem to have higher levels of anxiety (and its physiological correlates) and signs of behavioral rigidity. Beech and Fransella (1968) corroborate the anxiety consideration and suggest that self-acceptance is lower. Fransella (1975) has proposed therapy based on personal construct theory, understanding how the stutterer sees the world in which she or he lives. Many other writers have made similar statements about the overall adjustment and feelings of stutterers, and it seems appropriate to offer the following thoughts: In general, stuttering cannot be regarded as a symptom of a clinical emotional disorder or as a communication disorder resulting from internal emotional etiologies. As a result of therapeutic targeting, emotional feelings and adjustment procedures alone often will not address or ameliorate adequately the dysfluencies and dysfluency behaviors of stutterers. However, evaluation and management procedures for stuttering ought to provide for the feelings, attitudes, and adjustment behaviors the stutterer may have developed over time.

Psychosocial Theories

Learning theories   Learning theories deal with the conditioning of responses. In Pavlov's experiments, presenting food to a dog resulted in salivation. When a bell was sounded at the same time the dog associated its ring with the food presentation and, subsequently, would salivate when a bell was the only stimulus. In stuttering, if speech disfluencies become associated with anxiety responses, then speech and anxiety can become associated through learning. Van Riper (1982) traces back to at least the eighteenth century the view that stuttering is learned, and then he follows the various "habit" trends up into the nineteenth century. He states that by about 1850, habit theories were widely accepted in this country. In the opening decades of the twentieth century, learning theories were pushed back by Freudian and other analytical theories that regarded stuttering as a neurosis. However, in the 1930s, persons such as Bluemel (1960, 1935, 1932) proposed conditioned learning theories, and Knight Dunlap's (1942, 1932) use of negative practice was an example of interest in stuttering and learning.

Regardless of the persistence of learning theories, the 1930s became noted for the rapid development of pathophysiology theories of onset (see later), whether or not learning factors were involved in subsequent development. However, Wendell Johnson began to move away from his initial acceptance of pathophysiology and, in 1942, published the early statement of what became known as the diagnosogenic or semantogenic theory of stuttering. In a group study of 46 stuttering children and controls, Johnson reached the conclusion that stuttering develops after diagnosis, or labeling, and not before (Johnson 1955). Johnson set off an explosion of research and theory development in stuttering—one which is still going on. In brief, his view was that parents may have inappropriately high demands for fluency and overly concerned or negative reactions to normal disfluencies. As the child produces normal disfluencies, receives negative reactions, becomes anxious and struggles, a reinforcing cycle of stuttering behavior begins. According to Bloodstein (1986), Johnson was influenced by the European speech pathologist Emil Froeschels, by Bluemel's (1932) development of the concept of primary and secondary stuttering, and by the so-called general semantics orientation organized by Alfred Korzybski (1933).

In this interactional, or evaluational, theory of stuttering, three aspects (Perkins 1980a) have been the focus of casting stuttering as learned behavior:

- **Adaptation**—unreinforced repetitions of a response will lead to a reduction (or extinction) of the response. Over time, or repeated readings, stuttering will decrease.
- **Consistency**—when a response is associated with a particular stimulus, the reoccurrence of that stimulus will tend to precipitate the same response. Stutterers tend to stutter on the same or similar words, in the same or similar situations.
- **Spontaneous Recovery**—after adaptation, a latency period of non-stimulation will result in recovery of the original response. Stuttering will reappear.

Research and evaluation of the adaptation and consistency tenets articulated by Johnson have shown that the close linkage between stuttering and learning hypotheses actually is variable, and the same hypotheses seem equally applicable to nonstuttered disfluencies (Williams, Silverman & Kools 1969a, 1969b; Wingate 1966a, 1966b).

The diagnosogenic theory, according to Shames (1986), was the most widely accepted theory to explain the cause of stuttering. It also stimulated other theorists (Bloodstein 1958; Williams 1957); and Bloodstein (1986) notes that Wischner, Sheehan, and others (see later) studied with Johnson. The theories now attributed to these others were reorganizations, revision, or differing emphases on basic learning theory tenets. Overall, the diagnosogenic theory has been very difficult to verify or disprove because the center or core of the theory (the parental mislabeling of normal disfluencies) will already have occurred by the time the labeled "stutterer" is evaluated professionally. Van Riper (1982) has expressed the opinion that the semantogenic theory is actually a rudimentary cognitive learning theory (as opposed to conditioning). He states that parental misperceptions and interpretations are the root cause of stuttering and that the subsequent events which we regard as learning theory examples are actually the results of cognitive factors or functions. Johnson's strictures against direct therapy with children have been rejected in theory and (partly) in practice. The majority of writers and researchers no longer accept a central role for diagnosogenesis. Although there still are adherents, and research still is stimulated, Bloodstein (1986) wrote perceptively in stating, "Theories of stuttering are seldom abandoned because they have been disproved. Most often we just get tired of them" (p. 138).

Oliver Bloodstein (1961a, 1960a, 1960b) differed from Johnson in proposing that stuttering occurred not as a result of efforts to avoid stuttering, but as an effect of tension and fragmentation. These, in turn, were the results of "the person's efforts to talk well in the conviction that speech is a difficult, formidable undertaking" (Bloodstein 1979, p. 136). Tension shows most in speech prolongations, hard attacks, and tonic stoppages; fragmentation is displayed mainly in clonic (repetitive) behaviors and in silence. Bloodstein assumed that early tension and fragmentation behaviors differ only in degree from normal childhood disfluencies. This continuity hypothesis provides a frame of reference for diagnosis by eliminating the problem of differentiating abnormal (stuttering) dysfluency from normal (developmental) disfluency. However, the point on the continuum at which disfluency becomes dysfluency is not predetermined, and it cannot be said absolutely that the "nonfluent" utterances of children are different only in degree and not in kind. Perkins (1980a) has noted that many stuttering events are apparently not preceded by either expectancy or anxiety on the part of the stutterers.

Joseph Sheehan (1958, 1953) also departed from Johnsonian precepts, applying learning theory concepts expressed by Dollard and Miller (1950). This application concerned the area of conflict resulting from stimuli that are competitive in their valences. All stimuli are presumed to have valences, positive or negative. For instance, deciding to watch a favorite TV program or to study class notes are examples of positive and negative valences. We tend to approach positive valence stimuli and to avoid negative valence stimuli. When we cannot decide between stimulus valences, or if they are mixed (as they often are), an approach-avoidance conflict may emerge. The more nearly equal competing approach drives are, the greater the conflict and oscillation will be. Sheehan cast stuttering as an approach-avoidance conflict in which the stutterer desires the success of oral communication but wants to avoid the penalty of possible stuttering. The conflict can actually be a "double approach-avoidance" in which the desires to talk and not talk are accompanied by desires to be silent and to avoid silence. Approach-avoidance conflicts, according to Sheehan, can occur at five levels: word, situation, emotional expression, interpersonal relations, ego protection. Vivian Sheehan (1986) expressed that Joseph Sheehan's original formulations remained stable but that he had expanded applications and concepts. Until his death in 1983, Sheehan had become noted for his vigorous, pungent, and unremitting opposition to therapies that he felt were superficial and concerned only with symptoms. His criticisms of operant theory and therapy were especially strong. Overall, research in support of Sheehan's basic theory model has been minimal. There is little reason to doubt that many stutterers experience approach-avoidance conflicts. However, support relative to onset or to omnipresence in stuttering development has not been extensive. Van Riper (1982) felt that Sheehan failed to answer adequately issues of "onset, development, sex ratio, loci, and many other basic features of the disorder" (p. 299).

George Wischner was another learning theory respondent to Johnson's theory. Wischner (1952, 1950) applied the principles of Hull (1951), where the reduction of anxiety reinforces the behavior that caused the reduction. In application to stuttering the following was proposed: Fear and anxiety over speech result in stuttering that terminates in successful completion of the word, and in reduction of the anticipatory anxiety and tension. In other words, stuttering reinforces stuttering. As did Johnson, Wischner assumed that initial childhood disfluencies were normal and misdiagnosed. However, where Johnson assumed that stuttering occurred through the child's efforts to avoid stuttering, Wischner proposed that the child was trying to avoid or reduce anxiety and other emotional feelings antecedent to the stuttering events. Any punishment for having produced attention-getting avoidance behaviors occurs subsequent to their occurrence and does not alter the anxiety reduction (reward) referred to earlier. Van Riper (1982) questioned the latter assumption, pointing out that self-punishment by the speaker can occur during the stuttering process and negate or vitiate any feelings of success through stuttering. He also applied to Wischner the same remarks quoted earlier concerning Sheehan.

The final example of basic learning theory applications to stuttering is that of Brutten and Shoemaker's (1967) two-factor learning theory. They proposed that classical conditioning operates as stuttering dysfluencies are associated with the negative reactions and feelings related to their occurrence. On the other hand, associated behaviors of struggle and avoidance are instrumentally conditioned on the basis of individual stutterers' experiences and their perceptions of success and failure. Their theory assumes the importance of antecedent factors, assumes that dysfluencies emitted are not normal, and that the dysfluencies are representative of abnormal or disrupted variations of behaviors that originally were normal or appropriately organized. In an effort to explain the onset of stuttering, it would appear that Brutten and Shoemaker have been no more (or less) successful than have other theorists. Van Riper (1982) felt that their interpretation of stuttering development was valuable, however. Brutten (1986) has stated that the theory has retained basic value and validity, although changes must be made. For instance, although he rejects an all-encompassing pathophysiology (neuromotor) etiology for stuttering, he suggests that negative emotion (from conditioning) and neuromotor deficiencies could interact to produce negative effects on fluency. Brutten's epilogue would serve all theorists well: Theorists and theories must be sensitive to changes in data, correct their courses, and be willing to accept change.

Operant theory   Placing a section labeled operant theory in this chapter is somewhat misleading, since, as stated by Shames and Egolf (1976), "although this may resemble a theory of stuttering, it is erroneous to think of these ideas as a theoretical position about stuttering" (p. 17). What, then, is operant conditioning's relevance to stuttering? First, let us define our terms. Again from Shames and Egolf, "An operant is a group or class of responses that we regard as functionally equivalent" (p. 21). In this way, all the variously combined stuttering behaviors a person might have—repetition, prolongation, stoppage, silent avoidances, and so forth—are equivalent behaviors and constitute an operant. *Operant behaviors* are those behaviors that are influenced in their frequency of appearance by the results, or consequences, that the behaviors cause. If I speak to you as we pass, and you smile and reply, I am more likely to speak again when I see you and even when I pass others. However, if you ignore me or react negatively, those consequences will reduce the probability that I will speak to you (and perhaps to other passersby) in the future. However, if I must speak to you when I know the consequences will be unpleasant, then I am more likely to experience difficulty in speaking at all.

Operant formulations today stem primarily from the early and continuing work of B. F. Skinner (1958, 1938). The various operant applications to stuttering relate to a basic construct to explain simultaneously the occurrence of stuttering and the development of stuttering behaviors. This construct suggests that disfluencies increase if their consequences are rewarding to the speaker (parental attention, concern) and that disfluency struggles and avoidances increase if the consequences are punishing to the speaker (scolding, interruption, punishment). Therefore, a child's disfluencies that gain the attention, concern, and response from parents will be reinforced and tend to reoccur. However, if and when that attention becomes punitive, then the child will indulge in behaviors designed to avoid or suppress the disfluency. Variations of this concern with consequences, rather than with antecedent factors, represent operant orientations to stuttering. Most operant theories are, not theories, but structured views relating to the modification of disfluencies. In one sense, operant-oriented persons seek the key to effect changes more than the rationale to explain causes.

Operant procedures have had a tremendous impact on stuttering therapy since the early 1960s. Indeed, at times it has seemed as if data, counting, contingencies, reward, punishment (Daly & Cooper 1967; Daly & Kimbarrow 1978; Siegel 1976, 1970) would overwhelm therapy. An example of significant contributions to operant applications can be found in Flanagan, Goldiamond and Azrin's work (1958) on reducing stuttering through response-contingent consequences. Shames and Sherrick (1963) also suggested operant structure to explain and develop therapies of stuttering. Shames (1986) reviewed research and felt the findings suggest that "stuttering is reinforced on an individual basis in parent-child verbal interactions" (p. 255). This would be in accord with Shames and Sherrick's (1963) work relating Johnson's theory of diagnosogenesis to operant principles in which the consequences (parental concern/disapproval) of a child's normal disfluencies cause the development of stuttering dysfluencies. In 1986, Flanagan updated the 1959 view, stating flatly that "stuttering is an operant" (p. 231). However, he appealed to professionals to respond to stutterers as individuals and not as set pieces in a reward-fluency and punish-stuttering paradigm of rigidity. Shames (1986) has also maintained the validity of an operant view of stuttering, but he has felt that greater attention needs to be paid to antecedent events in stuttering and that the significance of emotions and feelings requires further exploration. However, Wingate (1976) regarded operant explanations as an "easy out" that just ignore all questionable aspects left unanswered. He argued that there is still no proof that stuttering initially is a response, that stuttering originates as normal disfluencies, and that the role of penalty and punishment in stuttering is, at best, confused. Research (Cooper, Cady & Robbins 1970; Williams and Martin 1974) has generated data in conflict with operant principles. It is quite appropriate to appreciate some of the values, organization, evaluation, and accountability that operant procedures have brought to therapy (or reinforced). It also is appropriate to suggest that some operant enthusiasts have fitted stuttering forcibly into too-narrow operant structures. The result of this has been embarrassing omissions and contradictions between problem and philosophy when stuttering has not conformed to all of the operant expectations.

Comment

In various forms and permutations, learning theories have been the most potent contributors in the history of stuttering theory and therapy. The past four decades have probably seen more knowledge and more advances than in all preceding eras. At times, struggles for theoretical dominance have distorted or retarded progress, and still can. In particular, any insistence on a solely learning explanation for stuttering operates to minimize growth and understanding. As we have come to accept the possibility and probability of mixed-effects causation with learning and other-area factors, it would appear that more knowledge and progress are open to us. In the next theory section, we examine pathophysiology theories from the time of their dominance to the present day, with the same reservations or additions in mind.

PATHOPHYSIOLOGY THEORIES

Pathophysiology is used to denote that an abnormality of physiology (normal function or performance) is responsible for stuttering. The term *physiological* to describe theories is used incorrectly, and *biological* or *organic* seems to include normal function also. Van Riper (1982) probably has the best overall review of what he calls organicity in stuttering. He notes that Aristotle blamed stuttering on a weak tongue, that Galen also blamed the tongue, and Francis Bacon suggested hot wine (!) to relax stutterers' tongues. Concerns with the nervous system seemed to surge in the nineteenth century. Other suggestions included breathing, auditory function, and body chemistry. The psychoanalytic theories of the early twentieth century (Freud was originally a neurologist) may have diminished physiology concerns but did not eliminate them. In the second decade of this century they began a strong return that peaked into dominance in the 1930s before crashing down before the wave of diagnosogenesis and other learning theories. For a while the displacement was nearly complete. This writer remembers submitting, in 1960, an article to a leading professional journal, suggesting that it would be appropriate to consider neurological factors in stuttering. Rejection was immediate and total, with an accompanying note from the editor that it was useless to submit such articles because in the face of published research it was "not worthy to beat the dead horse of neurological causation." In the following paragraphs we will review past and present information and try to determine whether we indeed have a moribund equine.

Cerebral Dominance

A landmark in pathophysiology can be noted in Samuel Orton's 1927 publication *Studies in Stuttering.* However, Lee Travis, in his 1931 book *Speech Pathology,* developed the cerebral dominance theory fully. Bryng Bryngelson (1935) also suggested a lateral dominance conflict. In cortical organization there is asymmetry in which different functions are associated with the right and the left cerebral hemispheres. Due to brainstem decussation (cross–over) of corticospinal and aberrant corticobulbar descending axons, cortical control of the body is contralateral; that is, the left hemisphere controls the right side of the body, and the right hemisphere controls the left side of the body. In most persons, language is dominant in the left hemisphere (even when the speaker is left-handed), so that the bilateral neuromotor coordinations for speech production are presumably under left-hemisphere dominance. Travis, and others, believed that stutterers tended toward equality of cerebral dominance, so that the refined timing and coordination required for speech was disturbed. This discoordination would be increased by emotional stress, since the limbic system involves and affects the thalamus and basal ganglia, which play a major role in timing and coordinating cortical neuromotor impulses.

Cerebral dominance was assumed for years to have passed away, as much a victim of its own excesses as of contradictory research. In its time, many stutterers were trained to shift manual laterality (a few had the offending arm set in a plaster cast), and to avoid bimanual activities such as piano playing or typing. Two of the stutterers with whom Travis tried manual dominance shifting were Wendell Johnson and Charles Van Riper. However, almost 50 years after the cerebral dominance theory proposals (Travis 1978) Travis reviewed more recent research, concluding that cerebral dominance reinforcement in therapy was still valid and that more research was needed.

Pyknolepsy and Perseveration

Other pathophysiology theories included the dysphemia theory of Robert West (1942) wherein a constitutional deficiency existed in the stutterer. One suggestion was that the deficiency might be a latent, variant, or subclinical form of pyknolepsy. Pyknolepsy is a very mild variation of epilepsy, usually without overt seizures or loss of consciousness, which is frequently outgrown before or during puberty. Hamre and Wingate (1967) reviewed the literature relating to West's theory and found at least five bases of noncomparability between stuttering and pyknolepsy. Jon Eisenson (1975a, 1958, 1938) suggested that stutterers have a basic tendency toward perceptual and motor perseveration. Research (Wingate 1966a, 1966b; Martin 1962) has provided little support for the perseveration theory. Other neurological dysfunction theories or possibilities are reviewed extensively by Van Riper (1982).

Genetic Bases for Stuttering

Early studies in stuttering reported high levels of stuttering "running in the family." Although these studies failed to utilize control groups, suffered from other design flaws, and reported incidence percentages ranging from about 24 percent to nearly 90 percent of stuttering among family relations, the studies were striking in their general agreement that heredity could play a role in stuttering (Van Riper 1982). What was even more striking was the ease with which some psychosocial theorists pointed to the age of the studies and the design flaws, generally failed to replicate studies, and explained away any residual doubts by suggesting that a family history of stuttering was literally that, just a history. Supposedly, stuttering in one family member sensitized the awareness of other family members to misdiagnose more readily the normal disfluencies of childhood. Others felt uncomfortable, but did nothing to accommodate. A few continued to search for further explanations. Studies by Bryngelson and Rutherford (1937), Wepman (1939), and even by Johnson (1959) that reported levels of family stuttering incidence many times that of the general population did not create particular obstacles for those who wanted stuttering to be only an interactional phenomenon. Wingate (1986a) refers to the subversion of (patho-)physiological points of view in general and the fact that it "has been essentially submerged for about 40 years" (p. 49). In his review of the predominance of psychological over the pathophysiological theories, Wingate details astounding and embarrassing occurrences of "experts" ignoring facts, of flawed studies, of experimenter interpretations contradicted by their own data and by the wish-to-believe orientation. Wingate's review of Gray's (1940) research, which supported the idea that genetic transmission actually was "social heredity" (diagnosogenesis), should become a classic example of placing wish fulfillment against the wall of harsh reality.

These attitudes were not shared by all professionals, however, and many were capable of revision and accommodation. Flexibility became necessary as evidence from well-designed studies started to accumulate on the side of hereditary predisposition. Andrews and Harris (1964), in a fascinating monograph that searched many aspects of stuttering, reported that stutterers had family histories of stuttering 39 percent, while less than 2 percent of the nonstuttering controls reported such histories. Unique contributions to verifying the importance of heredity in stuttering have come from research by Kidd, alone and in combination with others (Kidd 1983, 1980, 1977; Cox & Kidd 1983; Cox, Seider & Kidd 1984; Gladstein, Seider & Kidd 1981; Kidd, Heimbuch & Records 1981; Kidd et al. 1980; Kidd, Kidd & Records 1978). Female stutterers are more likely to have offspring who stutter, compared to children of males who stutter. However, males are genetically more susceptible to stuttering. Two models of transmission have been formulated, each one being sex linked. Howie's (1981a, 1976) research on twins and siblings indicated that if one twin from a single ovum (monozygotic) stuttered, then the chances were 77 percent that the other twin would stutter. Where twins came from separate ova (dizygotic), the probability of both stuttering was 32 percent. On the other hand, the probability of two sibling nontwins stuttering was 20 percent. Van Riper (1982) reported on knowledge of 14 married pairs of stutterers and noted that 20 of the 29 children born to these couples stuttered seriously enough to require clinical attention.

The research in heredity does not eliminate other factors. Effects of pregnancy, nutrition, teratogens, maternal age, birth trauma, environmental pressures, and other factors are not eliminated either as precipitators or contributors. There has been, overall, a shift to acceptance of the heredity factor in stuttering (Wingate 1986a; Wall and Myers 1984; Shames & Florance 1982; Van Riper 1982). It must be accepted that some or many stutterers, we do not really know yet, have a predisposition or susceptibility to stutter. We also do not know how strong this predisposition may be—whether some children are bound to stutter no matter what and others fall along a continuum of susceptibility, or if there are genetic subgroups yet to be described further.

Recent Pathophysiology

Although pathophysiology interests have never disappeared, their capacity to capture and influence a significant audience has been minimal until recent times. As learning and operant studies have revisited areas of existing knowledge, recast accepted information into jargon, and argued over reinterpretation of old data, new finds in pathophysiology have developed. Quinn (1972) found that about 20 percent of 60 stutterers showed reversed hemispheric dominance. Additional research has renewed the suggestion that cerebral dominance is a factor in stuttering (Moore 1986; Moore & Haynes 1980; Moore & Lorendo 1980; Moore & Lang 1977). Wilkins, Webster, and Morgan (1984) reported that stutterers showed right hemisphere interference with left-hemisphere activity during language-processing tasks. Stromsta (1986, 1964) reported and reaffirmed the existence of EEG (electroencephalographic) differences and suggested that in stutterers the "intraphonemic disturbances may have their basis in the relative difference in the timing of bilateral cerebral activity that we have observed to exist in stutterers as compared to nonstutterers" (1986, p.15). Many other hemisphere function studies have been performed, with some finding differences (Newman, Channell & Palmer 1986: Fitzgerald, Cooke & Greiner 1984; Cimorell-Strong, Gilbert & Frick 1983) and other researchers (Gruber & Powell 1974; Fox 1966) failing to find differences. This illustrates a problem pathophysiology (and stuttering research in general) has faced where replication of studies has generated both supporting and conflicting data. However, these conflicts have resulted in many professionals (especially in areas of psychological theory) behaving as if the original research has been "disproved" and no longer deserves consideration. Actually, assuming that all of the studies, on both sides, have been appropriately designed and adequately interpreted (an unwarranted assumption in many cases), the only reasonable interpretation is that not all stutterers display the characteristic, the deficit, or whatever has been measured. When combined with some of the attitudes and behaviors Wingate (1986) criticized, the research-difference muddle becomes worse. In fairness, it must be noted that all virtue and practice of the scientific method are not exclusive to pathophysiology, and recent disputes about the importance of attitudes and adjustments in stutterers reflect the same type of overbalanced viewpoint.

Other function areas of stutterers have received extensive attention. Several areas combine under stuttering and feedback systems. After World War II, the cybernetics work of Norbert Wiener (1948) excited interest in many fields, including that of communication disorders, an interest that continues to this day. Part of Wiener's developments explored servosystems, in which a system's output is monitored and subsequently used to alter the ouput of the system. The thermostat function in a heating-cooling system is a classic example. It is hypothesized that oral output in human communication is aurally monitored, while tactile, kinesthetic, and proprioceptive activity is physiologically monitored. It has been suggested that the frontopontocerebellar tract (and back to cortex) is a feedback example of a closed-loop or impulse-monitoring system. The feedback systems typically result in a variance signal based on output intentions, output results, and output effects. As a result, the speaker constantly modifies successive output signals in order to reduce the discrepancy of the next feedback variance signal.

Fairbanks (1954) followed Wiener's formulations and developed an early model of a speech communication servosystem. Others, particularly Mysak (1966, 1960) have extended feedback concepts. Cybernetics is not a theory of stuttering but a suggestion of how various factors might affect the system in different locations. Biological, learning, and other theories can and do make use of feedback concepts. Extensive and continuing research has tinkered with various feedback aspects—duration, rhythmic timing, loudness, frequency spectrum, tactile sensation, dichotic listening, kinesthetic feedback, and so on. Research in feedback has involved the use of various types of masking noise (Conture 1974; Adams & Moore 1972), delayed auditory feedback (Ham & Holbrook 1986; Ham, Fucci & Cantrell 1984a, 1984b; Leith & Chmiel 1980), and tactile and proprioceptive desensitization (Hutchinson & Ringel 1975), to name a few. Overall, feedback studies either have failed to differentiate stutterers and nonstutterers or have failed to develop strategies to detect differences, if they exist.

Over the years, research has noted respiratory anomalies in stuttering (Metz, Conture & Colton 1976; Starbuck & Steer 1954; Hill 1944a, 1944b). However, the prevailing conclusion today is that discoordinations in respiration are a concomitant, or a developed result, of stuttering spasms. Laryngeal function has received a great deal of attention, particularly with reference to vocal reaction or onset times. Adams (1984a) reviewed a number of articles and presentations on vocal functions in stutterers. With some exceptions, vocal response times of stutterers are slower. However, Adams cautions, exceptions do exist and we cannot make a blanket statement about laryngeal function and stuttering. Starkweather (1982a) provides a comprehensive review of laryngeal research in stuttering. In general, we find that stutterers tend to have slower vocal onset and termination times and to show various abnormalities of laryngeal function. Schwartz (1974) has identified laryngeal dysfunction (a disturbed airway dilation reflex) in the posterior cricoarytenoid muscle (regarded as the sole vocal fold abductor) as the cause of stuttering. However, few people have accepted this opinion, and supportive research is lacking. Curlee (1984) has noted that stuttering persists following surgical removal of the larynx (laryngectomy), and Irving and Webb (1961) reported that a prelaryngectomy stutterer was taught esophageal speech without recurrence of stuttering. Starkweather has suggested that present information leads him to support the concept that the larynx is involved in stuttering, as are respiration and articulation, but that there is minimal support for the idea that the larynx is the primary or causative agent in stuttering. As Curlee (1984) stated, "It is not clear how one subsystem of the mechanism could be more involved or more responsible for stuttering than other subsystems of the same mechanism" (p. 243).

Various researchers have investigated articulation in stuttering. Zimmerman (1980a, 1980b) reported slower onsets, slower achievments of peak velocities, and asynchrony of articulators in the fluent speech of stutterers. Distortions or aberrations of articulation and coarticulation have been observed during stuttering by many researchers. Stromsta (1986) has suggested that stuttering is neurophysiological in origin, with the "core effect" being sudden interruptions of formant transitions and the occurrence of abnormal terminations of phonation (p. 5). As with respiration and phonation, separating articulation from the rest of the vocal tract is difficult and debatable. Perkins (1980a, 1977, 1975) has proposed a discoordination hypothesis, in which he states, "We view stuttering as a discoordination of phonation with articulation and respiration" (1977, p.105). He based his hypothesis particularly on the fact that compared to usual voicing, whispered speech was accompanied by reduced stuttering, and "lipped speech" (soundless articulation) had the least dysfluency. Venkatagiri (1982) tested the discoordination hypothesis by evaluating stutterer and nonstutter reaction times in producing /s/ and /z/ sounds. Overall the two groups could not be differentiated, and the discoordination hypothesis was not supported. However, it was noted that severe stutterers did show longer reaction times on /z/ productions. Since phonation is involved, particularly with Perkins's hypothesis, the reader is referred to the statements by Adams (1984a) and Curlee (1984) discussed earlier.

Other pathophysiology research has included reports that the lingual tactile sensitivity of stutterers and nonstutterers differs (Fucci et al. 1985), that phonetic processing abilities differ (Perozzi 1970), that stutterers have slower reaction times for letter recognition than they do for figure recognition (Wilkins, Webster & Morgan 1984), and that sound fusion processing capacities of stutterers and nonstutterers differed significantly (Bonin, Ramig & Prescott 1985). Hannley and Dorman (1982) reviewed central auditory processing studies and suggested that small-N studies may contribute to some of the contradictory results. Adams (1984a) also found "equivocal questions" in auditory processing research. Again, we do not have a yes or no answer in this question area; we must consider whether the problem is only with our methodologies, with the possibility that one or more processing subgroups exist, or both.

Summary and Hypothesis

This section has traced a convoluted trail for pathophysiological theory formulation. From dominance to submergence and back to viability, the trail has been followed. At the present time, some professionals still avoid, reject, or question the concept of a pathophysiological basis for stuttering. Others cite limited or conditional consideration. Perkins (1980a) states that stutterers, as a group, cannot be differentiated biologically, except in the laryngeal area, from fluent speakers. Curlee (1985) concluded that stutterers, as a group, are biologically, anatomically, and neurologically normal. Wall and Myers (1984) find indicative, but incomplete, evidence of pathophysiology and call for more extensive research. Van Riper (1982) follows a somewhat similar course in writing that "the case for organicity in stutterers has only been partially supported"

(p. 353). It is possible that pathophysiology of stuttering can be regarded in several different ways:

1. It does not, per se, exist. Some stutterers have structural or physiological anomalies, but so do some nonstutterers.
2. Stutterers may exhibit physiological anomalies, but these are peripheral or concomitant results of the occurrence or the effects of stuttering.
3. Pathophysiology occurs variably according to a subgroup and/or severity categorization of stutterers so that some stutter for one reason, some for another, some for nonphysiological reasons, and some for a combination of factors.
4. "All" stuttering has a pathophysiological origin.

The third possibility, as an "eclectic elective," is attractive, and also rational. However, for purposes of stimulation and discussion, let us take the fourth proposition and propose a theory or hypothesis based on its implications.

A NEURAL INTEGRITY HYPOTHESIS

In the behavioral sciences, there have been prolonged struggles between advocates of social causation and those supporting constitutional or physiological causation. These arguments have cut across emotional disorders, crime and criminals, special education, and communication problems— just to name several areas. Within particular disorder categories, such as stuttering, theory struggles have been no less forceful and variable for the reduced area of concern. The disagreements intensify if we add in the area of cluttering (often described as a central language imbalance), dysfluency in psychiatric disorders, stuttering among the mentally retarded, and dysfluency in dysphasia and dysarthria. Where do we draw the line between "stuttering-stuttering" and other fluency disorders? When is it a neurological fluency problem, a neurotic fluency disorder, or stuttering? At the other end of the continuum, how do we explain the difference in degree, or kind, between so-called normal disfluency and abnormal dysfluency discussed in the first chapter? Are we not, perhaps, replicating the blind seers trying to describe an elephant depending on which part of the pachyderm we contact? It is suggested that fluency depends upon the **neural integrity** of the communicator, and the form and degree of fluency disruptions depend on the areas and severities of deficits in neural integrity, with external influences affecting the occurrence, timing, and future development of the fluency disruptions.

Neural integrity refers to the integration of the nervous system, in all its subdivisions and complexities. It begins with the embryonic disc development in fetal life, following earlier cell division after fertilization of the ovum. The first stage of neural integrity development may occur during the neural induction phase, starting at about the third week of fetal development. In this stage, the neural tube ectoderm begins differentiation into immature neurons and glial cells (Kallen 1979). It has been suggested that this stage is the time when neurons receive the genetic programming that will regulate their shape, size, sensitivity to stress, and other factors (Lund 1978).

The second stage of neural integrity rests upon the migration of neurons to the sites where they ultimately will develop into mature neural tissue. Rakic (1975) has suggested that neuronal migration provides for the future development of synaptic junctions among specific types of neurons and thereby lays the foundation for future function of the central nervous system. The mechanisms of neuronal migration may be chemical (Jacobson 1978; Lund 1978; Rutishauser et al. 1979) relating, for example, to cellular protein synthesis (Purpura 1977). It also may be assisted by glial cell fibers that physically help guide a migrating neuron toward its destination (Jacobson 1978). During migration, neurons develop their processes. Dendrites begin as small fiber tangles that finally develop and form dendritic spines that will be future synapse sites (Purpura 1977). Axons may develop from a fixed cell body and extend to a destination, or a fixed axon may elongate as its neuron cell migrates. Final synapses also seem to depend on interacting physical and chemical factors (Ramon y Cajal 1960; Vaughn, Henrickson & Grieshaber 1974).

The third and final stage of neural integrity begins soon after the initiation of neuronal migration and extends into the first two years of postnatal existence. This stage is the time when functional synaptic connections develop. It also is the time when inferior or inactive connections degenerate and preprogrammed cell death, referred to in the first stage, will occur (Kuffler, Nicholls & Martin 1984). We thus see that neural integrity extends, at least, over about the first three years of existence, with that cutoff being arbitrary, since certain aspects of nervous system development extend into the years of adolescence. At this point, it is appropriate to make several observations:

> Considering all the variables of parental health and age, pregnancy factors, birth events, and postnatal occurrences, it must be concluded that all living organisms carry deficits or differences in neural integrity in multiple sites, combinations, and degrees.

Differences in color awareness, motor reaction time, allergen sensitivity, emotional responsiveness, auditory perception skills, tactile sensitivity, pain thresholds, and on, and on, exist in all of us. These differences, to a great degree, relate to "how we are wired," or the nature of our neural integrity.

Neural integrity is a continuum in terms of adequacy or inadequacy, and the severity of integrity deficits or differences is a combination of the extent of an area loss, the number of areas concerned, and the connecting tracts among the areas.

This suggests that *normal, problem, disorder,* and *handicap* are terms expressing the factor of degree, and not kind (at least not directly). It does not reject the concept that kind is related to and affected by the degree possibilities and the area differences just cited. When we differentiate among fluency disorders to exclude certain ones from the "stuttering" rubric, we are simply restricting the semantic field to exclude certain labels on an arbitrary basis, whether that basis is carefully reasoned and functionally justified or not.

The appearance of a neural integrity deficit or difference will be the result of interaction between severity of the condition and environmental factors unfavorable to continued function or normal development of the function(s) associated with particular neural areas.

Such a statement allows for a mild loss of neural integrity in a particular function area to survive environmental events that would cause breakdown if the neural integrity were more seriously compromised, or if the environmental events were more extreme. It would also allow for children to outgrow problems as delayed integrity development occurs, as compensatory functions develop, and/or negative influences are mitigated or stopped.

Dysfunction development stemming from neural integrity deficits or differences, and precipitating factors, will be affected by the psychosocial influences of the environment and the response of the individual.

Principles of learning, reinforcement, conditioning, and so on, will tend to direct dysfunction development along certain typical patterns. Residual integrity of the organism may limit the effects of learning factors, but it will not eliminate them.

The particular form of dysfunction will be a combination of specific weaknesses in the overall neural system and conditioned experiences of the organism as it tries to function as if neural integrity was adequate in the functions involved.

Some stutterers will be primarily oral, laryngeal, or both, depending on system weaknesses and on their own trial-and-error efforts to resolve fluency disruptions.

Additional comments can be made with reference to therapy effects:

1. Intervention strategies at early ages may be able to take advantage of early

nervous system plasticity and effect alterations in area development and synapse formation, so areas of weak integrity are enhanced or compensated for.

2. Intervention strategies that utilize or emphasize neural functions or systems with greater levels of integrity may replace, complement, or facilitate further development of weaker integrity areas.

3. Intervention strategies emphasizing reduction of stress and limbic interference with planning and execution systems may enhance the performance of weaker systems.

The concept of neural integrity is not at all new. It is a partial relabeling of existing concepts, as well as a collection of previously known facts. The best and worst aspects of it are that the basic premise of neural integrity, at our present levels of science, cannot be proved or disproved. Where stutterers are found to be "not significantly different" from nonstutterers, either the manipulated variable itself is not significant, the detection methods are incorrect or too gross, or the subjects do not have integrity flaws or differences in those particular areas. The concept can be maddening at times, but it might provide a preliminary formulation to encourage the development of more focused, definable, and testable hypotheses and theories. Neural integrity permits diagnosogenesis, discoordination hypotheses, classical or instrumental conditioning, and other onset or development theories. It provides for linguistic deficit and difficulty in stutterers on an acquired or a developmental basis. The across-class variability or subgroup clustering of stutterers (and other disorder groups) also is not in conflict with this hypothesis. It also provides for the effectiveness, variability, relapse, and other effects of different therapy strategies. The point that it is not particularly verifiable and the point that it can be equated with intuitive empiricism must be admitted, in part. However, the neural integrity concept provides a quasi-philosophical frame of reference into which our present knowledge, existing conflicts and disagreements, and future research and therapy applications can fit.

LINGUISTIC CONSIDERATIONS

As in the discussion of operant applications there is, in the strict sense of the term, no linguistic theory of stuttering. Some who publish in the area of stuttering simply do not include linguistic factors in their considerations. However, others regard stuttering in the same way as phonology, once regarded as a speech function and now viewed as a language function, and suggest that fluency (or fluency disruption) has a linguistic base. The writer surveyed eight major introductory texts on communication disorders published between 1975 and 1986. Few of the texts discussed "language and stuttering" at all, and only one contained a specific section under causes of stuttering wherein linguistic factors were discussed. However, if one turns to texts and reference articles on stuttering, a different point of view is obtained. Most of these express interest in language factors, ranging from predominance to significant consideration in specified instances.

Discussions of fluency in Chapter 1 emphasized the importance of factors such as rate and rhythm, indicating the effects of language maturation on pauses, stress units, and other factors. Pearl and Bernthal (1980) suggested that at least some disfluencies (of normally fluent children) are related to sentence processing or to language construction points at which the child speaker determines the form of the anticipated response. Earlier Bloodstein (1974) suggested the possibility that early prestuttering phases in children could be noted where there are delays in the initiation of syntactic units. He thought that the noticed and labeled part-word disruptions of children are later, more molecular manifestations of the earlier, larger-unit problems. Bernstein (1981) overviewed linguistic research and felt it indicates that, as a normal part of development, children tend to have difficulty in planning syntactic structure. Stuttering, she suggests, can be identified by the form of the disfluency (not the cause) during this difficulty in planning. Several clinicians (Merits-Patterson & Reed 1981; Hall 1977) have noted disfluency increases among children as they progress in therapy for severe articulation disorders and/or language delay. This author has noted similar occurrences where, as children made rapid progress in language development, they began to show part-word, syllable, and phoneme fluency disruptions where none had existed previously. This is reinforced by Gordon, Luper, and Peterson (1986), who reported a relationship between syntactic complexity and the occurrence of normal disfluencies in five-year-old children. Recently, Homzie and Lindsay (1984) reviewed theories of stuttering and linguistic research. They concluded that language deficits contribute initially to the onset of stuttering and continue to be affecting factors as stuttering develops. Research for an underlying etiology of an organic nature is suggested.

Research about the linguistic aspects of stuttering and stutterers has contributed to concern over language involvement. Wall (1980) evaluated a small sample of stutterers aged 5.5–6.5 years and found they were less mature and efficient in their syntax. In another study (Stocker & Parker 1977), stutterers were significantly less adequate in the recall of meaningful verbal material. Overall, Gordon (1985) has compiled a summary of language-stuttering relationships. These include the consideration that stutterers may acquire language more slowly than do nonstutterers. She related this to the age of first words (Berry 1938), judgments by parents of their children's language development (Johnson et al. 1959), evaluations by clinicians (Van Riper 1982), auditory recall tasks related to linguistic information (Stocker & Parker 1977), mean length of utterance and language test scores (Kline & Starkweather 1979), predominance of one-word responses. (Silverman & Williams 1967), a higher number of grammatical errors and lower Peabody Picture Vocabulary Test scores (Westley 1979), and comparisons of clause and sentence complexity differences (Wall 1980).

The locus of occurrence of stuttering may be related to linguistic factors. Brown (1938) formalized an "initial triad" concept of difficulty in reporting that stuttering was more likely to occur on the first three words of an utterance. This was expanded to include the idea that stuttering was more likely to occur at the beginning of a clause (within a sentence) than on other words in the clause (Quarrington, Conway & Siegel 1962; Soderberg 1967). The significance of clause boundaries and stuttering has been reinforced in other research (Wall, Starkweather & Cairns 1981; Bernstein 1981). However, other factors also seem to be involved. Trotter (1956) noted that severity of stuttering was related to the conspicuousness of words, and research on pause occurrence (unfilled or filled) suggests that stuttering is more likely to occur on words of greater information uncertainty or unpredictability (Taylor 1966; Quarrington 1965; MacClay & Osgood 1959; Goldman-Eisler 1958). Wingate (1979a), in writing about the first three words of utterance, questioned the validity of the word uncertainty principle.

A great deal of research has centered around linguistic factors and stuttering. Schlesinger, Melkman, and Levy (1966) noted a significant increase in stuttering as word length increased. E-M. Silverman and D.E. Williams (1967) reported that stuttering was more likely to occur on longer words than on shorter ones, extending Wingate's (1967a) finding that stuttering occurred more often on two-syllable than on one-syllable words. Bloodstein and Grossman (1981) reported that more stuttering occurred on monosyllabic words than on polysyllabic words. Silverman (1972a) summarized five studies on word length and came to the conclusion that stuttering was more likely to occur on short words than on long words. However, Tornick and Bloodstein (1976) evaluated stuttering frequency on short sentences. They then lengthened the sentences by adding on to them, and they evaluated the frequency of dysfluency. When "same words" stuttered on were paired, more stuttering occurred on longer sentences than on short ones. Danzger and Halpern (1973) also found more stuttering on long words.

Other linguistic factors have concerned word frequency, abstractness, and meaningfulness or importance. Cohen (1953) reported that stuttering frequency and word weight were significantly correlated, and Danzger and Halpern (1973) found that more stuttering occurred on infrequently used words. Schlesinger and others (1965) reported a similar finding, but they also evaluated the effect of transition probability (predictability) of words on stuttering. Least stuttering occurred when the (Hebrew) words were high in both predictability and frequency. Stuttering increased on words that were high in use frequency but low in predictability. And it was greatest when both frequency and predictability were low.

Many clinicians have suggested that the meaning or critical value of words relates to stuttering occurrence. Lanyon (1968) disagreed with this idea and stated that low-information words were more likely to be stuttered, with sentence position being important. Peterson (1969) used semantic differential ratings of most-stuttered and least-stuttered words, and he could not support the concept that word meaningfulness was related to stuttering. However, Kaasin and Bjerkan (1982) had 26 stutterers give oral messages to listeners; they reported that stuttering occurred on 36 percent of the words critical to the message and on only 8 percent of the noncritical words. They also noted that since critical words fell in final positions in sentences, most stuttering tended to fall there also, instead of on the first three words. Earlier Soderberg (1971, 1967) stated that word length and information values are independently related to stuttering, but that longer words interact with information value factors. He felt that this interaction was a major factor in previous disagreements.

Danzger and Halpern (1973) found that word abstraction level was not significantly related to stuttering and that there was no significant variation among nouns, verbs, and adjectives. Blankenship (1964) reported that research on hesitations and stutterings indicated more problems with lexical items than with function words. Hannahm and Gardner (1968) suggested that more stuttering occurred on grammatical units that had a postverbal location. On a different track, Wingate explored "sound-mindedness" of stutterers. He reported (1967b) that stutterers were deficient in Slurvian skills—this, based on Tiffany's work (1963), and relates to phonetic manipulation capacities to take a phrase such as "scene owe weevil" and turn it into "see no evil." Wingate (1971a, 1969a) stated that stutterers seem to lack in the ability to manipulate phonetic features and to be aware of sound patterns. He felt that phonetic and prosodic factors may underlie the "apparent" grammatical features that many have associated with stuttering.

For over 20 years Marcel Wingate has developed the linguistic area of prosody as a significant factor in stuttering, even when many did not want to consider it. In 1966 (c) he suggested that adaptation on reading passages can be explained through increasing familiarity with prosodic values. In 1977 (a), he stated that research findings on the relationship between linguistic stress and stuttering are the most important source for explaining why certain words are stuttered on. After considering the "meaningfulness" factor (1979b), he concluded that too many persons have overlooked the frequent relationship between critical information words and utterance stress points. Similarly, he suggested that the essential feature in stuttering, on both the aspects of grammatical class and sentence position, was linguistic stress (1979a). Wingate reinforced prosodic significance and intuitive awareness of stress (1984c, 1983), but Weiner (1984b) reported that switching stress on a dual list of bisyllabic words resulted in no stuttering concentration on stressed or unstressed syllables. However, Wingate has continued to develop the significance of linguistic stress. Wingate (1988) has recently published a summary of his research and speculation concerning stuttering and psycholinguistics. This excellent source contributes significantly to discussions concerning developmental theories. However, it does not provide an answer to the question of whether linguistic factors are primary in their causation of stuttering, are a secondary causal factor after a neurophysiological etiology, or whether the linguistic factors are among a number of effects from deficient neural integrity. In a dual review of learning theory and stuttering (see this chapter on learning theory and Wendell Johnson), Wingate concluded that linguistic stress, and not adaptation and consistency, is central to stuttering.

Comment on Linguistics

The preceding review has indicated a central role for language in our overall view of stuttering. The fluency factors discussed in Chapter 1, combined with research on children who stutter, reinforce the significance of language considerations. This information does not necessarily support a conclusion that the onset of stuttering can generally be ascribed to linguistic deficits. Most writers have opted for variable significance of language function. Wall and Myers (1984) have reasonably suggested that an appropriate theory would involve a genetic factor that results in "a slightly incoordinated motor apparatus for speech" (p. 38). This substandard timing and coordination could be accompanied by linguistic problems stemming from language delay, with breakdowns tending to occur at clause boundaries (and stress points) where linguistic formulation and physiological execution vulnerabilities are greatest. Such a theory would allow for purely physiological stuttering to occur at the most likely trouble points—clause boundaries and stress points. Such a theory would be compatible with neural integrity, discussed earlier, and with learning theory factors that would be involved most with individual reactions to the hesitations and the dysfluencies that occur.

THEORY STATUS

The status of theory today is confused. As discussed earlier, many clinicians structure evaluation and therapy on the pragmatics of procedures that seem to work best, provide for convenient reporting in today's accountability systems, were taught during student training days, and appeal to the personal style or preferences of the clinician. Incongruities between predisposition and precipitation factors and development and maintenance factors have confused theories and therapies. This confusion has been intensified by theoreticians who have propounded single-model theories to cover both aspects (onset and development) when they actually, at least, related only to one. In some instances, but at critical points, specific theory proponents became disciples rather than clinical scientists, with the result that objectivity at times was replaced by ego territoriality and an insistence that facts must be interpreted to conform to the theory, instead of the theory developing, modifying and, if appropriate, self-destructing in response to the facts. Early preoccupations with pathophysiological theories and recent experiences with learning theories have provided examples of these unfortunate situations.

Research findings indicate significance for several factors. These factors include, but are not limited to, the following:

1. The significance of genetic and familial factors in occurrence of, or predisposition to, stuttering. Whether this is a universal or a multiple subgroup factor remains to be established.
2. The significance of pathophysiological factors in occurrence of, or predisposition to, stuttering. As in factor 1, the universality of pathophysiology and the degree to which it divides into subcategories requires further investigation.
3. The significance of learning factors in the precipitation of some stuttering (especially where these factors intersect with predisposing factors), and particularly in the development of stutterer reactions to dysfluencies.
4. The significance of linguistic factors in the development of fluency, differentiation between disfluency and dysfluency, and demarcation of significant areas, especially in prosody, where stuttering events are likely to occur.

This writer is suggesting a multicausality model for stuttering theory. Personal preference focuses the model toward a neural integrity loss due to genetic and/or external effects that result in otherwise inexplicable stuttering occurrences; but the model accommodates other precipitating factors as well. At this stage of knowledge, it is appropriate, at least, to say, "Learning, physiological, psychological, linguistic, and genetic variables all play a potentially important role in the breakdown of speech coordination" (Hanley 1986, pp. 39–40).

With the point of view expressed earlier, it is necessary to encourage certain developments. Research into the interactive aspects of the different factors affecting stuttering (rather than "proving" or "disproving" them) would help us identify and delineate stuttering subgroups. Such categorizations would aid significantly in prevention, early intervention, better identification of at-risk disfluent children, and formulation of prognostic indicators for children most and least likely to recover spontaneously from stuttering (see Chapter 1 discussion). We would be able to look more specifically at stuttering therapy procedures and determine whether all factor areas, some few areas, or only one area is significant in therapy. Design of a quasi-universal therapy model, or distinct models for different categories of stutterers (not just age based), might be feasible. Finally, issues of stabilization, maintenance, and relapse might relate, not only to therapy procedures, but also to the "type" of stutterer concerned.

The prior words are an expression of both wish and hope and, therefore, of conflict to a certain degree with reality. However, only those who desire a monolithic unitary theory structure should find it completely unacceptable. Consideration of multiple significance factors, and a willingness to revise our concepts as new data accumulate, can only, in the long run, benefit the clinician and improve the lot of stutterers seeking our help.

CHAPTER THREE
DIAGNOSIS
AND ASSESSMENT
Preliminary Considerations

SECTION INTRODUCTION

In the previous section an effort was made to review some of the things we know about stutterers and stuttering and to speculate about the factors associated with the onset and development of stuttering. We have been caught up in definition problems, lack of basic information about fluency, exogeny and endogeny in causation, as well as the need to view causation and development and maintenance as independent variables. In this section, we will discuss our practices as they apply to diagnosis and assessment.

The reader will notice that some of the practices in evaluation will relate to considerations raised earlier, in Section I, but that many of them will relate to therapy techniques, discussed in Section III. Since many of our therapy procedures are relevant to their effects on symptom suppression or fluency induction (and not to theories), it follows that assessment procedures will coincide with these orientations rather than with some of the definitions and theory concepts and questions developed in Section I. This is not as clinicians would prefer it, but it sensibly reflects the scientific trial approach to problem resolution. Until such time as our knowledge encompasses sufficiently the total construct or constructs of stuttering, we must function as best we can with the most effective tools we have developed. Diagnosis and assessment, perforce, must reflect this attitude.

OVERVIEW

Many of us, this writer included, transpose the words *diagnosis* and *assessment*. The former refers to identifying a state or condition, and the latter relates to a descriptive evaluation of what has been diagnosed. Many academic institutions have a course entitled "Diagnostic Procedures . . ." in which most of the content deals with assessment. Most of the time the transposition of terms, diagnosis to mean assessment, is acceptable as a semantic idiom. However, this is not the case in areas such as dysarthria/dyspraxia and dysphasia/dementia, where determining what the problem is can be as important as the evaluation process itself. The same distinction holds true, especially among children, with disfluency/dysfluency, or the separation of stuttering from normal fluency disruptions, and the evaluation of dysfluency once it has been diagnosed.

Adams (1984b, 1980) describes the differential separation of stuttering and normal disfluency in children as "vexing" and "intimidating." Only in the past ten years or so has any significant progress been made in establishing criteria and points of delineation in the differential process. Adams has contributed significantly to this progress (1984b, 1980, 1977), as have other clinicians (Starkweather 1987; Culp 1984; Wall & Myers 1984; Riley & Riley 1983; Gregory & Hill 1980; Gregory 1973). Not all agree with Adams and feel that diagnosis is not "as difficult as some writers have contended, even with young children" (Wingate 1984, p. 277). Similarly, Riley and Riley suggest that it is not particularly difficult to identify stuttering, but they point out that careful observation is required in order to determine appropriate treatment. Undoubtedly the reality lies somewhere between, and the clinician will see children where the diagnosis is clear and evaluation follows simple patterns. There will of course be the obverse: children who will not fit easily into diagnostic categories, and for whom evaluation is more complex.

ORGANIZATION

Developing a text diagnostic and assessment sequence for use with young people is complex because of several variables. These complicating variables include factors of age range, parent involvement, concomitant disorders, and clinical setting, to name several. Organization struggles with chronological sequences, symptom sequences, and procedural steps. Whichever route emphasis is chosen, the writer (and the reader) must deal with the interactions of the other two. After attempting several structural designs, this writer decided to divide diagnosis and assessment into two chapters. Chapter 3 considers preliminary aspects to evaluation and how other clinicians approach the process. Chapter 4 makes a longer presentation of methods and formats suggested by the writer. The topic areas are the following:

Chapter 3

> Overview of diagnosis and assessment
> Organization of the two chapters
> Nomenclature and Concepts:
>> definitions of basic dysfluency behaviors
>> definitions of associated behaviors
>> definitions of antiexpectancy behaviors
>> definition of basic measurement procedures
> Procedures followed by other clinicians

Chapter 4

> Psychological: reactions of client and environment; situation and person pragmatics
> Physiological: respiration, phonation, articulation, and general coordination
> Linguistic: syntactic, semantic, pragmatic
> Fluency and dysfluency: types of dysfluency; frequency and severity of dysfluencies

The topic areas in Chapter 4 are presented in the format of a complete diagnostic and assessment checklist or report form. The last section (fluency and dysfluency) provides graph forms on which measurements can be recorded for display, for use as baseline measures, and for replotting if measurements are performed again in the future.

Following the presentation of the checklist items, each major section is discussed with greater detail, information provided, and suggestions made. Where appropriate, separations by age are discussed. The total product is extensive and represents a potentially significant investment of time. Many clinicians will not have the required time available to follow the complete outline. Some will not need, or want, to complete the entire sequence. Thus a secondary reason for using the checklist or report form structure is that the reader can identify the portions or sections to be utilized, refer to the expanded discussions of the sections, and decide what procedures to follow and what others to omit, reduce, or alter.

Before moving to the checklist or report format, however, it will be useful to define a number of commonly used terms. This is done first, in the section following. After that is a brief review of some diagnostic and assessment procedures suggested by other clinicians. This provides the reader with other points of view and emphasis, giving alternative sources if the reader desires more information.

NOMENCLATURE AND CONCEPTS

In the following pages on diagnosis and assessment, and in subsequent therapy chapters, the reader will need to understand various definitions and concepts. Most of them will be consistent with those found in other clinical writings. However, variations in meaning do occur, and so some coverage at this point will provide frames of reference.

Disfluency   fluency disruptions usually not attributed to stuttering.

Dysfluency   fluency disruptions typically attributed to stuttering.

Block   used by some to refer to any stuttering event; others use it only to indicate a tonic stoppage. Used in this text, it refers to the latter.

Spasm   an author bias; some authors do not use the term because of semantic overtones suggesting neuropathology. Since its literal meaning refers to involuntary contractions of a muscle or muscles, it will be used here as an umbrella term for involuntary repetitions, prolongations, and stoppages in speech production.

Clonic   alternating contractions and relaxations of muscles or muscle groups.

Tonic   continuous contraction of a muscle or muscle group.

Repetition   stuttering spasms of a clonic nature where alternating contraction and relaxation of speech musculature results in repetitive productions. May occur at phrase or whole-word levels (WWR), at part-word or syllable levels (PWR), or at the phoneme or articulatory postures level (PR).

Prolongation   stuttering spasms of a tonic nature where respiratory, phonatory and/or articulatory movement proceeds at a slowed, elongated and (usually) tensed level. It may occur in voice or voiceless environments.

Stoppage   stuttering spasms of a tonic nature where occlusion of the vocal tract or fixation of an articulator results in complete stoppage of ongoing speech production.

Struggle   a term usually referring to exaggerated physical movements of the speech mechanism components and/or facial areas. Indicates excessive muscular tension and effort in attempting to overcome repetitions, prolongations, or stoppages.

Overflow   a term that encompasses *struggle* but also is used to include atypical limb postures or gestures, body postures or movements, during stuttering spasms.

Associated Behaviors

Struggle and overflow (see the list in the preceding section) are attempts to regain physical control of speech. The behavior definitions in the list that follows occur in response to the anticipation or occurrence of stuttering spasms and efforts to avoid or circumvent them.

Postponement   any behavior, vocal or nonvocal, used to delay the speech attempt. May be phrases, words, sounds, silence, gestures, movements, and so on. A temporal delay in the attempt to speak.

Starter   any behavior, vocal or nonvocal, used to facilitate movement/release in the speech production system, which usually occurs contiguously with the initial phoneme or syllable of a feared word. Most postponement behaviors can, with proper timing, be used as starters.

Release   any behavior, vocal or nonvocal, produced during a stuttering spasm in hopes of breaking out of the spasm or in timing the spasm release with the occurrence of the particular behavior. Changes in pitch, loudness, interjected sounds, gestures or body movements, and the like, may be used.

Retrial   stuttering has occurred, an effort has been made and terminated, and a new effort is attempted. May be a new effort to utter the word, repetition of several preceding words, and/or utilization of other behaviors described in this section.

Revision an attempt to revise a planned or uttered statement. Can actually occur after stuttering is completed and speaker revises statement in an effort to repeat it fluently. Shades into retrial, and also into circumlocution.

Substitution replacement of one word by (hopefully) a synonym. May occur prior to the attempt at utterance, during an attempt, as a retrial effort, or postspasm.

Circumlocution use of extra, usually less specific, series of words to avoid or resolve stuttering on a single word.

Antiexpectancy Behaviors

Properly speaking, all of the foregoing associated behaviors are of the antiexpectancy variety. However, they are aimed at actual or specifically anticipated moments of stuttering. The behaviors identified in the following list are aimed, in general, to reduce the overall possibility or probability that stuttering will occur at any time on any word.

Speech behaviors these will be alterations in modes of speech production. Habitual changes in loudness, pitch, variability, stress, rate, articulator contact strength, and so on may be adopted overall or on a situational basis.

Social behaviors these are changes in social communication behaviors and can include elective mutism or its verbal equivalent ("I don't know"), obsequious or submissive demeanors, aggressive behaviors, clowning style, and other supposedly protecting or distracting behaviors.

Measurements

Another nomenclature-concept area is that of some of the measures used in evaluating fluency and fluency disruptions. These measures also occur frequently as baseline data against which therapy progres is compared.

Words Per Minute (wpm) a classic measure of speaking rate, counting each word uttered, dividing the sum by the total talking time (TTT) in seconds, and multiplying the result by 60. A more accurate measure of fluency and rate can be obtained by counting syllables but otherwise following the same formula. Pause time can create misleading rate figures, but few clinicians possess the equipment needed to measure articulation time (TTT minus pause time).

Stuttered Words, Syllables Per Minute (SW/M, SS/M) dysfluency measure in which each stuttered word, or syllable, is counted and the sum divided by the total talking time (TTT) in seconds. The result is multiplied by 60. If using a syllable base, remember that every single repetition in a unit is counted.

Percent Stuttered Words, Syllables (%SW, %SS) dysfluency measure in which each stuttered word, or syllable, is counted and the sum divided by the total words or syllables uttered. The result is multiplied by 100. If using a syllable base, remember that every single repetition in a unit is counted.

Adaptation changes in the frequency and/or severity of stuttering over repeated productions of the same stimuli, repeated exposure to the same situation, or over time in a prolonged exposure. (Various adaptation formulas and reservations about adaptation measures will be considered later on when that section of the report form is discussed.)

Consistency the degree to which a stutterer is dysfluent on the same word, syllable, or phoneme during repeated exposures. (Consistency and its various aspects will be discussed later, also.)

Predictability   the degree to which a stutterer can predict or anticipate the occurrence of stuttering on a particular word, syllable, or phoneme. (There also will be later discussion of this topic.)

ALTERNATIVE DIGANOSTIC ASSESSMENT PROCEDURES

Every clinician evolves therapy procedures that "work best," usually starting with cut-and-dried methods and changing them as experience and increasing self-confidence develop. This development is channeled by the numbers and types of clients seen, equipment resources, support personnel availability, case load mix, time schedule, supervisor requirements, and other variables. The same situation occurs in diagnostic and assessment activities. As a result, it is impossible to formulate a procedure outline that can be transferred without change to the variety of professional clinicians and work settings. For this reason, the writer presents here a very extensive diagnostic and assessment program, of which individual clinicians will use selected portions. For the same reason, it is appropriate to sample summarized approaches suggested by other writers. It should be understood that the following is not a full coverage of all major programs, and each summary does not speak to the entire procedure and its variations.

Conture

Edward Conture (1982) urges the clinician to remember that stuttering is only one aspect of a whole person and that the aspects of the environment, personality, other speech areas, and so forth, should not be ignored. He also stresses that the clinician should project certain impressions and competencies to the client. Conture's coverage is generally in discussion form, suggesting areas rather than stipulating or prescribing specific procedures. The interview receives particular emphasis, with many useful suggestions. Typical areas of hearing, voice, articulation, reading, language, intelligence, neuromuscular abilities, and psychological factors are discussed. In fluency, Conture recommends the following six measurement areas:

1. What is the type or types of dysfluency?
2. What is the ranked mean and range of frequency for each dysfluency type?
3. What is the total mean and dysfluency range, and how does each type contribute to the percentage total?
4. What are the mean and range figures for dysfluency durations on a within-word basis?
5. What is the dysfluency adaptation factor?
6. What is the dysfluency consistency factor?

The foregoing six areas of evaluation lead Conture to consider several aspects of the evaluation:

1. Dysfluency nature, frequency, consistency.
2. Percentage of within-word, as opposed to between-word, dysfluencies.
3. The extent to which total dysfluency and within-word dysfluencies are inside the normal range for a particular client's age and communication skills.

The suggestion is made that within-word dysfluency rates above 2 to 3 ✔ percent per 100 words uttered indicate a fluency problem (although not necessarily stuttering). Children exhibiting some sound prolongations, good eye contact, and otherwise easy PWR patterns are candidates for follow-up monitoring. Those who obviously prolong as their most frequent behavior and have poor eye contact are regarded as good candidates for therapy. Some clinicians would feel that these criteria lower the "false failure" rate to unacceptable levels. Conture provides useful advice about decision making, trial therapy, parent counseling, and the consideration of client and environmental variables.

Culp

Delva Culp (1984) describes an assessment procedure directed at preschool children. A parent interview, utilizing a standard case history and fluency history is conducted. Basic evaluation procedures cover hearing, visuomotor, gross motor, articulation, and receptive-expressive language skills. Fluency data are collected in five separate speaking situations which follow, with 150 words collected in each situation.

1. **Monologue**—child is shown a story book and stimulated to talk or tell a story about it. Modeling and prompting are allowed.
2. **Dialogue**—any topic that will elicit speech.
3. **Retelling**—clinician uses cue pictures to tell a story (300 words or more). Cue pictures are redisplayed while child recounts own version. Several stories can be done in order to obtain a sufficient sample.
4. **Play**—use age-appropriate materials and have child lead the activity. Continue until an adequate sample is obtained.
5. **Pressure**—usually the preceding situation is continued, but the clinician provides pressure by interrupting, speaking faster, using more complex language, not paying attention.

Subsequently, the 150-word samples are analyzed for types and frequencies of dysfluency, and percentages are calculated. In a normative study, Culp noted that compared to normally speaking subjects, those with fluency disorders had significantly higher occurrences of PWR, WWR, and tense pause phenomena. She provides six areas of enrollment decision that include dysfluency percentages, dysfluency types, speaker self-concept, family history factors, and environmental concerns. These decision areas are quite broad, somewhat vague, and basically leave the decision up to the clinician as he or she considers all aspects of the situation.

Shine

Richard Shine (1980a, 1980b) has been associated with a widely used fluency reinforcement program, targeting children below eight or nine years of age. He follows many of Ryan's (1974, 1971) precepts in evaluation and therapy of stuttering. Shine uses the Ryan (1974) Stuttering Interview form, and Riley's (1980) Stuttering Severity Instrument (SSI) in his evaluation. Dysfluencies are recorded as WWR, PWR, prolongations (PROL), and struggle behaviors. Behaviors such as incompletions, interjections, revisions, extended pauses, and the like, are not counted except where they clearly are used as starters or are incorporated as part of the secondary struggle behaviors. The physiologic speaking process is evaluated in terms of respiration, phonation, and articulation. These areas are assessed constantly and are evaluated in terms of appearance during fluent speech and during periods of speech disruption. Shine also recommends a parent interview and observation of parent-child interactions (with particular reference to fluency) when parent and child are alone together.

Riley

Glyndon and Jeanna Riley (1984, 1983) advocate early intervention, stating that the possibility of providing therapy for young children "who will outgrow their stuttering anyway . . . is not a very strong argument against early intervention" (1983, p.44). They recommend an assessment program of two to three hours' duration. In addition to the usual components of a communication evaluation, the Rileys utilize two organized approaches, the SSI, or Stuttering Severity Instrument (Riley 1980), and the SPI, or Stuttering Prediction Instrument (Riley 1981). The SSI is probably the most widely used measurement instrument of dysfluency, particularly with children. Using spontaneous speech, or reading plus spontaneous speech samples, the form divides analysis into three categories: (1) spasm frequency, (2) spasm duration, and (3) associated physical behaviors. Each category produces measures that convert into scale scores. These scale scores are added together, and the total is related to severity of the overall problem. Child and adult scores are provided. Although reliability and validity data, as well as normative information, are provided, the scope and depth of the form are limited, and some of the subcategories are limited, or arguable. The SPI depends mainly on an extensive parent interview. The interview areas include family history of stuttering, onset-development history, most-least severity of dysfluencies, parental concern, child frustration, observed physical concomitants of dysfluencies, avoidances of words and/or situations, and negative reactions from the environment (siblings, peers, friends, and so on). It should be noted that in fluency evaluation, the Rileys suggest that the following be accepted and not utilized in dysfluency counts: whole multisyllable word repetitions, phrase repetitions involving two or more words, sentence rephrasing/revision, fluent interjections, and pauses that seem linguistically or otherwise appropriate to the moment.

Rustin and Cook

Lena Rustin and Frances Cook (1983) stress the importance of parent participation and provide specific suggestions for the parent interview. The fluency assessment activities with the client center around Ryan's (1974) Fluency Interview and utilize his classification system. The recorded verbal output is analyzed for stuttered words, words-per-minute rates, stuttered-words-per-minute rates, and percent stuttered words. Associated behaviors, physical coordination, and general communication factors are checked. If the child correctly identifies why he or she is being evaluated, then Rustin and Cook recommend extended probing of information, attitudes, and behaviors. They suggest trial efforts at fluency-inducing behaviors such as minimal response, slow rate, easy onset, short response units, and so on.

Gregory and Hill

Hugo Gregory and Diane Hill (1984) propose a complex, carefully planned structure for evaluation. Many clinicians will have difficulty using the entire approach due to factors of time and pressure of schedule, client fee costs, clinician time availability, and client time availability and willingness. However, the complete assessment program is well worth considering. Their program has two universal stages, followed either by therapy services or by in-depth assessment (followed by therapy). Initial contact is followed by a telephone interview. If elicited information indicates fluency or other concerns going back longer than one year, arrangements are made directly to schedule a comprehensive evaluation. Otherwise, the telephone interview would result in scheduling a screening evaluation. The telephone interview provides questions about the nature of the speech disruptions, when noticed, time span since awareness, any development changes in disruptions, child awareness, family reactions, and other areas of child development and behavior.

Following the telephone interview, the scheduled screening evaluation takes about one hour in its first stage and concentrates on fluency disruption, parent-child interactions, and a general speech, language, and hearing evaluation. One week after this assessment, the parents are interviewed on the basis of case history information, speech, language, and fluency development, and questions from the initial screening evaluation. The interview then converts into a feedback and counseling session to provide information, feedback, and recommendations to the parents.

As a result of the screening evaluation, intervention may be limited to the form of parent counseling or expanded to include counseling plus designated therapy activities to meet particular needs of the child. However, if a decision is made to provide a comprehensive therapy program (including both the parents and the child), then an in-depth evaluation of speech and language is scheduled. The in-depth assessment involves two two-hour sessions. The sessions cover the four areas of the screening evaluation (fluency, parent-child interaction, speech and language development, environment), but they probe more deeply and broadly in order to assess variables and related function areas and determine more exactly the therapy needs of the child. Trial therapy approaches are included as part of the sessions.

The Gregory-Hill approach is an excellent organization for diagnosis, assessment, and therapy planning. However, few (if any) public school clinicians can utilize such an approach. Not very many clinicians in other settings can utilize the full approach due to time and cost demands on both parties—the clinicians and the families. Nevertheless, the concept and content of this approach can be of value to clinicians in any setting and should not be passed by in a pragmatic hunt for "quicker and cheaper" methods. The latter all too often eventuate in use of an abbreviated test or form that supplies inadequate and incomplete information for decision making and therapy planning.

Wells

G. Beverly Wells (1987) has presented a very compact and useful guide to evaluation and therapy of stuttering, with varying emphases on different age groups. A comprehensive evaluation is recommended, with suggested questions provided for interviews with parents and with children who may be stuttering. Fluency assessment relies heavily upon the Riley SSI (cited earlier) and includes a number of physiological assessment points. She provides some very useful suggestions for evaluating the effects of syntactical complexity, psychosocial factors, and linguistic aspects as they relate to stuttering. On the basis of distributed results, children are placed into one of three categories or "profiles": Profile I, normal to advanced language status; Profile II, language delay with auditory-perceptual concerns; Profile III, second profile plus oral-motor and attending concerns. Therapy intervention is structured according to the profile of best fit.

Other

A number of other worthwhile presentations of diagnosis and assessment procedures are available. Wall and Myers (1984) have a useful discussion of differentiating disfluency from dysfluency. They also appropriately suggest awareness of symptom heterogeneity and warn against being misled by the averages of inferential statistics. Curlee (1984, 1980) also provides an extensive assessment presentation. (His criteria in case selection is presented in the next chapter.)

CHAPTER SUMMARY

This chapter has attempted to establish basic terminologies relative to stuttering in general so that they will be familiar in the procedures discussed in Chapter 4. Also, an effort has been made to indicate how other clinicians have approached the problem of diagnosis and assesment of stuttering in children. The next chapter continues the discussion of diagnosis and assessment begun here.

CHAPTER FOUR
DIAGNOSIS
AND ASSESSMENT
Forms and Procedures

ASSESSMENT PROCEDURES

Overview

The procedures in this chapter are organized into a preliminary section, a presentation of the diagnostic report form, and an extended discussion organized around the categories listed in the report form. Where appropriate, procedures or inquiry areas include age-related comments. Otherwise, it is assumed that the clinician will make necessary adjustments relative to the age of the client.

Organization

The organization of Chapter 4 has been explained in the previous chapter; however, our identification of the subject areas maybe useful to the reader at this point. The areas include the following:

- Overview
- Organization
- Preliminary considerations and preparations

- Sequence of the evaluation process
- Telephone interview form and procedure
- Stuttering evaluation form and procedure
- Dysfluency summary sheet and procedure
- Early characteristics of stuttering
- Listener judgment factors in fluency evaluation
- Evaluation of stuttering severity
- Assessment decisioning factors
    - Other clinicians
    - Recommended considerations
- Chapter summary

Preliminary Considerations and Preparation

It is assumed that the diagnostician will apply all procedures typical for any diagnosis and assessment activity. Any evaluations not mentioned, (hearing acuity, for example) should be assumed. Equipment adequate for purposes is also assumed. Beyond routine tongue depressors, facial tissues, and the like, the writer prefers the following:

1. Video-recording capacity, black-and-white or color. Take care that clinician seating or activity does not block the camera view of the child or the informant.
2. Audio-recording capacity. High fidelity broadcast standard equipment is not necessary. However, built-in microphones should be avoided, as they are too omnidirectional, often are of poor quality, and pick up too much ambient and recording machine noise.
3. Stopwatch, preferably digital. Slide bar or silent trigger switches are preferred.
4. Appropriate stimulus material, according to age and (if appropriate) reading level.
    a. Pictures and picture story books (both). Picture series that can be used to tell a story are helpful.
    b. Play material that can elicit commentary, for example, toy barns and animals, garages and vehicles.
    c. Text word lists, sentences, paragraphs, stories.
    d. Monologue topic cards covering 50–100 varied topics.
5. Digital counters. These come in mechanical and electronic forms and cover a wide range of complexity.

Sequence

The clinician is subject to the constraints of his or her work setting, and no diagnostic sequence will fit all settings. However, the following pages suggest a sequence that is maximally productive. The elements of the sequence are the following:

- Preliminary Telephone Interview
- Stuttering Evaluation Form:
    - Psychological Factors
    - Physiological Factors
    - Linguistic Factors
    - Fluency/Dysfluency Evaluation
- Summary and Decision Formulation

As stated, it is assumed that individual clinicians will utilize material provided here according to their job constraints and according to their needs. In certain sections of the chapter, especially when older children are considered, additional evaluation material is provided.

TELEPHONE INTERVIEW

The material in Figure 4–1 is based upon the Gregory and Hill (1984) procedure described earlier. It can aid the clinician in deciding whether or not to schedule an evaluation session, in planning the evaluation session, and in providing preevaluation suggestions or requests to parents. The interview form is divided into six categories: General Information, Fluency Concerns, Child Reactions, Environment Reactions, Other Areas of information, and Closing Activities. The six categories subdivide into 33 question or information areas. Since interview time could be from 15 to 60 minutes (average time is about 30 minutes), it is suggested the informant be contacted initially to arrange a call-back time when he or she will be able to spend the time necessary to answer all the questions. With minor revisions the form can be turned into (or appended to) a prediagnostic case history form that is sent and returned in the mail before the actual diagnosis is made. Also, the form could be adapted to an in-clinic interview outline, although certain values of early information would be lost in such an adaptation.

Telephone interviewing is a particular skill, since putting an invisible listener at ease can be difficult, visual cues from informants are lost, and some clients will not respond well to the impersonal aura of the telephone. It is often wise to spend a few minutes assuring clients that they are not being "treated by telephone." Since the legal complications (and psychological deterrence) of recording telephone conversations can be extensive, the clinician will need to develop the abilty to listen-write and talk-write to assure accuracy and minimize prolonged silences. As often as a "why, I never thought to look for that" rejoinder occurs, the clinician will want to reassure informants that "few of us do" and to suggest that in the time between the end of the interview and the occurrence of the diagnostic appointment, the informants do watch/listen for "that."

FIGURE 4-1. The disfluency prediagnostic telephone interview form.

Informant: _____ Date: _____

Client: _____ Clinician: _____

The following questions are to provide information that will aid in planning evaluation activities and in early decision development. Ask informant if he or she has 20-30 minutes available for questions (explain purpose). If so, continue with interview. If not, schedule a call-back time.

....

I. GENERAL INFORMATION

1. Child's birthdate: _____ Sex: _____

3. Names and ages of other children in the home: _____
   _____
   _____

4. Are both parents living at home: _____
   _____

5. Is mother at home full time: _____
   _____

6. Is child enrolled in: _____ public/private school; _____ preschool;
   _____ nursery/daycare; _____ other arrangement. Comment: _____
   _____

II. FLUENCY CONCERNS

1. When first noticed: _____

2. Who first noticed: _____

3. Others who noticed: _____

4. What was the problem like at first: _____
   _____
   _____

5. Since then, how has it changed: _____
   _____
   _____

6. What is it like now: _____
   _____
   _____

FIGURE 4-1 (continued)

7. How does it vary (time of day, different people, situations, etc.): _____
_____

_____

8. When trouble occurs, does the child:

_____ make faces; _____ make gestures or body movements; _____ stop completely; get stuck; _____ change loudness; _____ change pitch; show irregular, broken speech rhythm; _____ draw out, prolong sounds; _____ other: _____

_____

III. CHILD REACTIONS

1. Is the child obviously aware of the problem: _____

_____

2. If answer to 1 is no, do you think child is aware but covering it up: _____

_____

3. If answer to 2 is yes, how does the child label or describe the problem: _____

_____

_____

4. What kinds of reactions does child have when trouble occurs (none, surprise, frustration, irritation, fear anxiety, shame, etc.): _____

_____

_____

5. When trouble occurs, does child continue speaking, quit, etc.: _____

_____

6. Since problem developed, has child changed in willingness to talk, time spent in talking, etc.: _____

_____

IV. ENVIRONMENT REACTIONS

1. What has been done to try to help the problem; how well have they worked; how has the child reacted to them: _____

_____

_____

_____

FIGURE 4-1 (continued)

2. Have any persons outside the home reacted to or been involved with the child's speech problem: _____

   _____

3. Any problems with imitation, interruption, ridicule, etc., from other children:

   _____

   _____

V. OTHER AREAS

1. Describe general pattern of overall growth and development: _____

   _____

2. Discuss general health history: _____

   _____

3. Describe overall speech development (timing, course, present level): _____

   _____

   _____

4. Are there any speech/language problems now: _____

   _____

5. What is school performance like: _____

   _____

6. In general, what is behavior like, what kind of person is child: _____

   _____

   _____

VI. CLOSING

1. Do *you* have special questions or concerns: _____

   _____

2. Confirm, arrange, or postpone further scheduling for evaluation.

3. Encourage informant to continue thinking about topic areas, to observe the child and others interacting, etc.

....

On the bases of the foregoing information, you may recommend there be no diagnosis and assessment, or that one be scheduled. If scheduling is decided, indicate areas that require particular concentration and report if the informant was instructed to develop any special areas of information or observation prior to the appointment.

General Information is the usual background information. You may wish to expand or add certain information categories. Questions 3 through 6 try to sketch a picture of the child's environment, parental factors, and availability. Also, whether the child is in school, at home all day, or under another's care is important. Depending on the clinic location, you might want to ask whether traveling to the clinic is a problem, and whether it would become a problem if scheduled on a regular (therapy) basis.

Fluency Concerns attempts to chronicle briefly the history of the fluency problem. The question of when the problem was noticed (item 1) provides a rough measure of how long it has been evident. On the other questions it may be necessary to prime the informant with suggestions or examples. On items 7 and 8, routinely suggest that family members continue observing to augment and improve their data by the time the evaluation is scheduled.

Child Reactions is a very important category in terms of estimating therapy needs and modes. Similarly, the fourth section, **Environment Reactions,** is important. The halo effect (informant awareness of "good" answers) can operate strongly in this section, and so the clinician should be careful in phrasing questions or implying judgments.

Other Areas sections are in the nature of securing a quick overview of the child in general. Health, development, general behavior, and so forth, are of interest. In particular, the overall speech and language history is of concern. You may add to this section any comments made in response to questions from earlier sections.

The **Closing** section brings the interview to its conclusion. Thank and praise the informant for his or her effort, indicate that more questions will be asked during the evaluation, and be sure to ask whether the informant has particular questions or concerns. Be very careful to limit your judgments to three general categories:

1. At this time, an appointment for evaluation does not seem necessary; but a counseling and information appointment with the parents can be arranged.
2. There does not seem to be a critical problem, but a counseling and information appointment is desirable, and a recheck after three months would be wise.
3. An evaluation is needed and should be completed.

STUTTERING EVALUATION FORM

The material in Figure 4–2 is based upon years of fluency evaluation and the contributions of other clinicians. It is not that most elusive of things— a total evaluation instrument. There are no adequate substitutes for the experience, insight, imagination, curiosity, flexibility, and perceptiveness

FIGURE 4-2. Information and data summary form for stuttering assessment.

STUTTERING EVALUATION SUMMARY

The sections and subitems in this form can be used as needed. Specific items can be recorded as indicated or can be used as topic areas to elicit information.

....

PSYCHOLOGICAL FACTORS

These can be applied to school/home situations and use direct observation and/or elicited reports.

1. The child appears to be

    _____ unaware of speech disruptions at any time

    _____ occasionally aware and/or aware in specific instances

    _____ generally, consistently aware of difficulties

    _____ covertly aware, but pretends lack of awareness

2. If the child is aware, what are the behavioral reactions? Mark as many items as apply. To the right of any checked item, note any special variations or affecting factors. If possible, query parents, teachers, and significant others as to what they feel they have observed.

    _____ no observable reactions _____

    _____ pretense that nothing happened _____

    _____ changes in overall speech loudness, pitch, rate, etc. _____

    _____

    _____ alterations in amount of verbal output _____

    _____ signs of frustration, impatience, irritation _____

    _____

    _____ signs of embarrassment, shame, guilt _____

    _____

    _____ signs of anxiety or fear _____

    _____ overt identification that trouble occurred _____

    _____

    _____ specific behaviors to cope with specific disruptions _____

    _____

    _____

3. How do others react to speech disruptions of child? Below, leave blank unreported items, mark C if clinician-observed, and mark R if reported by parents, siblings, teachers, peers, significant others. A blank can have both C and R.

    _____ unaffected, unaware   _____ covert awareness

    _____ support, acceptance   _____ anxiety, concern

    _____ embarrassment, irritation   _____ assistance, concern

    _____ interruption, scolding   _____ imitation, ridicule

    _____ anger, punishment   other _____

FIGURE 4-2 (continued)

4. How do disruptions change as situational factors change? In the blanks, insert S if dysfluencies seem unchanged; insert W if they seem worse; insert B if fluency seems to improve.

   _____ general conversations with family or friends

   _____ reporting day's activities   _____ when being scolded or punished

   _____ arguments with siblings or peers   _____ when feeling unhappy or unwell

   _____ when feeling happy or excited

   _____ when being interrupted, corrected, disagreed with

   _____ talking with strangers   _____ when asking questions or permissions

   _____ reporting/reciting to class, peer group

   Talking with _____ father _____ mother _____ sibling _____ teacher

   _____ others

   Other special situations or people: _____

   _____

5. On the basis of observation and/or elicited information, which descriptors below describe parental and environmental communication patterns?

   _____ rapid rate   _____ slow rate   _____ competition   _____ nonresponse

   _____ emotional   _____ talkative   _____ demanding   _____ challenging

   _____ apathy   _____ interruptions   _____ extended silences

   _____ complex language   _____ other _____

   _____

   _____

6. In general terms, how does the child function in his or her environment? Descriptors below are ranged in contrasting pairs. Where child is reported "somewhere between," circle the slash mark separating contrasting terms.

_____ retiring/open _____	_____ neutral/affectionate _____
_____ shy/outgoing _____	_____ silent/talkative _____
_____ submissive/dominant _____	_____ isolates self/interactive _____
_____ accepting/argumentative _____	_____ whining/belligerent _____
_____ happy, depressed _____	_____ dependent/independent _____
_____ sensitive/insensitive _____	_____ anxious/confident _____

PHYSIOLOGICAL FACTORS

Respiration

1. Inhalation is _____ shallow, frequent   _____ phonation on inhalation

   _____ too extended   _____ clavicular, upper chest   _____ opposition

   _____ reversed

2. Exhalation is _____ air wastage before utterance   _____ air wastage during utterance   _____ excessive utterance per exhalation   _____ interrupted exhalations

FIGURE 4-2 (continued)

3. General patterns and effects of respiration: _____ irregular breathing cycles _____ phrasing interfered with   _____ poor coordination with phonation release _____ poor coordination with coarticulation factors   _____ poor coordination with linguistic elements, particularly those involving prosodic factors

4. How does breathing during dysfluencies differ from breathing during fluent speech?

_____

_____

Phonation

1. General phonation marked by _____ hard glottal attacks _____ breathy phonation   _____ strained phonation   _____ harsh, hoarse tone _____ vocal fry   _____ pitch problems   _____ loudness problems _____ other _____

_____

2. *s/z* ratio value (should be about 1.00) is _____ (pg 74)

3. During dysfluencies (check all that apply)
   Laryngeal spasms are _____ occasional   _____ frequent   _____ predominant
   Voiced prolongations are _____ occasional   _____ frequent   _____ predominant
   Silent stoppages are _____ occasional   _____ frequent   _____ predominant

4. Other vocal behaviors associated specifically with moments of stuttering:

_____

_____

Articulation
   _____ inadequate diadochokinesis   _____ inadequate rhythmokinesis
   _____ dysarthric articulator movements   _____ dyspraxic articulator movements
   _____ incorrect articulatory movement
   _____ exaggerated, incorrect preformations
   _____ inappropriate substitution/insertion of the schwa vowel
   _____ noticeable dysfluency occurrence on voiceless-to-voiced phoneme transistions
   _____ noticeable dysfluency occurrence by phoeneme class (stops, sibilants, etc.)
   _____ noticeable dysfluency occurrence by position (bilabial, linguovelar, etc.)
   _____ noticeable dysfluency occurrence on vowels
   _____ general articulation errors, without regard to dysfluencies

General Coordination
   _____ facial asymmetry   _____ muscle flaccidity
   _____ flattened nasolabial fold   _____ muscle fasciculations

FIGURE 4-2. continued

_____ tremors   _____ hypertonicity   _____ confused laterality

_____ gait abnormalities   _____ postural abnormalities

_____ other factors: _____

_____

LINGUISTIC FACTORS

Syntatic

_____ Name and results of formal test: _____

_____

_____ dysfluency frequency/severity seems related to syntactic complexity

_____ dysfluencies tend to occur among initial words of sentences/phrases

_____ dysfluencies tend to cluster around clause boundaries

_____ dysfluencies tend to cluster around prosodic stress points

_____ other: _____

_____

Semantic

_____ Name and results of formal test: _____

_____

_____ content words more frequently dysfluent, or

_____ function words more frequently dysfluent

_____ dysfluency frequency/severity related to semantic complexity

_____ dysfluencies increase as propositionality increases

_____ other: _____

_____

Pragmatic

_____ Name and results of formal test: _____

_____

_____ Observed effects of pragmatic factors (see 4, Psychological Factors):

_____

_____

Related Areas

_____ difficulties in auditory processing

_____ difficulties in auditory recall

_____ difficulties in attending

_____ other problem areas: _____

_____

_____

_____

of the clinician. The form can serve as a reminder and a guide, but it would be unusual if all its areas were needed in every evaluation or if it was not useful to add items to it in nearly every application. The form can be carried along and filled out, filled out subsequent to an evaluation, or used in other ways. Preferred tests or self-developed procedures can be integrated into its structure. Variations generated by client age, other speech and language problems, and the presence of cognitive, physical, or emotional problems will alter how the form can be used and add information areas to it.

Psychological Factors

This area, the first in Figure 4–2, provides exploration of some psychosocial aspects of communication disruption. The first item queries the child's awareness. For a generation or more it was believed widely that young children had little or no awareness of their fluency disruptions. Oddly enough, the people who articulated this myth found no contradiction in also warning that the same unaware children were so perceptive, discerning, and sensitive that adults must inhibit explicit and implicit reactions to dysfluencies (or disfluencies) because these reactions would create the "vicious cycle" of stuttering development. How a child so perceptive could be simultaneously unaware of fluency disruptions was never explained satisfactorily. Bloodstein (1960a, 1960b), in summarizing 418 stutterers from preschool to midadolescence, reported that "all" persons showed awareness to some degree, many engaged in conscious anticipation of stuttering, and that some (even among the youngest) displayed acute emotional reactions. He categorized four levels of awareness:

1. Little overt reaction and apparently no self-concept as a stutterer.
2. Awareness of self-stuttering, but no particular reactions are observable.
3. Reactions in the ranges of frustration, irritation, anger, and so forth.
4. Reactions of fear, embarrassment, guilt, shame, and so forth.

Thompson (1984) reported on 48 school-age stutterers, primarily in grades K–7. She stated that in general these children were aware of their stuttering and, furthermore, most of them were willing to talk about it. It has been suggested that primary school age stutterers were not particularly concerned about their fluency problems, and Culatta and others (1985) have reinforced this finding. These findings do not mean that all children will be aware of stuttering, and it would be inappropriate to extend Thompson's findings down to the two-year-old to four-year-old age group without qualification. Nevertheless, extra time and gentle questioning of a child may elicit admissions of awareness, an awareness that had not been realized previously by the parents. Remember that children early on become cautious about exposing problems to adults; and also they may lack the language descriptors adults are used to and familiar with. These reports of awareness are interesting in view of Cooper and Cooper's report (1985) of a ten-year survey (1973–83) of about 674 speech and language pathologists. In response to the proposal that there is no such thing as a primary unaware stutterer, almost 66 percent disagreed, while another 13 percent were undecided. Interestingly, 29 percent agreed that kindergarten and first-grade children should not receive therapy (21 percent were undecided), and 48 percent felt that first and second graders should not hear the clinician use the words *stutterer* or *stuttering* (18 percent were undecided).

Item 2 under Psychological Factors in Figure 4–2 raises questions concerning the stutterer's reactions to stuttering occurrences. These reactions divide into those associated with specific occurrences of dysfluency and those general attitudes toward speaking per se. F.H. Silverman and Williams (1968) studied kindergarten and first-grade stutterers and nonstutterers in story-telling activity. They found the stutterers to be lower in their mean length of response (MLU), in variability in response length, in the average of their five longest responses, and in structural complexity of language. The stutterers were higher on one-word responses. Subsequently, F.H. Silverman (1976) reported that second-grade and third-grade stutterers used about 10 percent fewer words in story telling, while in grades 4, 5, and 6 they dropped to 25 percent fewer words. Devore, Nandur, and Manning (1984) failed to differentiate young stutterers and nonstutterers on the basis of communication attitudes. As noted earlier, Thompson (1984) reported that school-age stutterers did not show marked negative feelings or avoidance behaviors concerning speech.

It would be a potential error to assume much more than the following: most children have significant awareness of fluency disruptions, and that complicating reactions to dysfluencies develop over time. The clinician should observe closely and not hesitate to probe. Subsequent sections of the evaluation form provide for a variety of speech complexity and situation variables. Client behaviors, as well as dysfluencies, should be noted in all of them. In addition, the clinician should query and probe informants for their observations and remembered incidents. Where feasible, instructions to "view anew" and report back to the clinician later can help the process (particularly during therapy) as the informants reobserve with an augmented frame of reference.

Item 3 of Psychological Factors deals with the issues of how others react to the child's stuttering. This will be reinforced in item 5 when the parent and home situation is viewed. On a number of occasions I have inveighed against past overemphasis on parents and other environmental-social factors, particularly in the onset of stuttering. These objections should not lead to the conclusion that psychosocial factors are felt to be unimportant. As we approach and cross a hypothetical border in stutterers (eight to ten years of age), external social forces appear to become much more significant. Cooper and Cooper (1985) reported that about two-thirds of 621 speech and language clinicians agreed that a child's peers would tend to react more negatively to stuttering than they would to other speech disorders. This is reinforced by Thompson (1984), who reported that about 75 percent of 48 school-age stutterers had apparently been ridiculed because of their stuttering.

I have found, interviewing parents or others, that a strong halo effect operates. When queried about reactions, informants are quick to say, "It's okay . . . I just ignore it . . . we wait . . ." and so on. If the clinician persists, or uses the cross-hatch questioning technique (Emerick and Hatton 1979), more revealing answers usually eventuate. I will often accept the no-reaction answers briefly but return with questions such as these:

> "Many stutterers report unfavorable experiences. Where do you think _____ has had them?"
> "Stuttering can be frustrating to the listener as well as to the speaker. Haven't you observed or experienced this?"
> "Siblings can be pretty tough on each other at times. Haven't you observed this happening?"
> "People outside the family can show a real lack of understanding at times. Hasn't this happened to _____ ?"

Leading questions in many other forms can be shaped. It may also be helpful here to instruct informants to reobserve and report back later.

Item 4 confounds with the pragmatics item under Linguistic Factors of Figure 4-2. In questioning parents about their child, I usually say something like the following:

> "Quite commonly the amount of trouble a child has while talking changes when the people, the situation, or feelings change. Sometimes there is more speech difficulty, or less, and the trouble also may change in its form. In the following (subitems from item 4), what kinds of changes, if any, have you observed?"

If questioning the client, rather than parents, essentially the same approach can be used. Where the interview setting is in school, some situations can be dropped and others added. For adolescents, for example, peer relationships and situations often need to be expanded. As before, the informant can be instructed to consider/observe further and report later. Where possible, clinician observation variables actually in operation can be compared to informant statements. Aside from assessment values, item 4 provides foundation information if a stress hierarchy is to be structured in subsequent therapy.

Item 5 relates more to preschool and early elementary children, although it can function at almost any age. The item aims at securing a picture of how the parents and the overall home environment create positive and/or negative influences for the speaker. There has been a great deal of research on parents, and our philosophy has suffered from trying to balance inconsistencies in reported family socioeconomics, family histories of stuttering, numbers of siblings, which child stutters, accuracy of labeling, tests and procedures used, and so on.

Allan and Williams (1974) stated that families of stuttering children are more emotional in their interactions, less effective in decision making, direct fewer statements to the stuttering children than to their fluent children, and show noticeable similarities to the functioning of disturbed families. Crowe and Cooper (1977) evaluated parents of 36 school-age and 14 college-age stutterers on stuttering attitudes and knowledge about stuttering. Compared to parents of nonstutterers, these parents were significantly less accepting in their attitudes and significantly less informed in their knowledge about stuttering. Riley and Riley (1979) reported that slightly over 50 percent of their child sample had disruptive communication environments, unreasonable parental expectations of the children, and other negative factors. A series of studies on preschool and school-age stutterers are summarized as follows (Moore & Nystul 1979; Fowlie & Cooper 1978; Yairi 1973; Kasprisin-Burrelli, Eyolf & Shames 1972; Goldman & Shames 1964; Kinstler 1961):

> Parents display a "more negative manner" to stutterers than to nonstuttering siblings.
>   Mothers reject stutterers overtly less, but covertly more; accept them covertly less and overtly slightly less; reject them more than they accept them.
>   Fathers tend to be more conventional and rigid; mothers tend to be more democratic or liberal, so that the environment climate is unstable.
>   Mothers felt their stuttering children were more introverted, anxious, fearful, insecure, and sensitive.
>   Parents, particularly fathers, of stutterers tend to set generally higher goals for their children and specifically to have higher speech adequacy expectations.
>   Adolescent stutterers perceive their parents as not being like "other parents," with mothers differing more than the fathers do.

Not all studies have established parental differences or patterns. Bourdon and Silber (1970) failed to separate young stutterers and nonstutterers in terms of how they perceived their parents. Similarly, Cox, Seider, and Kidd (1984) could not differentiate families in terms of parental factors, family anxiety levels, speech attitudes, or parent and child perceptions of each other's behaviors or traits. Finally, Meyers and Freeman (1985a, 1985c) failed to support the hypothesis that mothers of stutterers are more dominating (Moncur 1955). They did, though, note that when a stuttering child displayed physical concomitants and struggle, the listening mothers tended to show nonverbal reactions such as immobility, looking away, and changing facial expressions.

Literature reviews have concluded that stutterers' parents do not present typically neurotic or psychotic traits. However, many seem to be more competitive and perfectionistic, overconcerned about their children, and more inclined to dominate their children and to set unrealistically high goals (Bloodstein 1969). It has also been concluded that parents tend to be marked by low social dominance and that the mothers in particular tend to be passive and/or permissive (Quarrington 1974). We simply do not have an adequate description of family environment characteristics, or we must accept the suggestion that no stereotype or stereotypes exist.

Most of item 5 in Psychological Factors, Figure 4–2, deals specifically with the speech and language environment of the home. This is a direct reflection of, or reaction to, the preceding review of parent research. It does seem feasible to set model questions about parental traits and behaviors except as they relate to communication. This does not imply that the clinician should be oblivious to environmental relationships, and prior items 3 and 4 will supply some information there. Also, the following item 6 can be applied to the family members as well as to the child. With adolescents it can be self-administered with reference to the home and to the client.

Item 6 under Psychological Factors concerns the behavior of the client in his or her environment. Figure 4–2 provides only a bipolar adjective checklist, but many additional areas can be considered. Clinicians may also want to use personal observation, information forms, attitude scales, personality tests, and other methods to assess client adjustment and behavior. Andrews and others (1983), in their extensive review of stuttering research, surveyed a few studies dealing with the intelligence of school-aged stutterers and found they supported the view that stuttering children are less intelligent than are their nonstuttering counterparts. This differential, in both verbal and nonverbal tasks, fell at about six months of educational progress. The Cooper and Cooper study (1985) of clinician attitudes reported a shift, in the past decade, away from beliefs that stutterers have particular personality characteristics. However, agreement percentages ranged from 42 to 81 percent (all but two above 50 percent) for the belief that most stutterers have the following: psychological problems, distorted perceptions of their own stuttering behaviors, feelings of inferiority, characteristic personality traits, distorted perceptions of social relationships, and the need for more clinician psychological understanding than do other communication disorders. About 81 percent agreed that stuttering was the most psychologically devastating of the communication disorders.

Personality differences between stutterers and nonstutterers have not been established, except where certain behavioral characteristics could be attributed to developments as a result of stuttering, rather than the other way around. This may be a finding of dubious value as far as assessment is concerned. There is a danger that many clinicians will feel that personality adjustment factors are of minimal or no importance. However, the prevalence of adjustment problems in the general population is actually fairly high (in terms of prevalence figures on mental health). When the stress of fluency disruptions is added to the picture, behavior and environmental adjustment are appropriate concerns in dysfluency assessment and therapy programs. Adams (1969) reviewed about 20 references concerning the psychology of stutterers. Overall, he concluded that grouped findings suggest that nonstutterers and stutterers differ significantly in several areas of psychological characteristics.

Although Devore, Nandur, and Manning (1984) failed to differentiate young stutterers and nonstutterers on the basis of communication attitudes, selected projective drawings did separate them, and these drawings changed significantly during therapy for the stutterers. Duncan (1949) reported that stutterers tended to feel their parents were disappointed in them, that their homes lacked real love and affection, and that parents did not understand them. Woods (1974) compared stuttering and nonstuttering third-grade and sixth-grade males on self-ratings and peer ratings of social acceptance. Overall, the nonstutterers were rated significantly higher in acceptability, and the stutterers' self-ratings were significantly poorer than the self-ratings by the nonstutterers. Riley and Riley (1983) cite high self-expectations as a complicating factor among stuttering children. This included self-blame, anxiety, withdrawal, dependency, and poor ego strength.

The authors just cited have also commented on how some children use stuttering to manipulate situations and their general environment (Riley and Riley 1983, 1979). This phenomenon has been noted frequently. Some children perceive clearly that certain behaviors tend to secure attention, excuse failures, ward off punishment, delay actions, facilitate permissions, and so forth. Behaviors can include whining, tantrums, headaches—or stuttering. Parents can be loathe to "upset" the child, and some children use this with the precision of an Ellis RET (rational emotive therapy) counselor. I have observed it in children below the age of three, even to the extent of their applying such behavior (or trying to) against therapists using operantly based fluency programs. Our refusal to respond or to allow the behavior to continue was a great surprise to the children, as well as a revelation to the observing/participating parents. A few tested further by transiting into temper tantrums, but clinician support of the parents helped them weather the storms!

An extension of manipulative behavior occurs often as the child matures, and that extension is what I call the stutter crutch. This term refers to the use of stuttering as an excuse, an alibi, a rationalizing agent. This behavior is probably strongest among adolescent stutterers, where academic and social interactions expand considerably. At times, the crutch system is difficult to separate from understandable avoidances due to anxiety and embarrassment. At times, the logic becomes tortuous and fragile:

Q: How are things in your classes?
A: Not so hot.
Q: How come? What's the problem?
A: Aah, I don't turn in my homework stuff like I should.
Q: You don't! Can't you figure them out?
A: Oh heck, yeah, sure. But, you know, if I do, then she asks questions about it in class and I know I'm gonna have trouble, you know, when I talk.
Q: But doesn't she hassle you when you don't turn it in?
A: Not much. She used to but I always had so much, you know, so much trouble, now she just yells at me and I just duck my head.

Physiological Factors

The section Physiological Factors breaks down into four areas of function concerning the physiology of communication: **Respiration, Phonation, Articulation,** and **General Coordination.** In the fourth section there is a separate consideration of cluttering. Now that we have moved away from the myth that stuttering is only a socially induced problem, we find that old myths die hard and many practicing clinicians were trained in "social cause only" environments. In the Cooper and Cooper (1985) study referred to before, only 30.5 percent of 674 speech and language pathologists agreed that most stutterers have some underlying physiological impairment, although nearly 90 percent accepted the proposal that multiple coexisting factors were involved in most stuttering.

Andrews and others (1983) cited three studies of EEG differences in stutterers, with conflicting results. Cerebral lateralization may very well differentiate between acquired stuttering and so-called idiopathic stuttering, since a number of studies suggest right-hemisphere activity of stuttering during language-processing behaviors (see the pathophysiology section in Chapter 2). Various studies suggest that recognition and recall of syllables, words, and messages are likely to be less adequate among stutterers than nonstutterers. A majority of studies indicate that stutterers have slower vocal and manual reactions times. Wexler and Mysak (1982) have speculatively separated types of dysfluency, relating one group to physiological, or neuromotor, factors, and the others to linguistic factors.

One host of studies has suggested few or no differences between stutterers and nonstutterers in a wide range of physiological functions. However, another host of studies has reported positive findings across a number of capacities or factors. In-between studies report confused results, and a number of researchers have found nonstutterers to be as poor in performance as the worst stutterers, while some stutterers performed about as well as did the best of the nonstutterers. With children, there is also the possibility that some physiological patterns will develop as a result of habituation processes due to the stuttering, rather than exist due to an underlying neurophysiological etiology. Since most of our studies are on adults, not children, we must be very careful in establishing assumptions about what children who stutter can or cannot do in terms of function.

Respiration   Items 1 and 2 of Respiration in Figure 4–2 relate primarily to respiratory behaviors during speech and during dysfluencies. Bloodstein (1969) suggests looking for antagonism (opposition of inhalatory and exhalatory muscles), irregularity, prolonged inspiration or expiration, interruptions of exhalations by sudden inhalations, efforts to speak on inhalation, and respiratory stops. Other possibilities are cited in the evaluation form.

The clinician will want to separate vegetative (life) respiratory patterns from those involved in communication. A stutterer may have abnormal speech respiration due to habituation but still present a normal vegetative pattern. It is possible that abnormal patterns will be limited only to moments of dysfluency (and adjacent times), with fluent speech exhibiting adequate patterns. At the opposite end, some stutterers will have a total respiratory pattern that is inadequate and/or distorted. Issues of vital capacity and related measures are so rarely involved that no specific measurement procedures are presented here. However, useful references on speech respiration are easily available (Zemlin 1980; Hixon 1973).

Phonation   In the Phonation section, item 1 asks about the general presence and function of the voice. Blood and Seider (1981) noted that about 1 percent of their stuttering population had phonatory disorders as well. In addition to this, as stutterers develop toward and into adolescence, we are more likely to find the development of habitual vocal alterations in pitch, loudness, and inflection as part of an overall antiexpectancy pattern of behavior. In item 2, the s-z ratio is suggested for evaluation. Have the client take a maximal inhalation and then, on signal, produce the desired phoneme (/s/ or /z/) for the maximum time possible. Time production to the second. Best results are obtained by having the client produce one phoneme three consecutive times, average the results, and then repeat this with the other phoneme. Production should be "normal" in its effort, and not underproduced or overproduced. Divide one average into the other in order to establish the coefficient value.

Research has indicated that stutterers tend to have longer vocal onset times (VOT) and vocal termination times (VTT), that is, the time it takes the vocal folds to initiate or terminate vibration with reference to an arresting or releasing consonant. Adams, among others, has been interested in this phenomenon (Adams and Hayden 1976). Voicing differences have been noted particularly where stutterers must shift back and forth between voiced and voiceless productions, especially if such shifts occur at clause boundaries and/or at prosodic stress points. Adams and Reis (1971) constructed two reading passages, one in which all sounds were voiced, and the other loaded with off-on voicing requirements. Stutterers produced significantly more dysfluencies in reading the off-on passage and had significantly more adaptation (reduction in dysfluency frequency) with the all-voiced passage. Runyan and Bonifant (1981) followed a similar design with 22 elementary-age stutterers. Overall, the groups did not differ significantly on either the quantities or qualities of dysfluencies on the two passages. However, slightly more than one-third of the stutterers had more dysfluencies while reading the off-on passage. Adams (1984b) recommends evaluating sustained phonation and VOT performance.

Item 3 on the evaluation form targets laryngospasms, or dysfluencies that are localized at the vocal folds. These usually will be tonic stoppages (vocal arrests) or prolongations. Observation across situations and with different types of material are useful in checking for spasm types. In addition to laryngeal spasms, look generally for strong glottal attacks during fluent or dysfluent utterances. Glottal attacks are part of every speaker's speech pattern and physiologically involve complete vocal fold adduction prior to initiation of the breath stream. It occurs commonly in utterances such as

"Well, I don't know about you, but I'm going!"
"Hey! Watch out for the dog!

Hypertense vocal function can be indicative of overall tension levels, as well as emphasizing laryngeal stuttering. Some clinicians want to divide stutterers into three spasm groups: oral, laryngeal, orolaryngeal. Such a division, for some therapies, might be useful. Schwartz (1976, 1974) has stated that the problem of stuttering is solved: It is known now to be due to discoordination of adductor and abductor muscle combinations in the laryngeal system linked to distortion of the infantile airway dilation reflex (to keep the infant's air passageway clear). However Schwartz's proposals have been questioned in terms of their adequacy, specificity, substantiation by research, and value (Ham 1986; Ingham 1984; Sheehan 1980; Gregory 1979). Nonetheless, several therapies target the airflow-phonation situation.

General articulation　"Children who stutter are more likely to have articulation problems." How many times have we heard that, or similar statements? Blood and Seider (1981) reported that 16 percent of 1,060 stutterers (14 years of age or younger) also had articulation problems. Williams, Silverman and Cools (1968) have evaluated stutterers in grades K–9 and reported similar results, especially at lower grade levels. If we added "minimally acceptable" to those actually having difficulty, then it would be probable that a large number of children who stutter will not be typical in their articulation of phonemes. For all preschool and early-grade children (first through third), formal articulation tests should be a part of every evaluation. Because so many are available, no specific one is recommended here, but it should be comprehensive. Also, articulation in spontaneous speech should be checked.

The articulation section of Figure 4–2 also concentrates on two other aspects: articulator structure and motor function, and phoneme articulation as it relates to dysfluencies. These two general areas will be looked at separately.

Articulation function   The first items under Articulation in Figure 4–2 relate to diadochokinesis and rhythmokinesis. Diadochokinesis involves *diado-* (successive) and *-kinesis* (motions), in which opposing muscle groups perform alternate functions. Finger tapping, foot patting, and jaw clicks are examples. M.H. Cooper and G.D. Allen (1977) compared normal speakers, treated stutterers, and in-treatment stutterers on the timing of repeated utterances. There was considerable variation and overlap; but, overall, normal speakers were the most accurate timers, and treated stutterers were more accurate than were those still in treatment. Diadochokinesis can be tested in many ways, but isolate sounds /p /, /t /, and /k / are typically used for bilabial, lingualveolar, and linguavelar productions (with mandibular involvement). Then, two-phoneme and three-phoneme combinations are tested. Table 4–1 provides abridged data and test procedures reported by Fletcher (1972), plus age extensions downward added by Riley and Riley (1983). Diadochokinetic rates, like the *s/z* ratio, will usually be more accurate if three trials are averaged. A little practice to clarify signals and timing may be useful. Rhythmokinesis is diadochokinesis wherein a rhythmic pattern is superimposed on the successive productions. The clinician instructs the child to imitate her or his production. Any simple patterns can be used, with stress points added if desired.

Other articulator function points are raised in this section of Figure 4–2. All of them can be answered by performance of an adequate peripheral speech mechanism evaluation. This should be performed for every client, at any age, in any setting. There are a number of commercially available evaluation forms, and hundreds of individual forms have been designed. A form is supplied at the end of this chapter, but individual preferences are encouraged.

Articulation dysfluency   This part of the articulation section suggests that the clinician apply phonological classifications to analysis of dysfluencies. Clinicians may lack time to do an in-depth job of this while preparing the initial assessment report. However, later review and analysis of recorded or transcribed speech efforts can provide a treasure of information as the clinician plans therapy. This is particularly true for younger

TABLE 4–1. Children's Production of Measured Numbers of Single or Sequenced Syllables.

AGE	AVERAGE TIME				
	$p\wedge$*	$t\wedge$*	$k\wedge$*	$p\wedge t\wedge$**	$p\wedge t\wedge k\wedge$***
6	4.8	4.9	5.5	7.3	10.3
7	4.8	4.9	5.3	7.6	10.0
8	4.2	4.4	4.8	6.2	8.3
9	4.0	4.1	4.6	5.9	7.7
10	3.7	3.8	4.3	5.5	7.1
11	3.6	3.6	4.0	4.8	6.5
12	3.4	3.5	3.9	4.7	6.4
13	3.3	3.3	3.7	4.2	6.4

Source: Adapted from S.G. Fletcher, *Journal of Speech and Hearing Research,* 1972, 763–770.

* = 20 productions, ** = 15 productions, *** = 10 productions

Note: Riley and Riley (1983) have added ages four and five to the measure, with $p\wedge$ averaging about 2.5 seconds for ten productions (5.0 for 20), $p\wedge t\wedge$ averaging about 5.3 seconds for ten productions (7.95 for 15), and 10.6 seconds for five-year-olds (only) on ten productions of $p\wedge t\wedge k\wedge$. Fletcher's instructions involved the examiner first modeling the performance, then having the child and examiner perform dually for several seconds, having the child utter alone for several seconds, and finally telling the child to perform until told to stop. The child is to wait for starting signals and then "go as fast as you can."

children where control of stimulus material can be very important in various modes of fluency reinforcement therapy. It may also be useful with older children who might develop phoneme-related spasm occurrences.

General coordination   As long as we have unresolved issues surrounding neuromotor aspects of stuttering, our applications of general physiological factors in assessment will vary greatly. Previous sections have indicated VOT and VTT differences in many stutterers, and other timing research studies tend to report similar results. Finkelstein and Weisberger (1954) administered the (then) Oseretsky Test of Motor Proficiency to 15 stutterers, ages four to ten, and to matched controls. Overall, the stutterers were superior to controls, averaging a chronological age of about one month less and a motor age of about seven months more than the nonstuttering controls. This anomalous result was not supported by Riley and Riley (1980), who reported that 69 percent of a large sample of child stutterers (ages 5–12) displayed motor production problems or neurological soft signs. Much earlier, Bloodstein (1969) suggested looking for rapid hand tremors and eye movement irregularities (vertical jerking, prolonged fixations, other inappropriate movements). Cross and Luper

(1983) evaluated stutterers of 5, 9, and 18 years of age on their finger movement and vocal reaction times in response to auditory stimuli. All subjects decreased reponse time with age, but at all ages the stutterers took significantly longer to respond (both types of response). The end-of-chapter peripheral mechanism examination form has a number of general coordination evaluation points that might be useful for this section. In school settings, conversations with physical education staff may elicit interesting information about a client's general coordination.

Cluttering   At times we seem to create problems for ourselves as we define disorders too rigidly and, as discussed earlier, wind up with embarrassing nonconformities to deal with. The whole issues of dysarthric and dyspraxic patterns of "stuttering" have not been dealt with adequately. Also, dysfluency among the mentally retarded has received comparatively scant attention, as have a number of other problem categories. St. Louis (1986) has edited a text paying particular attention to the atypical-stutterer categories.

Overall, cluttering has received minor attention in research and even less in diagnosis, evaluation, and therapy. Our primary references have been European (Luchsinger and Arnold 1965; Weiss 1964; Froeschels 1952), and progress in differentiation has been slow. According to St. Louis, Hinzman, and Hull (1985), cluttering and stuttering were first differentiated about 1830. Perkins (1978) regards cluttering as a symptom of a "central language imbalance" that includes dysfunctions in articulation, language, fluency, behavior, general neuromotor function, and cognition. European literature, in particular, discusses divisions such as clutterers, clutter-stutterers, and stutter-clutterers, and stutterer subgroups.

Research has suggested that clutterers have less accurate and organized performance than do stutterers in semantic, syntactic, and pragmatic aspects of language. St. Louis, Hinzman, and Hull (1985) found that both stutterers and clutterers, compared to controls, were marked by higher frequency of phrase and word repetitions. However, compared to stutterers, the clutterers were much lower in sound/syllable repetitions, prolongations, and struggle behaviors. Linguistically, they were below the other groups in completeness and complexity of utterances. Dumke and others (1963), reported that clutterers used more filler sounds and phrases, hurried motor rhythms, tended to accelerate (festinate) on longer words, and had below-average musical ability.

A still useful guideline, but one to be applied with full awareness of human variability, was supplied by Darley (1964). He summarized extant resources and suggested that in comparison to stutterers, clutterers

- Are less aware of their dysfluencies.
- Become more fluent when attention is paid to speech.
- Are most dysfluent in free, spontaneous speech.

- Are more fluent when speaking with strangers.
- Are more fluent in brief, rather than long, utterances.
- Are helped by repeating previously dysfluent utterances.

Several clinicians have noted that while stutterers tend to improve under delayed auditory feedback (DAF) conditions, clutterers tend to become more dysfluent. This author has observed this phenomenon in several therapy situations but knows of no research to support the concept.

The significance of cluttering should not be overlooked. Curlee (1985) notes that differentiation procedures (from stuttering) are not particularly adequate. He states, "In addition, there is no known practical advantage or usefulness in making this distinction" (p. 316). While the label *cluttering* does nothing for us clinically, an awareness of the conditions thought to characterize cluttering should suggest several approaches, all practical and useful. These could include the following:

1. More extensive testing of diadochokinesis and rhythmokinesis.
2. Finer evaluation of coarticulation and dysfluency.
3. Sensitivity to possible dysarthria/dyspraxia fluency problems (Canter 1971).
4. Closer observation of overall neuromotor coordination.
5. Greater sophistication in the assessment of language functions.
6. Testing specifically for festinating characteristics and conditions affecting it.
7. Specific activities to increase and decrease pressure on and awareness of speech.
8. Specific activities aimed at monitoring and self-correction of speech.
9. Use of delayed auditory feedback.
10. Environmental checks on behavior, intellectual functions, and academic performance.

Therapy approaches could be modified or enhanced in a number of practical and useful ways. Cluttering will be considered further in Chapter 15, when we look at complicating variables in therapy.

Linguistic Factors

The section of Figure 4–2 devoted to linguistic factors covers several topic areas of evaluation. Because we are focusing on young children and extending down to preschool years, the attention is appropriate. The section is divided into the subsections Syntactic, Semantic, and Pragmatic, plus one called Related Areas. It is assumed that the clinician will use formal tests when appropriate, and space is provided to identify such tests. No tests are suggested, since there are so many variables and aspects to direct test selection. As a general rule, the younger the client, the greater the tendency to evaluate by observation and interview. There is, however, a need to test both comprehensively and in depth across linguistic areas.

Riley (1980) evaluated stuttering children, ages five to twelve, and reported that 27 percent had auditory perception problems, 31 percent central language processing difficulties, and 36 percent displayed attending problems. Blood and Seider (1981) determined that 10 percent of 1,060 school-age stutterers also had language problems as well, and Wall and Myers (1982) suggested that about 35 percent of stuttering children are language delayed. Language consideration should be eclectic, subset groups can be looked for with expectations of different factors combining among different stutterers, and assessment should include free speech as well as controlled-structured utterances (Adams 1984b; Homzie and Lindsay 1984).

Syntactic factors have been of interest to researchers for many years. We have long accepted that stuttering tends to occur among the first three words of an utterance (Brown 1938) and to be affected by the grammatical type and the information value of words (Brown 1937). We have also found that initial consonants and longer words are more likely to be dysfluent (Trotter 1956; F.H. Silverman 1972a; Danzger and Halpern 1973). E-M. Silverman (1974) reported that nonstuttering four-year-olds were more likely to be disfluent on initial words, just as are stutterers. Tornick and Bloodstein (1976) found that sentence length and disfluency were correlated. However, the word-sentence length effect, compared to information value effect, has been questioned (Peterson 1969; Soderberg 1971, 1967; Kaasin and Bjerken 1982). Pearl and Bernthal (1980) studied the effect of grammatical complexity on the disfluencies of three-year-old and four-year-old children, concluding that the issue itself is complicated and that factors other than grammatical complexity alone will affect the occurrence of disfluencies.

As children mature, language delay will appear to drop rapidly in significance. However, bearing in mind the limited language skills (compared to possibilities) needed for general social adequacy, the clinician should not assume an age-level cutoff for language weaknesses or fail to consider the foundation language skills in older child stutterers. Do not assume that for different ages the same "rules" or value weights apply to syntactical factors and the distribution of dysfluencies. Each stutterer should be evaluated to determine, not confirm, the rules in operation.

Semantic considerations deal broadly with the content and meaning of communication in terms of how the symbols (oral or graphic) relate to concepts they represent. We might assume that dysfluency and semantic factors can be related, and Westley (1979) reported that kindergarten and first-grade stutterers and "highly disfluent" normals made significantly more incorrect responses on semantic tasks than did fluent normals. Greater stuttering on content words has been reported by some (F.H. Silverman 1972a; Williams, Silverman, & Kools 1969b; Blankenship 1964), and on function words by others (E-M. Silverman 1974; Helmreich and Bloodstein 1973; Bloodstein and Gantwerk 1967).

Semantic effects may also occur in terms of response length. E-M. Silverman and Williams (1967) studied kindergarten and first-grade children in story telling tasks. The stutterers were lower in MLU, in variability of response length, in the average of the five longest responses, and in structural complexity. They were higher in one-word responses. F.H. Silverman also reported (1976) on the performance of 68 stutterers and their controls in story-telling tasks. In second-grade and third-grade children, the stutterers used about 10 percent fewer words (nonsignificant), while at grades 4, 5, and 6 the stutterers used at least 25 percent fewer words (significant at the .05 level). Whether the reduced length represents problems in internal resource and word finding (Weuffen 1961) or conditioned efforts to minimize verbal output and hence stuttering, less effective communication may result.

The link between complexity of reading material and stuttering in reading has also been considered. Blood and Hood (1978) reported a positive correlation between difficulty of reading material and the type and frequency of stuttering dysfluencies. Cecconi, Hood, and Tucker (1977) reported similar results in evaluation of nonstuttering children reading at progressive levels of difficulty. The question of whether stuttering children have more difficulty in general with reading is not clear. Janssen, Kraaimaat, and Van der Meulen (1983) evaluated 44 elementary-age stutterers and matched controls on standardized reading tests. The two groups could be differentiated on the bases of reading rate and errors, but not on the basis of comprehension. Interestingly, disfluency and reading ability were significantly associated within the nonstuttering group, but not among the stutterers (except for rate). Conture and Naerssen (1977) could not differentiate school-age stutterers and nonstutterers on the basis of reading ability. Nevertheless, bearing in mind research cited earlier, that child stutterers typically display some educational delay and intellectual limitation, greater difficulty with reading should not be a surprise and ought to be checked.

Pragmatic aspects of language relate to factors and situational variables that may affect language fluency functions. Factors include the number of people involved, the type of communication, and many other considerations, including internal ones known only to the speaker concerned. Pragmatics also has an evolving definition relative to the things a speaker does, in an extralinguistic sense, during the communication process. Prutting and Kirchner (1987) have presented an excellent summary (and measurement protocol) of this aspect. It is interesting relative to this book's earlier preoccupation with definition that they noted a recent text in pragmatics that devoted 53 pages to defining the subject area! This book uses pragmatics in the much older and looser concept of situational and personal variables (however, the clinician is not prevented from evaluating pragmatics in other contexts). Many clinicians recommend observation of parent-child interactions on the grounds that this important relationship may influence a child's dysfluency. However, Trotter (1960) had young children tell stories with the mother present and with her absent, and he reported no effects on words spoken, stuttering frequency, spasm type, and overall severity of stuttering. Later, Martin, Haroldson, and Kuhl (1972) compared preschool children in talking with their mothers, and then with a peer. Neither the number of words uttered nor the disfluencies produced differed, as a group result, for the two situations. In a different view, E-M. Silverman (1973) compared a structured interview and preschool classroom speech in four-year-olds. The interview produced considerably more disfluency, even though types and extents of disfluencies remained comparable.

We simply cannot predict what factors are going to affect, if they do at all, the dysfluency severity or patterns of a stuttering child. But, there are possibilities that can be explored. In the Pragmatics portion of Figure 4–2, clinicians are referred back to item 4 under Psychological Factors, the first section of the form. This item suggests a range of persons, situations, and emotional factors that might relate to dysfluency production. In addition, the clinician can usually accomplish several of the following:

1. Observe client as he or she talks to different members of the family.
2. Observe client in peer interaction and various types of speaking situations in the classroom.
3. Introduce strangers into the diagnostic situation.
4. Vary language complexity of stimulus materials.
5. Vary language complexity of clinician communications to the client.
6. Send the client on "errands" to reliable observers who can report later and/or have client make telephone calls to prepared recipients.
7. Role play different situations.
8. Increase clinician speech rate.
9. Interrupt, complete statements, disagree with things the client says, and so on.
10. Use topics likely to generate stress ("tell me about your happiest/saddest experience").
11. Disagree, criticize, or otherwise exert stress on the client.

In the following list general suggestions are offered relative to testing areas in general linguistic functions. They are not intended to replace formal tests or subtest items, although they can provide sufficient material for evaluation and planning purposes:

1. **Naming**. Have child point to items in the room, body parts, stimulus objects, and pictures. Complexity can be increased. Repeat by having child name the things you point to. Note any patterns, phonemic or linguistic, in dysfluency or performance levels.

2. **One-word Response**. Using similar material as in suggestion 1, ask questions that can be answered with one word:

    What color is the rug?

    How many cars are there here?

    What is the boy doing?

3. **Multi-word Responses**. Using stimulus material, ask simple questions that can be answered in two or three words:

    Where do you buy eggs?

    Who works in a hospital?

    Where do you live?

4. **Monologue Response**. This can be graded somewhat in complexity. Stimulus material can be used and/or topics can be introduced:

    What do you think these people are doing?

    Tell me how to prepare your favorite sandwich.

    Tell me the story of _____ (TV show, movie).

    What do you do on the weekends?

    Tell me about your after-school job.

5. **Conversational Response**. This calls for the clinician to be able to hold up one end of a social conversation. Any age-appropriate topics can be used.

In evaluation of the monologue and conversation samples, the clinician will want to pay attention to dysfluency occurrences as they relate to noun-phrase and verb-phrase distinctions, conjoined sentences (where grammatical units, such as conjunctions, link sentences), to adjoined sentences (linked sentences where the linkage is logical and relative), and to relative clauses embedded in the sentence. Distribution of dysfluencies by these various elements can be calculated on the bases of frequency, percentage, type, and severity.

Related language aspects include word finding, auditory perception, auditory processing, and attending problems. These have generally been covered in other sections of the evaluation form. The auditory and attention areas may have particular significance in client self-awareness, self-monitoring skills, and ability to profit from progressively incremented levels of therapy complexity such as ELU (extended length of utterance) and GILCU (gradual increments in length and complexity of utterance) programs.

DYSFLUENCY DATA SHEET

The last section of Figure 4–2 is the Dysfluency Data Sheet (DDS), which requires little additional test material or procedures. It is structured so that it can be separated physically from the rest of Figure 4–2 and used independently. The DDS form is too detailed and complex, and it offers too many alternative measures for every clinician and for any one particular client. It is assumed that a clinician will select preferred items from the DDS form, varying the selection with different clients. The form provides for indicating whether the subsequent data are drawn from reading, directed monologue, or conversational speech. If more than one mode of speech is utilized, their data should be treated on additional copies of the form—although it is assumed that items P (adaptation) and Q (consistency) will utilize reading material even though alternatives will be discussed.

    Item A requests a total of the client's TTT in seconds. This can be as simple as timing a series of reading passages. It can also involve more complex, subjective timing of monologue and conversational speech, from which the following time segments would be omitted:

1. Speech by any person other than the client.
2. Pauses that are obviously due to thought formulation or external distractions, and not part of ongoing speech or dysfluency problems.

There will be an unavoidable error factor due to 2 above. However, experience will help the clinician, and the error factor usually is not of a magnitude to affect results meaningfully (in a clinical sense). One limiting factor overlooked by many clinicians is that of the representativeness of speech observed during assessment activity. F.H. Silverman (1975) queried elementary-age, secondary school age, and adult stutterers ($N = 115$) about how "typical" their speech had been while they had been performing tasks in a "therapy room." About 65 percent of the subjects reported, subsequently, that their speech had not been typical. One cannot assume that fluency will be less adequate than usual. Indeed, it is possible to speculate that clutterers or clutter-stutterers might be better in such situations. This emphasizes the importance of soliciting information from parents, teachers, and other sources to compare descriptive differences. In particular, the child can be used as an information source.

    Item B involves counting the number of words uttered, or the number of syllables produced. Prosek and Runyan (1983) have related rate to listener perception of stuttering. Edited speech samples of fluent speech from nonstutterers and treated stutterers were identified easily by listeners as to stutterer and nonstutterer classifications. The tapes were then reedited to alter segment and pause durations of the treated stutterers (increasing apparent rate) and resubmitted in a listening design. Listeners' accuracy in identifying stutterers was reduced significantly. Word counts are relatively simple (see subsequent caveat), but syllable counting can be tiresome. Some clinicians randomly select ten examples of 10 consecutive words each and count the number of syllables. The ten sample

DYSFLUENCY DATA SHEET

Client Name: _____   Age: _____   Sex: _____

Clinician: _____   Date: _____

Data taken from: _____ reading _____ monlogue _____ spontaneous speech

A. Total Speaking Time: _____ seconds.

B. 1. words uttered _____   2. syllables uttered _____

    3. wpm rate _____   3. spm rate _____

C. Total of:

    1. phrase repetitions _____   2. word repetitions _____

    3. syllable repetitions _____   4. sound repetitions _____

    5. sound prolongations _____   6. tense pause/stoppages _____

    7. grand total of all dysfluencies (C1 through C6) = _____

D. _____ % repetitions = $\dfrac{C1 + C2 + C3 + C4}{B1} \times 100$

E. _____ % prolongations = $\dfrac{C5}{B1} \times 100$

F. _____ % tense pause/stoppage = $\dfrac{C6}{B1} \times 100$

G. _____ % total dysfluencies = $\dfrac{C7}{B1} \times 100$

    Enter D, E, F, G percentages on Graph I, according to the alpha legends.

H. _____ % phrase repetitions = $\dfrac{C1}{C1 + C2 + C3 + C4} \times 100$

J. _____ % word repetitions = $\dfrac{C2}{C1 + C2 + C3 + C4} \times 100$

K. _____ % syllable repetitions = $\dfrac{C3}{C1 + C2 + C3 + C4} \times 100$

L. _____ % sound repetitions = $\dfrac{C4}{C1 + C2 + C3 + C4} \times 100$

    Enter H, J, K, L percentages on Graph II, according to alpha legends.

M. Duration of prolongations. Count those lasting:

1. _____ 1 second or less   2. _____ 1–2 seconds   3. _____ 2–4 seconds

4. _____ 5+ seconds   5. _____ seconds, mean of three longest

N. Duration of tense pauses/stoppages. Count those lasting:

1. _____ 1 second or less   2. _____ 1–2 seconds   3. _____ 2–4 seconds

4. _____ 5+ seconds   5. _____ seconds, mean of three longest

   Enter M1–5 and N1–5 on Graph III, according to alpha-number legends.
   Note that M5 and N5 are entered on the upper right-hand side.

O. Number of repetitions:

In each category below, count every repetition per unit and add them.
Also, note how many repetitions are in the longest repetition unit.

1. Sounds: _____ average $= \dfrac{\text{total all sound repetitions}}{C4}$

   _____ number in longest repetition unit

2. Syllables: _____ average $= \dfrac{\text{total all syllable repetitions}}{C3}$

   _____ number in longest repetition unit

3. Words: _____ average $= \dfrac{\text{total all word repetitions}}{C2}$

   _____ number in longest repetition unit

4. Phrases: _____ average $= \dfrac{\text{total all phrase repetitions}}{C1}$

   Enter the results of O on Graph IV, according to number legends,
   using a dot for the averages and an *x* for the longest units.

P. Adaptation:

For each of five readings, or for five measured spontaneous productions,
enter the number of stutterings below.

1. _____   2. _____   3. _____   4. _____   5. _____

_____ % adaptation between P1 and P2 $= \dfrac{P1 - P2}{P1} \times 100$

_____ % adaptation between P1 and P5 $= \dfrac{P1 - P5}{P1} \times 100$

Enter the results of P1 through P5 on Graph V, according to number legends.

Q. Consistency:

For each of the five readings, record the total stuttered words (TSW) and the stutterings that recurred from reading to reading.

	Reading				
	1	2	3	4	5
TSW	____	____	____	____	____
1		____	____	____	____
2			____	____	____
3				____	____
4					____

Consistency is calculated by: $\dfrac{R_y \text{ stuttered words also stuttered on in } R_x}{\text{TSW on } R_x} \times 100$

_____ % R1/R5 = $\dfrac{R_5 \text{ stuttered words also stuttered on in } R_1}{\text{TSW on R1}} \times 100$

_____ % R_4/R_5 = $\dfrac{R5 \text{ stuttered words also stuttered on in } R_4}{\text{TSW on } R_4} \times 100$

Wingate (1984) recurrence method:

Count stuttered words as indicated below:

TSW R_w

_____ words stuttered on once $\times$ 0 =   ____

_____ words stuttered on twice $\times$ 2 =   ____

_____ words stuttered on three times $\times$ 3 = ____

_____ words stuttered on four times $\times$ 4 = ____

_____ words stuttered on five times $\times$ 5 = ____

_____ ---------------- TOTALS ---------------- ____

_____ R_m = TSW $\times$ N_r, where N_r is the total number of readings.

_____ R_r, the recurrence ratio = $\dfrac{R_w}{R_m}$

The closer R_r is to 1.0, the higher the consistency, or recurrence.

I. Percentage Distribution of Types of Dysfluencies.

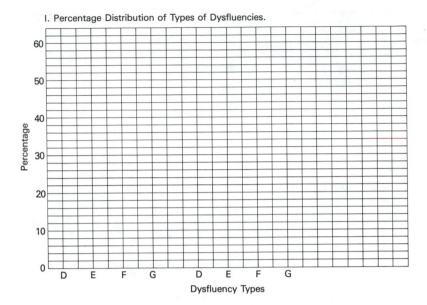

II. Percentages of Repetitions by Occurrence Category

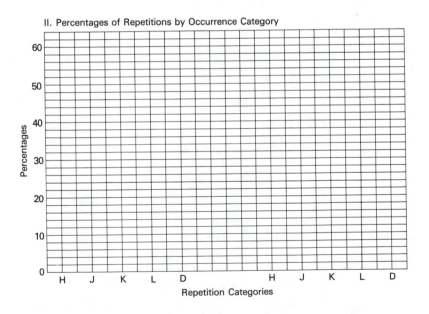

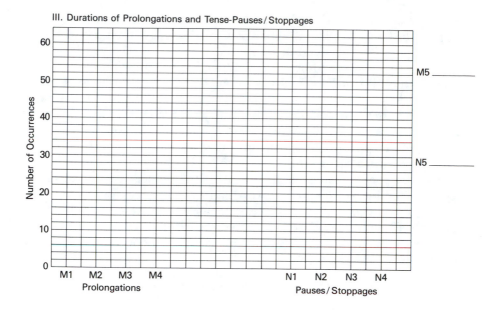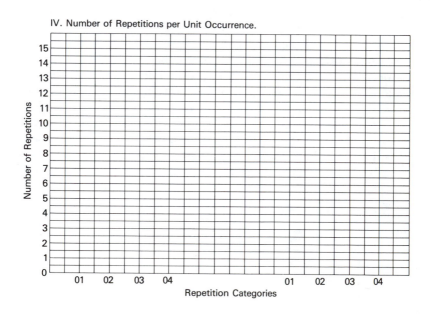

III. Durations of Prolongations and Tense-Pauses/Stoppages

Number of Occurrences

M5 _____

N5 _____

M1 M2 M3 M4   N1 N2 N3 N4
Prolongations   Pauses/Stoppages

IV. Number of Repetitions per Unit Occurrence.

Number of Repetitions

01 02 03 04   01 02 03 04
Repetition Categories

counts are added and then divided by 100 to arrive at an average sylla-bles-per-word weight. The number of words actually uttered is counted and multiplied by the weighting factor (for example, 125 words × 1.73 weight = 216 syllables) to obtain the derived approximation of the sylla-ble total. In both word and syllable counts there is a *caveat*, however: Ex-actly what do you count? If you count repeated words and syllable repeti-tions that occur in dysfluencies, you will secure relatively accurate rate statements in terms of motor production but lose accuracy in terms of meaningful or appropriate productions that occurred within the confines of the timed interval. By the same token, calculation of percentages of various occurrences would be thrown off. For instance, assume an utter-ance or a reading passage had 98 words and 154 syllables and took a stut-terer 63 seconds to read or say. Also assume the stutterer had 3 phrase repetitions (8 words or 12 syllables), 7 word repetitions (11 syllables), 17 interjected sounds (17 syllables), and 52 syllable repetitions. Counts and calculations could vary, as follow:

	TTT	WORDS	SYLLABLES	WPM	SPM
Limited Count	63	98	154	93.6	146.4
All-item Count	63	113	246	107.4	234.0

In terms of saying what he or she wanted to say, the stutterer had a sylla-ble-per-minute (spm) rate of 146.4. However, the production rate was 234 spm. Many clinicians prefer to use the limited count on the grounds that therapy progress will be more meaningful in that TTT figures can be re-lated to wpm and spm figures as the frequency and unit duration of spasms decrease over time. I prefer the limited count, but the all-item count can have research and therapy applications.

Item C involves the first breakdown count of dysfluencies. This re-quires the clinician to decide how he or she is going to mark dysfluencies. One method is to transcribe utterances into double-space or triple-space format and write coded designations above each stuttered item. The other approach is to use a sheet with various spasm-type codes, and arrange blanks, such as

WWR ⦀⦀⦀_____   SounR ⦀⦀⦀⦀⦀ ⦀_____
PWR ⦀⦀⦀⦀⦀ ⦀_____   TePa/St ⦀⦀⦀⦀⦀ ⦀⦀_____
SyR ⦀⦀⦀⦀⦀ ⦀⦀⦀⦀⦀_____   Prol ⦀⦀⦀⦀_____

The first system is best in the long run because material is then available for second-look analyses of phonology, syntax, grammar, and prosody, as well as for adaptation and consistency measures. For more limited pur-poses, the second method has greater efficiency.

Counting dysfluencies in item C is simple. In each category, only unit occurrences are totaled, that is 17 repetitions of the syllable /sʌ/ in *sunlight* counts as one occurrence of syllable repetition. The seventh category under item C is the sum of the previous six categories. The following judgment guidelines are offered:

1. PWR or broken-word repetitions are counted under category 3, syllable repetitions.
2. Sound repetitions do not include consonant + schwa repetitions; these also go under category 3.
3. Sound prolongations will usually be vowels or continuant consonants (everything but stops). Occasionally some stutterers will distort and prolong stops.
4. Category 6, tense pauses and stoppages, can occur prior to sound initiation or within an utterance.

It is recognized that stutterers can combine more than one spasm type in a dysfluency. In order to facilitate baseline measures, assign each spasm to one of the six categories on the basis of its most predominant form. However, later in the outline, there will be an item allowing the clinician to indicate the prevalence of mixed-spasm patterns.

Items D, E, F, and **G** begin the calculation sections, which are to be recorded in the spaces provided and then transferred for graphic display. These first four measures, spasm types by percentage, are calculated easily. If the B1 words uttered were 127 and item C had the following results

C1	3	C2	7
C3	24	C4	6
C5	4	C6	7
	C7	51	

Then the calculation of item D would be

$$\frac{3 + 7 + 24 + 6}{127} = \frac{40}{127} = 0.31 \times 100 = 31\%$$

so that D percent would indicate that 31 percent of the words uttered were repetitions of one sort or another. The percentages for items E, F, and G would be calculated along the same lines (for example, prolongations percentage is C5 divided by 127, multiplied by 100). The clinician then turns to the end of the form and locates Graph I, Percentage Distribution of Types of Dysfluencies. Under the first *D*, mark the percentage with a dot. Repeat this process for E, F, and G. A second series of D,E,F,G is provided so that measurement later on (for instance, during therapy) could provide visual comparison to the baseline measure. Another use, in evaluation, would be to calculate one on reading and one on spontaneous speech, or performance before the clinician and performance before a small group. Graph points can be connected by lines and/or bar graph shadings can be added.

Items H, J, K, L (the I is eliminated to avoid confusion with graph numbers) follow a similar formula pattern, except that we are looking only at repetitions. Using the figures of the previous example for item D, we could calculate H as follows:

$$\frac{3}{3 + 7 + 24 + 6} = \frac{3}{40} = 0.08 \times 100 = 8\%$$

So we can say phrase repetitions comprise 8 percent of the total repetitions. The calculations for J, K, and L would yield respective percentages of 18, 60, and 15. These figures are to be entered at the end of the form on Graph II, Percentage of Repetitions by Occurrence Category. Methods of recording are the same as before, and two entry possibilities are provided.

Items M and **N** each have five subparts. Both are duration, not frequency, measures. It will be easy for most clinicians to simply count (without timing) durations of one second or less. With a little practice, most can do the same to prolongations and stoppages in the range of one to two seconds. Longer durations should be mechanically or electronically timed, preferably with a stopwatch. Clinicians should realize that items M and N, and especially N (tense pauses/stoppages), will involve nonvoice intervals. Working from audiotape will introduce uncertainty and variability into the timing process; that is, one can be flexible in when to start timing. Experience will help in doing this. Analysis as soon after the session as possible may help also, and video records will help most of all. The count data are entered on Graph III, Durations of Prolongations and Tense Pauses/ Stoppages. Only one recording opportunity is provided for each. However, this can be overcome if desired by, for example, using a red pen for the first measurement and a different color when a remeasurement is taken. Please note that M5 and N5, the averages of the three longest durations in each category, are separated from the other count measures.

Item O returns to that most frequently observed stuttering phenomenon, repetitions. The average number of repetitions per unit occurrence and the largest number of repetitions in a single unit are often used in enrollment decisioning and in therapy progress measures. Item O is divided into four categories: **phrase, word, syllable,** and **sound** repetitions. In each category, the number of repetitions in each occurrence unit is counted. For instance, if a client said, "Whe- whe- whe- whe- when I go to be- bed, I ca- ca- can't sleep fuh- for a long tuh- tuh- time," the clinician would count ten repetitions across four units, so that O2 would be 10/

4 = 2.5, and the longest unit would be four. The results are entered on Graph IV, Number of Repetitions per Unit Occurrence. It is suggested that each average be marked on the graph with a dot, and each longest repetition marked with an *x*. Differing colors can be used also. A remeasurement capacity is also provided.

Item P deals with a favorite constant in stuttering, adaptation. Adaptation in stuttering is the decrease of a measured variable over time of continued speaking and/or repeated productions of the same material. Its significance, or lack of it, in stuttering has been discussed elsewhere and will not be debated further here. Johnson and others (1963) state that adaptation was named and first reported by Johnson and Knott (1937) when 2 to 123 repetitions of a reading passage were measured. The typical number used today is 5. Spontaneous speech can be used, but Coppa and Bar (1974) reported that although both stutterers and nonstutterers adapted, only the stutterers achieved significance. Earlier, Cohen (1953) compared adaptation in reading and in spontaneous speech, finding adaptation in both modes, but "considerably less" during spontaneous speech. Disfluency and dysfluency adaptation in nonstutterers and stutterers (five to eight years of age) was evaluated by Neelley and Timmons (1967). Both groups displayed adaptation, but the stutterers' scores were higher. Further, the material used may affect adaptation. Adams and Reis (1971) compared adaptation on an all-voiced and a mixed voiced and voiceless, reading passage, finding greater stuttering adaptation on the all-voiced passage. Similarly, Adams and others (1974) reported that adaptation is facilitated as speaking requirements reduced needs for prompt phonation onset and for complete articulatory constriction in sound productions.

In item P, data are collected most easily by having the client perform five consecutive readings of an age-appropriate passage that is phonetically distributed. If spontaneous speech is used, it will be necessary to analyze five time periods containing the same number of words (time lengths will vary). For reading passages, use a clinician copy and mark each stuttered word with a 1 on the first reading, a 2 on the second, and so on. This is done in case the same performance is to be used for **item Q, Consistency.** Such marking on spontaneous speech is usually not feasible.

When stutter counts have been made, enter the five totals in P1 through P5. The form provides only for calculating adaptation comparing P1/P2 and overall adaptation comparing P1/P5. Any other adaptations can be calculated using the formula in item 5. If the stutterer stuttered 27 times on the first reading, and 18, 15, 10, and 8 times on the successive readings, the following calculations could be made:

$$P1/P2 = \frac{27 - 18}{27} = \frac{9}{27} = 0.33 \times 100 = 33\%$$

and:

$$P1/P5 = \frac{27 - 8}{27} = \frac{19}{27} = 0.70 \times 100 = 70\%$$

The P1/P2 comparison is provided because the greatest adaptation usually occurs between the first two readings, tending to increase as stuttering is more severe (Quarrington 1959), so that it may create a false perception of overall adaptation. Tate, Cullinan, and Ahlstrand (1961) also criticized the straight percentage method of calculation. Nonetheless it is in majority use today.

Adaptation scores may suggest stutterer reaction to stress, and can be used to remeasure during fluency reinforcement or symptom modification therapy. The most popular measure, stuttering spasms, has been used in these examples. However, you could use TTT (total talking time) on reading, or number of avoidances, or type of spasm, duration of spasms, or almost anything else you wished to measure.

Item Q in Figure 4–2 concerns the consistency of stuttering, or the degree to which stuttering recurrs on the same words. Many studies have been done in this area, with disagreement over what is typical. We do know that dysfluencies in repeated utterances tend to recur on the same words (Bloodstein 1960a, 1960b; Neelley and Timmons 1967; Williams, Silverman, and Kools 1969a). Statements of typical consistency have ranged from 36 percent (Hamre and Wingate 1973), to 48 percent (Hendel and Bloodstein, 1973) and up to 65–75 percent (Johnson and Knott 1937). Bloodstein (1960a, 1960b) suggested that consistency effects can be observed at every age level; subsequent research has confirmed this. Neelley and Timmons (1967) reported consistency effects in stutterers 5–8 years of age at higher levels than those displayed by nonstutterers. Williams, Silverman, and Kools (1969a) reported that elementary-age stutterers and nonstutterers exhibited consistency in their production of dysfluencies and disfluencies. The stutterers had a higher consistency percentage, though this might be due in part to the fact that stutterers started out at a much higher dysfluency percentage level (thereby making consistency occurrences more feasible). Exactly what contributes to consistency is not clear. Prior sensitization, "Jonah" words, prosodic stress points, clause boundaries, and word position and length may be some of the factors. It has been reported that eliminating previously stuttered words or rearranging sentence structure reduces consistency (Brutten and Gray 1961), but Avari and Bloodstein (1974) reported that stutterers 10–14 years of age still had significant amounts of stuttering occur on words adjacent to previously stuttered words that were blotted out on the rereading.

The procedure in item Q of Figure 4–2 (consistency measurement) is to follow that suggested for item P, five successive readings, marking each stuttered word with the number of the reading. Because two methods of analysis are provided, two raw data modes are set out. In the first method, the standard percentage method, the following example is provided:

12345	123	1			12345	234	5
I	am	not	sure	how	many	times	I

123	1345		3		12345	12	4
have	seen	the	movie.		It	has	been

5	12	1234	2	
my	favorite	show	for	years.

This fragment of a reading passage has each stuttered word marked according to the readings in which stuttering occurred. These occurrences are then transferred to the Q item form that follows. Note that the TSW (total stuttered words) for each reading is recorded:

Reading	1	2	3	4	5
TSW	10	10	9	7	6
		8	9	5	4
2			7	5	3
3				6	4
4					4

The first blank line on the form displayed in Figure 4–2 records stutterings in the first reading (R1) that recurred on each successive reading. In the second reading (R2) eight R1 stutterings recurred, on R3 there were nine recurrences of R1 stuttering, and so on. The second blank line compares the second reading (R2) stutterings to successive readings. Seven stuttered words in R2 also were stuttered on in R3. The rest of the form is filled out similarly.

Using the preceding example, R1/R5 consistency would be

$$\frac{\text{R5 stutterings also in R1}}{\text{all R1 stutterings}} = \frac{4}{10} = 0.40 \times 100 = 40\%$$

and the calculation of R4/R5 consistency would be

$$\frac{\text{R5 stutterings also in R4}}{\text{all R4 stutterings}} = \frac{4}{7} = 0.57 \times 100 = 57\%$$

This method, although widely used, is open to several errors or mis-interpretation factors (Ham 1986; Cullinan 1963; Tate and Cullinan 1962), and thus several more complex alternatives have been proposed. Nevertheless, many (indeed most) tend to use the simpler percentage method. Wingate (1984d) has suggested a procedure that typically begins with consecutive readings (usually five) of the same passage, with each stuttered word being marked with the number of the reading. The next step is to establish a weighted value (Rw) for recurrent (consistent) stutter-ings. Unlike the previous formula, one simply counts how many readings a particular word was stuttered on. A word stuttered on in readings 1, 2, 3, or in 3, 4, 5, or in 2, 3, 4, or in 1, 3, 5, and so on, has the same recur-rence value of 3. The recurrence values can be no greater than the num-ber of readings. The total recurrence score for any reading is multiplied by the number of that reading, for example:

13	words stuttered on, one time only	=	0
5	words stuttered on twice, multiplied by 2	=	10
7	words stuttered on three times, × 3	=	21
4	words stuttered on four times, × 4	=	16
2	words stuttered on five times, × 5	=	10
31	——————— TOTALS ———————		57

The recurrence weight, or Rw, is 57. The formula to obtain this, which we already have done, is:

$$Rw = 2n_2 + 3n_3 + 4n_4 + 5n_5$$

where the number category is used to multiply the number of recurrences in that category. Then a maximal recurrence, or Rm figure, is obtained by multiplying the total number of words stuttered (T) by the number of readings (ΣR), or

$$Rm = T \times \Sigma R$$

In the previous example, 31 total stutterings occurred, so we have

$$Rm = 31 \times 5 = 155$$

We are now ready to calculate the recurrence ratio, or Rr, in which

$$Rr = Rw \div Rm = 57 \div 155 = 0.37 \times 100 = 37\%$$

In the Wingate procedure, recurrence values can range from zero (no re-currence at all) to 1.00 (total consistency). Please note that 1.00 would not mean that every word was stuttered on in a passage, only that in each reading the same words were stuttered on every time. Space precludes a simulated comparison between the recurrence ratio and the popular method, but Wingate (1984d) makes such a comparison, with noticeable differences. On Figure 4–2, and in this discussion, some of the original recurrence symbols have been altered for (what is hoped to be) greater clarity and consistency between the two.

The uses of consistency, or recurrence, are extensive, both in assessment and in therapy. As noted, many factors can affect it, and we can expect considerable individual variation. It can be part of the final decisioning process and also be of value in selecting therapy approaches and varying applications of particular therapy techniques.

RELEVANT TOPICS

In using Figure 4–2, or in any type of diagnostic and assessment organization, it seems appropriate to consider several topics that relate to evaluation. One topic is that of what is characteristic, or typical, of early fluency disruption. A second topic is the degree to which listener perception is related to accurate identification and labeling procedures. The third topic concerns the factors involved in severity judgments, particular with reference to ranking or scaling severity. These three topics are discussed briefly in this section, and the chapter then ends with a section on decisioning factors.

Early Characteristics of Stuttering

What we respond to in diagnosing stuttering is at the core of evaluation and differentiation. Boehmler (1958), among many others, indicated that sound and syllable repetitions were more likely to be labeled as stuttering than were revisions or interjections. Children, in general, show considerable variation in fluency within a group and, individually, over time (Yairi, 1982). This also was noted by Wingate (1962a, 1962b, 1962c), who stated that research has established that although children generally display considerable variation in their fluency disruptions, certain forms are frequently found among children who are called stutterers. Yairi (1972) compared 92 elementary-age stutterers with nonstuttering controls, dividing each group into "high" and "low" fluency subgroups. For the two nonstuttering subgroups, disfluency percentages for seven categories were almost uniformly proportional relative to overall disfluency— a case of same-but-more as they became worse. However, as stutterers became more dysfluent, they tended to increase the percentage of WWR, PWR, interjections, tense pauses, and disrhythmic phonations. The proportion of phrase repetitions and utterance revisions decreased as dysfluency levels increased. Also, the PWR percentage for both nonstuttering groups was small, compared to the PWR percentage for either of the stuttering groups.

E-M. Silverman (1973) speculated that stuttering children might display more disfluency "runs" (extended disruption on a single word) and "clusters" (dysfluencies on one or more contiguous words), compared to four-year-old nonstutterers. Culp (1984) evaluated children at three, four, and five years of age. Compared to nonstutterers, the stutterers were significantly higher in PWR, WR, disrhythmic phonations, and tense pauses. The stutterers were also higher, but not significantly so, on phrase repetitions and interjections; whereas the nonstutterers were higher only on the number of revisions. Yairi and Lewis (1984) approached the diagnostic timing element by evaluating two-year-old and three-year-old "stutterers" within 60 days or less of the time of initial diagnosis by parents. Compared to controls, these children were three times more disfluent, had more PWR and prolongation phenomena and had significantly more repetitions per unit of occurrence. Wall and Myers (1984) suggest that the label is more likely to be applied as severity or struggle increases, as the phonologic-linguistic unit disrupted is smaller, and the more frequently a disruption occurs, whether on a per-unit basis or across speech in general.

It seems that we are looking for increased amounts of dysfluency, longer durations per unit of occurrence, possible shifts in dysfluency types as severity increases, sound and syllable repetitions (including PWR) as opposed to WWR and phrase repetitions, prolongations, tense pauses and stoppages, and evidence of disrhythmic phonation. In the next section we consider how well we listen for these phenomena.

Listener Factors

In each stuttering or diagnostic and assessment class I teach, the students always seem to want to know, "What does it sound like . . . look like?" as we cover different problems. Judges, even naive ones, are reasonably accurate or consistent in differentiating stuttering from nonstuttering. The problems will tend to arise when we ask these questions:

- Exactly at what points did stuttering occur?
- Exactly what happened during the stuttering spasm?

Curlee (1984) reviewed a series of studies concerning accuracy of listener judgments when identifying moments of stuttering. He concluded that identifications are likely to be inconsistent and subject to influence by a number of factors. Although cautious in generalizing from adult chronic stutterers to children, he stated that "it seems plausible that a large proportion of children's speech disruptions would be judged ambiguously as stuttering or as normal disfluencies" (p. 230). Curlee continues to note several studies where interjudge agreement on frequency of stuttering is high (generally 90 percent or more), but again he indicates much poorer agreement on specific moments of stuttering. In his summary, Curlee concludes that we do not fare well in identifying particular moments of stuttering, and that our "empirical foundation . . . on the speech of children who stutter is not secure, particularly with regard to younger children who have not been stuttering long" (p. 233).

We can compensate for some of the problems cited previously by using several judges, by having one judge reevaluate the same material several times, and by building our experiential frames of reference. Although Curlee's comments are appropriate and improvment in accuracy is needed, this author believes that the majority of stuttering children can be differentiated from nonstutterers on the basis of frequency, severity, and types of stuttering (Johnson 1955; F.H. Silverman 1974; Yairi 1983, 1972).

Severity Concerns

As we differentiate stuttering from nonstuttering phenomena and identify particular spasm types, we also have the question of defining severity. In overall assessment of severity, Lewis and Sherman (1951) indicated that spasms of longer duration, increased frequency, slow and/or labored rate, lip tremors, and the number of different anatomical areas involved all increased perceptions of severity. Hood (1974) based severity scaling on a molecular analysis of stuttering behaviors, and Riley (1972) combined frequency with duration and concomitant behaviors evaluations. Frequency is used most often and correlates well with overall severity factors. Johnson, Darley, and Spriestersbach (1963) recommended eight categories of dysfluencies. Young (1961) reduced these to five by combining WWR and PR (phrase repetitions), placing "broken words" under "prolonged sounds," and placing "incomplete phrases" under the "revision" category.

With reference to the foregoing categories, establishing severity levels is difficult, in part, because of the different behaviors that are measured. Berry and Silverman (1972) established that the Lewis and Sherman nine-point scale (1951) was ordinal, rather than interval, in nature (that is, the severity distances between progressively ranked items were not equivalent) and recommended eliminating the "very mild" and "mild" categories. Van Riper (1982) also criticized the scale and devised a different scale, presented in Table 4–2. Its applicability to children has a number of debatable points, and it is presented here simply as a reference point for evaluating stuttering. Its degree of applicability will go up as the stutterer approaches adolescence. Beech and Fransella (1968) provide an extended discussion of five-point, seven-point, and nine-point equal-interval scales that provide minimal definitions, a seven-point scale with precise definitions, and direct magnitude estimation procedures. Overall, they prefer a seven-point scale with minimal definitions.

TABLE 4–2. Profile of Stuttering Severity

SEVERITY LEVEL	PERCENT OF STUTTERING	TENSION- STRUGGLE PRESENCE	SECONDS OF SPASM DURATION	PERCENT OF POSTPONEMENT- AVOIDANCE
1	Under 1	None	Under 1	None
2	1–2	Rare	About $1/2$	Under 5
3	3–5	Mild	About 1	5–10
4	6–8	Severe	About 2	11–20
5	9–12	Very severe	About 3	21–31
6	13–25	Overflow to eyes, limbs	About 4	31–70
7	25+	Overflow to trunk	5+	70+

Source: From C. Van Riper, *The Nature of Stuttering,* 1982, p. 201.

Research has shown that identifying and rating the severity of stuttering frequently has a poor interjudge reliability. Also, the type of task, the stutterer's pattern, the clinical setting, and a number of other variables can affect speech fluency. Sampling a reading passage and a few minutes of spontaneous speech will be informative, but only to a limited point. In using the various measures suggested here, the clinician should apply information gained in Linguistic Factors, Figure 4–2, and also in item 1 of Psychological Factors. Data from these areas will supply dysfluency information to amend or extend the limited coverage of various other measures and calculations. In addition, they will provide insights into the attitudes, feelings, reactions, and general behaviors of the speaker and of the speaker's environment. In the long run, these last information areas will be at least as important and useful as the more precise data counts favored today.

DECISION FACTORS

The goal of every diagnosis and assessment process is to reduce the residual diathesis (the unknown, the *x* factor) to a level sufficiently low to allow us to identify the problem and make appropriate decisions. With children, identification can be more difficult than with adults, and the recommendations also need to be considered carefully. This section summarizes comments and/or criteria from a number of clinicians (in part repeating material from Chapter 3), and ends with this writer's own summary.

Conture (1982) has suggested that children be enrolled for therapy if their speech typically is marked by prolongations and if they tend to avoid or shift eye contact. If the child displays the prior behavior to a limited extent and otherwise has predominantly easy PWR dysfluencies with good eye contact, Conture recommends further monitoring and a future follow-up. If the dysfluency pattern is mild and rather typical, Conture suggests parent counseling as the clinical response. Adams (1984b, 1980) has proposed the following criteria: PWR and prolongation occurrences above 7 percent, PWRs marked by three or more repetitions per unit occurrences, substitution of the schwa vowel in repetitions, prolongations that last for longer than one second, and initiation/maintenance problems with airflow during repetitions and/or prolongations. Adams suggests that fluency be regarded as acceptable if none, or only one, of the prior behaviors is confirmed. A *borderline* label is used if the child displays two or three of the behaviors, and *incipient* or definite stuttering is assumed if all, or all but one, of the behaviors is confirmed.

Curlee (1980) suggested seven points of decision relative to identifying a stuttering problem:

- PWR of two or more per unit on 2 percent or more of the words uttered. Additional signs are increases in loudness, pitch increments, during repetitions.
- Involuntary stoppages or hesitations longer than two seconds in the flow of speech.
- Prolongations of greater than one second duration on 2 percent or more of the words uttered. Additional signs are increases in loudness, pitch increments, or abrupt terminations.
- Visible struggle signs.
- Noticeable emotional reactions or avoidance behaviors.
- Client complaints about effects of speech disruptions.
- Marked variations in frequency/severity with changes in speaking tasks or situations.

Curlee revised this list somewhat (1984) in suggesting later that a stuttering decision could be involved when

- PWR above 2 percent; with use of the schwa vowel, rate increase of repetitions, and airflow interruptions being added causes for concern.
- Prolongations of 1 second or more on more than 1 percent of words uttered; additional concern over loudness/pitch variation, and overabrupt terminations.
- Excess effort or struggle during dysfluencies.
- Client self-labeling or admission of problem, and/or overt emotional reactions to dysfluencies.
- Observable effects on frequency/severity of changes in speech situation factors.

Culp (1984) established five separate speaking situations (see Chapter 3). She suggested enrollment if a child met one or more of the following criteria:

- Dysfluency rate of 10 percent or more across one or more of the five situations; 7 percent on two or more; 5 percent across all five situations.
- Tension in speech and/or a "significant number" of disrhythmic phonations, tense pauses, and/or multiple-unit PWRs or WWRs.
- Quantitative or qualitative significant disfluency" (p.48), plus one or more of the following:
  - Poor concept of self as a speaker.
  - Discoordination of the speech mechanism.
  - "Subtle language problems."
  - Family history of dysfluency.
  - Parent and/or teacher who demonstrated significant concern.

Overall, the reader will note a general consistency among the clinicians just cited. For decisioning procedures, this writer has developed a checklist of factors that support a decision to enroll a child for therapy, (see Table 4–3). Various weighting systems to use with it have been devised over the years, but one that some individual client will not confound or invalidate has never been found. Individual variations and interaction among the various items frustrate a fixed value system, and there is no re-

TABLE 4–3. Decision Factors in Stuttering Evaluation

CATEGORY OR QUALITY

Environment
    High level of concern, anxiety, stress in parents, teachers, others
    Family/school environment judged to be negative, stressful
    Family/school environment nonsupportive, apathetic
Child
    Self-labeling, poor attitude, negative behavior, low self-esteem
    Awareness, concern, anxiety about speech
    Awareness, frustration, confusion about speech
Dysfluencies
    Average of three or more repetitions per unit occurrence
    PWR frequency about 2 percent of words uttered
    Prolongations over one second on 2 percent or more of utterances
    Tense pauses and stoppages over one second on 2 percent or more of utterances
    Substitution of shwa vowel for appropriate vowel sounds
    Disrhythmic phonations
Struggle
    Articulator distortions, preformations
    Facial grimaces, contortions
    Head, neck, eye contact irregularities
    Body, limb concomitants
    Interjected sounds, words
Associated Behaviors
    Avoidance behaviors specific to moments of dysfluency
    General avoidance behaviors

turn of value from devising (if one could) a horrendously complicated formula of weight values.

CHAPTER SUMMARY

The overview of Chapter 3 referred to Adams's (1984b, 1980) description of the separation of disfluency from dysfluency as "vexing" and "intimidating," and this author suggested that perhaps this was somewhat of an overstatement. At the end of about 80 manuscript pages dealing with diagnosis and assessment, I am compelled to agree with the thrust of Adams's statement. It is not that the separation of disfluency from dysfluency is so complex, since we tend to focus on the "easy" items and avoid those difficult to clarify. The vexation comes with the whole complex of interacting factors: child, parents, environment, articulation, language, fluency, cognition, adjustment, and so on. This chapter has actually omitted or skimped a number of subject areas, yet it has still managed to provide most clinicians with sufficient assessment considerations and procedures to overflow almost any evaluation schedule, no matter how generous. Deciding what to use and how to apply it, as stated previously, will depend on a number of factors. The extended detail provided in these two chapters will perhaps make these decisions informed and appropriate ones.

CHAPTER FIVE
CONSIDERATIONS
AND CONTROVERSIES
IN THERAPY

This final section of the book will be longest and most complex. It concerns a variety of approaches to three broadly designated age groups and thus requires a more extensive introduction here.

The first therapy chapter, Chapter 5, was originally to be a short commentary, appended to this Section III introduction, about factors affecting therapy. It developed a demand-life of its own, became a chapter, and displaced by one all the subsequent chapters. This displacement was repeated as the author attempted to make a few comments about therapy planning. The result was the addition of one more previously unplanned chapter, now Chapter 6. We then come to Chapter 7 (originally Chapter 5), which concerns language factors as they relate generally to therapy of stuttering and includes a review of some specific therapy approaches that emphasize linguistic planning. The next chapter (8), involves parent counseling and aspects of environmental manipulation, as sole therapy and as adjuncts to more complex programs of therapy. Chapters 9 and 10 discuss attitude, motivation, and emotions in stuttering—first, in terms of our concern with them; second, in terms of procedures and techniques that might be applied in therapy. Chapter 11 deals with relaxation and desensitization, again as sole therapies and as therapy adjuncts. The next two chapters, 12 and 13, review therapy procedures across a matrix of overlapping areas: rate control, rhythm, unison speech, masking, breath-stream management, breath chewing, ventriloquism, easy onset, and singing. In Chapter 14, symptom modification procedures are presented as a sequence, rather than as isolated procedures. This has been done to conserve text space, because it is felt that symptom therapy is less likely to be used with many of the children's age ranges defined in the next chapter. Chapter 15 surveys a variety of topics covering special therapy procedures, group therapy, use of punishment in therapy, and the issue of cluttering versus stuttering. Finally, Chapter 16 discusses the troublesome areas of transfer, maintenance, and relapse.

The purposes of the various chapters include the survey of a wide range of methods and techniques of stuttering therapy. Except as occasional examples, program sequences of particular therapy will not be developed or recommended. Research concerning various approaches will be cited, but there is no intent to survey all research, to identify "best" approaches, or to declare how techniques should be altered or improved. The reader is expected to regard the chapters as information and resource material, subject to their own additions and alterations. As rapidly as therapy is changing, the chapters cannot be regarded as a last word on current therapy practice, and they are certainly not intended to mandate any particular form of therapy.

OVERVIEW

As noted in the section introduction, this chapter began as a brief area to more or less set the scene for subsequent chapters discussing therapy procedures. It was to be a bridge between evaluation and therapy, a review of age factors affecting therapy, consideration of therapy settings, exploration of clinician philosophy, and mention of other factors or concerns relevant to therapy. Now as a chapter on its own it attempts to deal with some of the "But what about . . . ?" questions that will come up as subsequent chapters are read.

In therapy of stuttering, separate books have been devoted to the topic of children who stutter (Wall and Myers 1984; Prins and Ingham 1983; Luper and Mulder 1964), to the topic of operant procedures in stuttering (Ingham 1984; Shames and Egolf 1976), to therapy in school settings (Leith 1984a), and to the subject of atypical stutterers (St. Louis 1986), to controversies in stuttering therapy (Gregory 1979), and so on. This chapter, and subsequent ones, cannot possibly cover all topics, or cover any one of them to great depth. However, certain areas have been selected for discussion.

The *age of the client* is commented on, since there still is some lingering, disappearing debate about early intervention with stuttering, and more current and active debate over the forms of that intervention. As children mature into early school ages and then adolescence, the stuttering and the psychodynamics change, and so does therapy. The next section concerns the therapy *environment* in which emphasis may be home and clinic, clinic and home, clinic, and school. The shifts in emphasis affect the type of therapy and the way in which it is applied.

The third section deals with two aspects that may affect therapy, both of them *stereotypes*. One stereotype concerns that of the stutterers and what we think they are like, even though research often contradicts these perceptions. The other stereotype has to do with the clinicians and how they view themselves, relative to working with stutterers. The fourth section, a more extensive one, concerns the general *forms of therapy*. Whether direct or indirect therapy is best with children, and at what ages, is considered. Also, the simmering and periodically reerupting controversy over "fluency" and "symptom" therapy will be considered at some length.

Since the remaining chapters of this book generally shy away from established programs of therapy, the fifth section of this chapter summarizes briefly a number of programs that have been described in the literature. These descriptions are meant to illustrate the different ways in which techniques can be put together and to provide the reader with sources he or she may want to consult. The sixth and final section presents a few comments about technique modification and eclecticism.

CLIENT AGE

Age in therapy is a factor to consider as techniques are reviewed in various chapters of this book. With wide variations, the following aspects can be affected by the age of the client:

1. The characteristics and severity of dysfluencies.
2. The importance, and availability, of significant persons in the client's environment.
3. The attitudes and behavior of the client.
4. The degree to which therapy can, on the basis of age, utilize certain techniques, utilize some with modifications, or not be able to utilize specific procedures.
5. The level of client autonomy and insight.
6. Transfer and spontaneous generalization of therapy.
7. Maintenance needs and relapse probabilities.

At one time age was a determinant of whether or not direct therapy should occur at all. Most clinicians now favor early intervention, before school age, as soon as there is demonstrable dysfluency or inappropriate parental concern about dysfluencies. This early intervention shift is due partly to the maturing concept of preventing more serious problems in the future. However, in stuttering it also concerns the amount and duration of therapy required, the permanence of therapy effects, and the degree of fluency obtained. Rubin (1986) states that when stuttering children "or their families are seen early enough, recovery is complete in 100% of the cases" (p. 483). He feels that, unlike many programs discussed in this chapter, a 100 percent fluency criterion is reasonable and attainable. Nevertheless, it is accepted generally that "the earlier, the better" applies to stuttering.

Childhood, however the age limits are defined, is a state of continuous change. Skeletal structures and physiologic processes are growing and developing. Neurological characteristics and capacities undergo change. Some of the changes are a function of preprogrammed organic and neurological integrity factors, some are effects from nutrition and teratogens, and some reflect the compensatory efforts of the organism to cope with the normal (and supranormal) stresses in its environment. The result of this is that the stutterer at 4 years of age is not the same at 6 years of age. He, or she, has changed structurally, neurologically, functionally, cognitively, and emotionally. The combinations among all these factors predict a constant factor—change. The stutterer at 17 and at 19 years of age may show minimal changes in most areas, but this is not true at younger ages. As we respect the age factor in changing the stutterer, we also should be wary of categorizing stutterers within a set age range. (This has been discussed earlier under developmental tracks in stuttering.) An example of variation possibilities within an age range exists in Conture's (1982) summary on 15 stuttering adolescents, ages 12 to 14 years. Their severity of stuttering in %SW averaged 16.5 but varied from 1.0 to 43.0 percent. In considering the most frequent types of dysfluency, clients split so that 55 percent were predominantly PWR and 45 percent produced sound prolongations. The male-female ratio (typically 3.5 : 1) was 14 : 1, about 45 percent were first children, and 67 percent had articulation problems. The possible combinations of all these factors could produce three stutterers of identical ages who presented totally different problem patterns.

With that caution in mind, therapy can be divided into three age categories: preschool, elementary school age, and adolescence. For practical purposes, when age groupings are discussed in this text, the following will be applied:

- Group I—ages 3 to 6 years, preschool.
- Group II—ages 6 to 9 years, elementary.
- Group III—ages 9 to 16 years, preadolescent and adolescent.

It should be emphasized that the ranges cited in the preceding list are approximate and indicative, not prescriptive. Some children at 10 or 11 years can be regarded as Group II types behaviorally, while a child of 7 years may resemble older children in Group III. From another point of view, the children could be divided into the following groups:

- Group I—strong home and parent involvement, milder patterns, less struggle, few avoidance or attitude problems.
- Group II—home and school involvement, more severe problems, more struggle, peer problems, avoidance and attitude problems.
- Group III—school, peer, and home involvement, mature stuttering patterns, significant avoidance and attitude problems.

In the therapy chapters following, some procedures tend to sort themselves by age of the clients. Other procedures are applicable at any age, with only the factors of approach, intensity, clinician control, and the like, varied. At all times the clinician should avoid using procedures, as opposed to designing programs to contain procedures. In the later sections on stereotypes, on therapy orientation, and on technique modification, this flexibility mandate is further emphasized.

THERAPY ENVIRONMENT

Environment as a factor relates mostly to the place where therapy occurs; it has already been alluded to under the age factor. Therapy in a private-practice location, a therapy center, or a university clinic often involves variations in the frequency/duration of sessions, the availability of ancillary support systems and specialist assistance, and the participation of family members. The fact that a procedure worked excellently in a laboratory setting does not mean it will be as effective in a clinical or a school environment. Similarly, what went well during in-school or in-clinic sessions may not be nearly as successful at home or in the reality of the outside world. Before blessing clinicians with laboratory success methods, designers should consider the variables imposed by the therapy environment. Before clinicians transfer session-successful performances to the outside environment, the unique characteristics of each client's environment need to be considered. Therapy in school settings often mandates an entirely different set of circumstances. The author conducted a number of in-service training sessions for public school clinicians and asked their opinions about therapy needs in school settings. In one session a clinician stated firmly and succinctly:

> I don't have any specialists with me. I don't have any equipment more complicated than my own personal cassette recorder. I do have three children I

can see together for 20 minutes each session. The parents work and the classroom teachers are helpful but darn busy with their own problems. Now, what can I do to help these kids?

In various chapters, separate mention is made of applications in school settings. Other approaches are targeted to other particular environments. Not all techniques are adaptable to all situations, but most of them have flexible possibilities or transferable characteristics that allow their use in nearly all therapy situations.

STEREOTYPES: CLIENTS AND CLINICIANS

Large areas of human behavior and interaction are based on stereotypy. The stereotype provides for economy of evaluation and reaction time, increases potential efficiency, and may facilitate learning. It also contributes to faulty evaluation and inappropriate reactions, reduces efficiency, and may hinder the learning process. What is stereotypy? In one sense, it is a generalization transformed into dogma,

> a simplified and standardized conception or image invested with special meaning and held in common by members of a group. (Stein 1967, p.1394)

Stereotypes cover such concepts as Scots are stingy, the French are lovers, Orientals are inscrutable (whatever that is), and so on. Because of stereotyping, most motorists will not pick up hitchhikers, children may be frightened of police officers, and many students believe that teachers enjoy giving tests! There are "good" and "bad" stereotypes, and all of them violate the basic tenets of the semantic differential. Most of our psychological tests of adjustment, dysphasia tests, neuromotor evaluation forms, and so on, function by comparing test results to a stereotype model. If there is "enough" coincidence between the test score or profile and the standardized stereotype, then the subject is identified with that stereotype label. By the same process, labels can cause stereotyped images of a person's characteristics: "a good boy," "troublemaker," "learning disabled," "Broca's dysphasia," "hysterical dysphonia," all carry descriptive connotations. This is true of stutterers and stuttering. It also applies to clinicians.

Stutterers

Research into whether or not stutterers are stereotyped generally has shown that they are, and that the traits ascribed to stutterers are undesirable and do not differentiate among ages or types or degrees of stuttering. Yairi and Williams (1970) reported that when 127 public school clinicians rated stuttering boys as to their traits, about 65 percent of these traits were undesirable. Woods and Williams (1976) evaluated seven groups in their assignment of traits to child and adult stutterers and non-stutterers. The groups were parents of stuttering children, parents of children with other speech problems, parents of normally speaking children, elementary teachers, adult stutterers, public school clinicians, and college students. Results indicated that the various groups had a strong, negative stereotyped image of stutterers, and that these traits were attributed to children as well as to adults who stuttered. Even the stutterers rated stutterers as tense, insecure, and submissive types who were afraid of talking. Earlier, Woods and Williams (1971) had asked school clinicians to rate stutterers' traits. With agreements ranging from 25 to 75 percent, the clinicians rated stutterers as rigid, self-critical or defensive, having emotional concerns, being shy or insecure, and being nervous or fearful. Classroom teachers and speech and language clinicians were singled out for further investigation in a replication study with different groups (Woods 1976, 1977). A stereotyping pattern again was prominently displayed. Woods reported further that expansive-restrictive traits of quiet, passive, hesitant, self-derogatory, guarded, introverted, and withdrawn characteristics were among the primary traits identified.

Adams (1984a), in a review of literature on stuttering theory, research, and therapy circa 1977–82, stated that until 1977 the literature on stuttering was almost unanimous in supporting the concept that stutterers comprise a homogeneous group that could be evaluated and treated accordingly. This has been discussed several times already in this text, the most recent note being the points of adolescent diversity reported by Conture (1982). In spite of Adams's optimistic comment, research indicates that stereotyping continues to be a problem. Turnbaugh, Guitar, and Hoffman (1979) had 36 clinicians fix traits for fluent speakers and for mild, moderate, and severe stutterers. They reported that the clinicians separated stutterers and nonstutterers on the basis of negative traits, and that only the polar extremes of severity (mild versus severe) failed to lump the stutterers as an homogeneous group. The same researchers (1981) suggested that negative stereotypes do exist and are applied, but that there is opportunity for the stereotype to change during continued contact where the listener can observe other traits of the speaker.

Stereotyping and presumed homogeneity may not only contaminate the therapy we use but also affect the research upon which theory and therapy are based. Rentschler (1984) observed that most comparative research on stuttering assumes that the stuttering experimental group is homogeneous. By manipulating selection criteria stringency, he demonstrated differences, or subgroupings, within the stuttering population. White and Collins (1984) have suggested that stutterer stereotyping by clinicians is the result of cognitive inference and social categorization, and that stereotypes tend to continue because the clinician does not stop to compare occurrences of nonstereotypic behavior with the stereotype that is currently being expressed. Since most clinicians are poorly prepared to provide therapy of stuttering (see next section), the persistence, or even the creation, of stereotypes will be affected most by the training-program classroom teachers and clinical supervisors responsible for the education and training of the student clinician. Shames (1986) has pointed out that clinicians may be working with different kinds of stutterers. The challenge is, not to develop a single explanation of or a monolithic therapy of stuttering, but to learn how to do a better job of matching client and therapy in order to be more effective. The degree to which we operate with stereotypes will handicap meeting that challenge.

In the preceding discussion of stuttering stereotypes, it is necessary to avoid stereotyping stereotypy. We cannot deny that many different groups or categories of people have shared, in-group characteristics. This is true of stutterers also. For example, Gregory, Shanahan, and Walberg (1985) reported on 278 high school seniors with speech disabilities. They were compared to their peers and found to be older, to have additional disabilities more often, and tended to be from linguistic minority groups. These students were also lower in achievment, had poorer self-image, were less motivated, and had lower career aspirations. This does not mean that all high school students with speech problems fit the pattern just described. In the evaluation section past, and in some of the therapy chapters, traits of commonality are assumed. Such assumptions are valuable, or necessary for effective, economical function. However, when commonalities are assumed to be universal constants, when the client must adapt totally to the therapy, when we assume that "all stutterers" think, feel, or behave in certain ways, then the client suffers and the clinician is burdened with an unwarranted handicap.

Clinicians (Characteristics and Competency)

Is there such a thing as a clinician stereotype? What is a stutterer-clinician like, and what should one be like? The available literature does not provide a reassuring picture of clinicians or of therapy. Costello (1980) has stated that, all factors considered, the training of clinicians in therapy of stuttering is mediocre at best (p. 322). Published research seems to support her contention. Leith (1971) surveyed 50 graduate clinical training programs and reported that overall there were two clinicians for every available stutterer. Even worse, if stutterers were divided into four age groups, then the clinician-client ratio went to nine clinicians per stutterer. The result can be that few if any clinicians ever have a training opportunity to initiate therapy and bring it to a dismissal point, assuming they have an opportunity to work with stutterers at all. Research has indicated that the majority of our masters degree graduate student clinicians do not experience therapy with stutterers, some have never even observed therapy of stuttering, and a large number have not even had a graduate-level course devoted exclusively to stuttering.

When we consider the training problems, didactic and experiential, in stuttering, and add to them the issue of stereotyping discussed previously, it is not surprising that many clinicians are hesitant to approach therapy of stuttering. Blood and Seider (1981) reported that of school-age stutterers who also had other communication problems, 83 percent were being seen by public school clinicians, not for their stuttering, but for the other problems. Thompson (1984) in her survey of east-central Ohio schools reported that clinicians felt insecure in working with stutterers. She stated that clinician perceptions of stutterers is distorted and that clinicians are reluctant to schedule evaluations of stuttering and to provide therapy. She placed the blame squarely on university training programs. The stutterers themselves may not profit from the problems evidenced by clinicians. E-M. Silverman and Zimmer (1982) surveyed ten males and ten females who stuttered and stated that there was essential unanimity among them that "school therapy" did not help them. Their opinions were that therapy relief was not obtained until after they graduated from school and obtained outside therapy.

Wingate (1971b) stated that many clinicians, especially those in the public schools, are afraid of dealing with stuttering. He suggested that the reasons for fear include the "mystery" surrounding stuttering, the idea that the clinician may cause psychological harm to the stutterer, clinician doubts about the efficacy of therapy, and the belief in stereotyped traits that have been associated with the label of *stuttering* (see previous section). It is clear that university programs are all too often perpetuating stereotypes or failing to discredit them. They also have difficulty in providing adequate numbers of stutterers for experience, in total and among various age levels. Based only on personal observation and many conversations with clinicians, the author feels that universities also fail to provide an adequate foundation of therapy procedures and, what is more important, fail to prepare students to intermingle and adapt procedures into programs of therapy according to the needs of clients. We must realize that student clinicians will have questions based on ignorance, inexperience, and fears drawn from stereotypy. A recurrent question this author is presented with by student clinicians, who have become aware of their own disfluencies, is whether or not they can "catch" stuttering! Kimbarrow and Daly (1980) evaluated the fluency of student clinicians before and after providing intensive therapy for stutterers. They were compared to clinicians who did not work with stutterers. The researchers reported that while overall disfluencies reduced significantly among the student clinicians over the six-week period, there was a substantial increase in the occurrence of PWR and sound prolongation disfluencies. Exactly what these results mean is not clear, but in over 35 years of working with stuttering the author never has seen, or heard of, an instance when a clinician metamorphosed into a stutterer. The reverse often has occurred. Nevertheless, fears of clinicians do not have to be logical in order to be real.

Part of our problem, aside from reasons discussed previously, may be that we are not defining adequately the what and how content of clinical training with stuttering. The clinicians in the field say that their preparation is not adequate, and this inadequacy is reflected in their feelings about therapy of stuttering. This was supported by clinicians when Cooper and Cooper (1985) reported that in the last decade there has been almost no change in the number of clinicians (75 to 90 percent) who disagreed with statements that they worked well with and felt secure in working with stuttering children. Dopheide (1987) surveyed 22 clinicians in varied work settings. He asked them to assess which competencies they supported, as preparation for therapy of stuttering. In sum, the clinicians favored ability to evaluate situation effects on fluency, ability to determine the importance of significant others, evaluation of client awareness and of associated behaviors, and familiarity with stuttering theories. The agreement among clinicians on each of the foregoing items ranged only from 20 to 30 percent of the 22 participants, while 9 other suggested competencies fell below a 10 percent agreement level. In remediation procedures, 11 competency suggestions fell below the 10 percent level of agreement; and of the 11 competency statements that garnered 20 to 50 percent support, only 3 secured agreement from more than 25 percent of the clinicians:

1. Adjust therapy directness/intensity to the status level of the problem (50 percent).
2. Deal with the child's negative feelings about self and speech (45 percent).
3. Be familiar with many different therapy approaches (45 percent).

The last percentage figure tends to boggle the writer's mind. The clinicians all had at least two years of experience, and CCC-SLP (or equivalent) status. Nevertheless, the agreement levels among full-time clinicians is surprisingly low. Others have suggested competency or skill areas they feel are important for therapy of stuttering and other problems.

Lay (1982a, 1982b) reminded us that specific therapy procedures are only part of therapy. The self-management skills, the self-confidence projection, and the personal therapeutic relationship are all important to therapy. This emphasis on interpersonal skills has been echoed many times by Cooper (1977, 1976) as well as by others. Dalton (1983a) discusses clinician competence and characteristics. She agrees with Van Riper (1975) that clinicians should have a solid foundation of information about stuttering and should have contact with people who stutter. She concludes that our greatest lack in training clinicians is in the counseling skills across the whole range of communication disorders, not just in stuttering.

> Whether this be called "work on attitudes," "counselling" or "psychotherapy," these skills too need to be learned and provision for their learning should be made part of a therapist's basic training. (p. 223)

In addition to the counseling role, which will be discussed further in this and other chapters, there is the question of whether the clinician can go beyond the primitive, simplistic counting of behaviors or timing of responses and actually deal with the multivariate communication behaviors of the client. Shames and Florance (1982) point out that with any one client, the clinician must be able to shift from being a teacher and demonstrator (clinician centered) to being a reinforcer and responder (client centered). I would add the role of being a counselor for problems ranging from mild to severe, and the ability to deal with or refer appropriately for problems not central to communication but affecting therapy of stuttering. Conture (1982) states that clinicians must be able to handle multiple inputs simultaneously and deal with different events, each with its own characteristics and serial time sequence. He concludes that if a clinician cannot do this, then he or she should not be with stutterers.

The profession of speech and language pathology has failed to establish what it requires every undergraduate student to do in her or his clinic orientation course. Students may be required to submit written lesson plans that stipulate goals, establish rationale, and explain procedures. With stuttering, we have not agreed on what adequate preparation is (goals), have not generated an accepted rationale for what we do or fail to do, and apparently have insufficient stutterers and/or program resources to train with the goals and rationale we do express. As a result, the title of this chapter applies directly to the clinician who is supposed to provide therapy to the stutterer.

ORIENTATIONS TO THERAPY

Background

Another consideration, or controversy, interwoven through subsequent chapters is the form of therapy. As a single topic, this could occupy several hundred pages of text. The author has selected two or three aspects, assigning the rest to brief discussions in various therapy chapters or leaving them to writers such as Gregory (1979), Ingham (1984), and Shames and Rubin (1986). The topics that will be addressed are those of direct versus indirect therapy, operant versus interpersonal therapy, and fluency versus symptom therapy. The last two are intermixed for reasons that will become clear. Issues relative to counseling and psychotherapy are discussed in another chapter.

The therapy that we use is a major determinant of therapy outcome. However, the procedure is only part of the picture and, as Conture (1982) has suggested, procedures by themselves are not therapy, although we have many procedures that we can call on. Wingate (1984d) presents an extensive, but not exhaustive, list of therapy procedures that can be used. These include alterations in voice, easy onset, singing, "sounding," chanting, monotone, rhythm, prolongation, reduced rate, dialect, unison speech, masking, DAF, breath chewing, ventriloquism, and prosodic reading. Others could be listed. But we need to be careful in selecting a procedure and not be overly impressed by a journal article reporting that X punishment or reinforcement, or insight development, resulted in 99.9 percent reduction in dysfluencies. What works in the laboratory may not fare as well in therapy groups or in complex social situations (Murphy 1977). Nearly 20 years ago Slorach (1971) reported a renewed interest in group therapy and in relaxation therapy and a trend toward use of intensive therapy. We find all of these procedures in use today, as they were a century ago, and therapy goes on. With a host of procedures and programs available, clinician choice becomes highly significant.

Adams (1983) indicates that one of the variables that can affect the outcome of therapy is the clinician who makes an erroneous assumption about the client and/or about the stuttering. As a result of this error a wrong or less-adequate therapy is structured. One must expand this to include several subvariables that can lead to poor therapy decisions:

1. Overcommitment to a theory that cannot account for stutterer subgroups and intraclient variations.
2. Overacceptance of stutterer stereotypes.
3. Overdedication to one school or form of therapy.
4. Overreaction to fears of stuttering, and selection of therapy to reduce clinician fears rather than address the client's problems.
5. Overresponse to every "new" therapy procedure or technique that is published.

Choices should be made thoughtfully and flexibly, for sound clinical reasons. In the subsequent paragraphs several major areas of choice are reviewed.

Direct and Indirect Therapy

There is a potential semantic boggle here. Some clinicians divide client-centered therapy into three categories: direct, indirect, and nondirect. However, current literature on stuttering among children tends to regard indirect therapy as therapy with persons other than the stutterer, and direct therapy as therapy with the stutterer personally. How direct direct therapy can be is a variable, and this will be commented on subsequently. For the moment, however, indirect/direct therapy will equate with environment/client therapy.

A generation or more of speech and language clinicians, many of them still working, were taught that children should not receive therapy of stuttering because this would probably exaggerate the problem. Instead, parent counseling and environmental manipulation was to be used. In this approach attention was to be directed away from dysfluencies. Such inexcusable neglect of other valuable therapy approaches has fortunately been reduced greatly as clinicians have become aware of the values of early, direct intervention. As Conture noted (1982), "It is not the age of the child with the problem, but the age of the problem with the child" that makes a difference (p. 42).

Adams (1984a) summarized information indicating that direct treatment of stuttering in young children has taken hold firmly and that clinicians realize they can concentrate on speech behaviors without fear of ruining the child. When, then, is indirect or direct therapy appropriate, assuming there are no practical constraints? There is no validated answer. However, assuming that parents are available, the clinician should look at the situation and assign the child and the parent, each, to one of the subcategories listed:

FLUENCY PROBLEM	ENVIRONMENTAL CONCERN
1. No fluency problem.	A. No parental concern.
2. Noticeable disfluency, few classical signs.	B. Concern appropriate to the level of the problem.
3. Dysfluent, mild, or inconsistent.	C. Inappropriately low concern.
4. Dysfluency, mild and consistent.	D. Inappropriately high level of concern.
5. Moderate to severe dysfluency.	

A designation of 1-A receives no therapy and no follow-up. Designations of 1-D, 2-D, 3-A, 3-C, or 3-D would probably be targets of indirect (environmental) therapy ranging from one counseling session and a follow-up to a scheduled program of counseling. The child in 3 might or might not receive therapy for general speech support, fluency enhancement, and parental interaction or observation. The combinations of 4 or 5 with A, B, C, or D call for direct therapy intervention with the child, targeting dysfluencies, and the appropriate and feasible attention to the environment. As you have just seen, indirect and direct therapy often is not an either/or proposition. Actually, as Ramig and Wallace (1987) report, a combination of indirect and direct therapies will produce better results in terms of degree of fluency and permanence of results. Overall, "the vast majority of contemporary therapies for children who stutter include both indirect and direct manipulations, with a decided emphasis on the latter" (Adams, 1984b, p. 273).

Dual Controversies

The section title "Dual Controversies" refers to a confusion that has arisen over certain forms of therapy. Until about the 1960s, the prevailing forms of therapy tended to deal with the modification of stuttering spasms and/or the feelings and objectivity of the stutterer. Therapy design, conduct, and measurement was often loosely structured so that progress was reported in terms such as "better," "little changed," "more tolerant," "less severe" and so on. A number of researchers, such as Goldiamond (1960), began to apply learning theory principles of Skinner (1958, 1938) to therapy with stutterers. Rather than utilize so-called traditional methods of symptom control, emphasis was placed on reinforcing fluency and punishing stuttering. Many successes were reported as operant-conditioning clinicians utilized modern technology and ancient methods to achieve results.

The confusion stemmed from the mutual identification many placed on operant conditioning and fluency therapy. As we will see, operant conditioning does not necessarily have anything to do with fluency or with stuttering. Both events, fluency and stuttering, are behaviors, and most behaviors can be modified through the use of operant principles. Nevertheless, advocates of symptom and of fluency approaches tended to assign operant conditioning to fluency reinforcement, and loose structure to symptom modification. Much of the following discussion will help the reader follow this forced dichotomy. (The artificiality of the separation is considered again later on.)

The reader will recall that operant conditioning is based on a simple model, namely, that the consequences or results of certain behaviors affect the frequency or likelihood that the behavior will occur again. If a *stimulus* (S) results in a *response* (R), the future occurrence of R will be affected by the *consequences* that follow. If a student asks a question in class and the teacher responds pleasantly and reinforcingly, there is an increased probability that the student will ask other questions in the future. On the other hand, a negative or sarcastic reply by the teacher will decrease the likelihood of future questions. The teacher's reactions are "contingent consequences," and they are the factors affecting the future occurrence of R. There can be four contingencies: positive reinforcement, negative reinforcement, extinction, and punishment. *Postive reinforcement* (Rf+) is any event that will increase the future occurrence of R; *negative reinforcement* (Rf−) is any event whose termination increases future occurrence of R; *extinction* refers to the elimination of a response by removing a previous reinforcer; and *punishment* is any event that interrupts or decreases the occurrence of R. The important aspect, aside from an appropriate contingent response, is the consistency and timing of the occurrence.

Along with the description just provided, operant conditioning applied measurement principles. The behavior to be changed had to be accurately identified, its pretreatment frequency (or other measures) established, and response counts conducted during therapy to provide a semicontinuous measure of R frequency in order to compare it with the pretreatment baseline frequency. Criteria defining the success of therapy varied from zero occurrence of R to some arbitrary, permissible frequency of R occurrence. With these definitions, and with awareness of the forced association of fluency reinforcement and operant conditioning, let us continue and examine the dichotomy of fluency reinforcement and symptom modification. In applying operant principles to therapy, several factors should be emphasized:

1. The operant, or target behaviors, should be identified clearly and therapy procedures should deal directly with the targets.
2. Reinforcing or aversive stimuli should be applied systematically so that the recipient can develop an association between them.
3. Baseline measures are extremely important, as they help define the operants and provide the necessary data by which progress can be monitored and change assessed.
4. Similarly, behavioral counts during the therapy process are important. Occasional score totaling is inadequate and undermines the ability to assess the effectiveness of methods being used.
5. Operant procedures tend to be reliable as long as they are applied within the context of the stimulus-response situation. Transfer stability is less certain and will be discussed later.
6. Operant procedures provide continuous feedback to the clinician for support of decision making. Decisions may be relative to moment-to-moment response in therapy or about overall directions of the therapy program.

Fluency and Symptom Approaches

Guitar and Peters (1980), with conference panel assistance, prepared a Speech Foundation of America (SFA) report on contemporary therapies of stuttering. They separately defined stuttering modification and fluency-shaping therapies. Stuttering modification includes

> reducing avoidance behaviors, speech related fears, and negative attitudes toward speech [and] . . . helping the stutterers learn to modify the form of his stuttering. (p. 13)

Reference, for examples, is made to Van Riper (1973), Sheehan (1970), Luper and Mulder (1964), and previous SFA publications (1978, no. 12, 1974). Fluency-shaping therapy is defined as therapy based on operant conditioning and programming principles . . . [so that] some form of fluency is first established . . . , reinforced and gradually modified to approximately normal conversational speech . . . , [and] then generalized to the person's daily speaking environment. (p. 13)

For examples, reference is made to Ryan (1974), Webster (1974), and SFA (1970, no. 7). The author would add Brutten (1986), Ingham (1984), and Costello (1983) for more recent examples.

Referring to page 20 of the Guitar and Peters publication, the author has developed a summary (Table 5–1) comparing aspects of the two therapy approaches. Such summaries often elicit objections from clinicians who do or do not conform to the pattern presented. However, they represent the results of observations, clinical conversations, and readings to provide a general summary of how the approaches often differ. The basic, schismatic difference between the two approaches is that the modification approach works with the moment of stuttering and the shaping approach works with the nonstuttered speech of the client. All of the differences are a result of tradition, habit, and selection. For instance, conditioning/programming principles are 100 percent applicable to modification methods, while motivation, attitude, and avoidance behav-

TABLE 5–1. Stuttering Modification versus Fluency-Shaping Therapy

STUTTERING MODIFICATION	FLUENCY SHAPING
Attitude, Speech Fears, Avoidances	
Major interest and focus	Little or no attention
Client Analysis and Evaluation of Stuttering Behaviors	
Major interest and focus	Little or no attention
Modification of Stuttering Spasms	
Primary goal of therapy	Not dealt with
Alteration of Speech to Establish a Fluency Pattern	
Not dealt with	Primary goal of therapy
Development of Self-monitoring Skills	
Emphasized	Varies from little to much emphasis
Establishment of Baseline Measures	
Usually in qualitative terms	Usually in quantitative terms
Measurement of Progress	
Usually in qualitative terms	Usually in quantitative terms
Therapy Structure	
Emphasis on rapport, motivation, teaching, counseling	Emphasis on conditioning or programming principles, use of punishment and/or reward contingencies
Attention to General Speech Skills	
Usually minimal attention	Usually minimal attention
Transfer	
Usually planned	Usually planned
Maintenance	
May be planned, but often left to the client	May be left to the client, but often planned with evaluation systems provided

iors can be (and have been) dealt with in an operant therapy mode. This also is true for other comparisons made in Table 5–1. Communication between therapy modes, and opportunities to profit from them, becomes impossible when an "authority" states that attitude is not important in therapy, or that operant design destroys the clinical relationship. Both types of statements are dogmatic evangelism and, like most generalizations, are not necessarily true. The sum total of this comparison, as noted before, is that fluency therapies admit to and accept therapy goals that involve the emission of uncontrolled dysfluencies, that symptom therapies admit to and accept goals that involve the emission of uncontrolled dysfluencies, and that both aspire to goals that involve speech devoid of uncontrolled dysfluencies.

In the controversies that have boiled around operant conditioning therapy and classical interpersonal therapy, rational dialogue has been damaged by extreme-example criticisms and too-rigid postures. A thorough, rational, and readable explanation of operant principles was published by Shames and Egolf (1976). This text aims primarily at applying operant principles to the interview structure of stuttering therapy. They note that so-called laboratory principles and practices of operant conditioning cannot be transferred, unchanged, to the interpersonal structure of clinical therapy. Different clients have different histories, different needs and behaviors in the present, and different goals in the future. Different therapy environments alter establishment and transfer requirements. Different clinicians vary in their histories, capacities, and goals. Different therapy settings encourage, alter, or proscribe various therapy procedures. Shames and Egolf discuss a number of concerns (pp. 28–33) in the therapy controversy:

1. Operant therapy deals solely with observable behavior, including that of the clinician.
2. Advance selection of certain behaviors (and exclusion of others) by which to measure progress restricts clinical judgment and flexibility. Shames and Egolf note that operant principles mandate consistency, and any shifts in emphasis should be done carefully and only after cautious judgment.
3. There is preoccupation with count data that ignores timing, emotion, situation variables, and the like.
4. Transfer of in-clinic results is not an expected product of operant procedures, unless specially designed transfer programs are used.
5. Operant procedures do not generally deal with issues of emotion in stuttering or the feelings of the stutterer.
6. Many clinicians do not like the idea of being manipulators. Shames and Egolf note appropriately that therapy of any type is manipulation, and the only question is how much manipulation there is to be and the form that it is going to take.
7. Operant therapy does not tell the clinician what to manipulate, only how to go about it. The specifics in various therapy programs are variable fill-ins riding on the infrastructure of operant procedures.

Shames and Egolf (p. 32) note a basic, irreconcilable difference between operantly based and stuttering modification therapies:

> Stutterers should not be asked to accept their stuttering, to learn to live with their stuttering, and to modify it into more socially acceptable forms. The goal . . . is speech that is free from stuttering.

Indeed, this basic difference noted by Shames and Egolf highlights another aspect of controversy. Modification therapy has been attacked because it asks the stutterer to accept stuttering, learn to live with it, and modify it. This philosophy has been contrasted with the behavioral modification goal of stutter-free speech. However, *stutter-free* in the ELU program Shames and Egolf described involved a discharge criterion of 1 percent or less SW (p. 57). Shine (1980a, 1980b) accepts stuttering frequency up to 0.5 SW/M. Other operantly based programs express similar criteria. As a result, it seems that operantly treated clients in fluency programs may have to accept stuttering and learn to live with it!

Using the Shames and Egolf success criterion, the author could stutter 50–60 times during a class lecture and still meet the fluency requirement. This split-personality approach to therapy goals is exemplified by Guitar and Peters (1980) in their comparison of symptom and fluency therapies. They define three levels or types of speech behavior outcomes of therapy (p. 125):

- **Spontaneous fluency.** This is achieved without monitoring or control, minus tension and struggle, and with no more than "an occasional number of repetitions and prolongations."
- **Controlled fluency.** The results are similar to that of spontaneous fluency, but the speaker must monitor speech production, may control rate, and may use pullouts and preparatory sets.
- **Acceptable stuttering.** There are noticeable, though not severe, dysfluencies, but the speaker is comfortable. Controls and monitoring may be used.

Guitar and Peters state that both fluency and symptom therapies aspire to the first outcome, spontaneous fluency, and both therapies are oriented to accept the second outcome, controlled fluency. The difference lies in therapy emphasis—fluency and speaking manner in the one, and fear reduction and symptom control in the other. The third outcome possibility, acceptable stuttering, would be a program failure in fluency therapy and a limited program success in symptom therapy. The sum total of this comparison leads to the conclusion, noted previously, that fluency therapies often accept residual stuttering as part of their definition of fluency. If symptom modification is to be labeled as "stutter acceptably" or "stutter fluently" therapy, as some fluency therapy adherents have done, then semantic justice might suggest that fluency therapy be relabeled as "stutter less", not stutterless, therapy.

The discussions centering around operant, or fluency, therapy and symptom therapy have been "enthusiastic" at times. Wingate (1980) challenged directly the operant concept that stuttering is learned behavior, stating that there has been no research to prove this. Further, he argued that all the operant therapy studies have achieved is to indicate that in some instances stuttering frequency can be reduced by associating the stuttering with some signal—and this in no way proves that stuttering is learned. On the other hand, Rubin and Culatta (1986), in 1971, stated that a stutterer does not "have to stutter" (p. 467) and that organic factors are not included among the reasons for stuttering. Since they have proved neither statement, and there is evidence to the contrary, their objection to what they call "stutter better" therapy, especially when "both he and the clinician know that he is capable of complete fluency," is suspect. The previous statement also is presumptive and without support. Culatta (1976) rejected symptom therapy as having no logical basis and for approving the development, or modification, of pathological behavior, stuttering (see the earlier discussion of Guitar and Peter's outcomes of therapy). Ryan (1979) commented that operant principles have not been welcomed by "speculators and philosophers who see no value in collecting quantitative data." Even worse, Ryan feels, are the "pseudobehaviorists" who "use some of the terminology, none of the basic procedures, and all of the old nonbehavioristic therapy activities" (p. 131). Similarly, Rhodes (1973) spoke sarcastically of therapy that produced the "happy stutterer" and wrote that the assets of operant therapy outweighed any of its liabilities and that "it's harder to argue with numbers than it is with speculation and theories" (p. 93). In one of these statements (p. 91) that tend to haunt one in the future, Rhodes avowed:

> Therapeutic strategies and techniques which do not have as their major objective the generation of fluency (or, if you wish, nonstuttering speech), are unsatisfactory, unacceptable, and may be **unethical.** [emphasis added.]

Contrary opinions concerning fluency therapy were not lacking. Sheehan (1979) was not impressed by operant methods or results. He argued that most of the techniques were resurrected from the diseased pile of failed therapy methods and the magical parchments of therapy charlatans. Techniques aside, he also objected to the fluency orientation itself, stating that it was a role denial and a distortion. A comment this writer heard from a symptom clinician compared fluency therapy to teaching a cat to walk on its rear legs—"It's surprising at first, but it isn't normal and it usually doesn't last." Sheehan may have made a tempered contribution to the debate when he wrote, "'Traditional' is always the other fellow's therapy. 'Innovation' is always our own—no matter how hoary, ancient, and bearded" (p. 188). Murphy (1977) supported therapy with the "whole person," and noted that behavioral programming "always stands in danger of choosing trivial goals, because it is the trivial goals that can be most readily translated into testable, operational statements" (p. 30). Cooper (1984, 1971a) concluded that operant therapy, while efficient and effective within a certain range of behaviors, does not deal with the abstracts such as self-concept and client-clinician relationship. Conture (1982) felt that the last 20 years have seen "a rush to be clinically quantitative, to count and assess behavior" in various behavioral structures. He argued that this has caused clinicians to stop paying attention to the client's behavior. "We can easily set up charts to depict behavior change over time, but we cannot as easily explain to ourselves and others what behavior needs to be charted" (pp. 82–83). However, as we examine polarized viewpoints, it is wise to remember that there will always be another viewpoint. Stromsta (1986) either clarifies or confuses further the issues by identifying himself as a symptom therapist and then rejecting a great deal of what has been regarded as symptom therapy. He states that what most clinicians call symptoms are actually reactions to a real or basic symptom, the intraphonemic disruptions in the forward flow of speech. "Recognizing, practicing, and suppressing complicating behaviors is little more than a negative approach; it offers nothing to stutterers in terms of identifying and alleviating the core behaviors of stuttering, the original impetus for the complicating behaviors" (p. 116).

Summary

A byproduct of heat can be light, and there is some light growing out of the controversies that have been discussed. Moderate voices have suggested combinations of behavior modification and psychotherapeutic procedures (Cooper 1971a), and more and more behavioral therapists are finding values in amalgamating cognitive therapy aspects into their structures (Maxwell 1982), and utilizing a wider range of behaviors (such as thematic content and symptom modification) in operant frameworks (Costello 1980). Wells (1987) has recommended combining "the best of each treatment approach" (p. 46); and Egolf, Shames, and Blind (1971) long ago described a therapy sequence of operant applications to eye contact and thematic content, with Sheehan-type approach-avoidance therapy added.

The settlement of the debate is particularly critical when we remember this text's emphasis on stuttering among young people, since operant purity has been strongest (and the results most impressive) in dealing with the young. Starkweather (1980) makes the point that the child who stutters is a different kind of stutterer from the adult who stutters. With due notice to variability, it is safe to generalize that the form and intensity of the core stuttering spasms differ; presence and degree of associated behaviors constitute a difference; motivation, attitudes, and awareness are usually not the same; psychosocial interactions show extreme differences;

and environmental expectations and reactions usually are different. Where stuttering, and the conditions surrounding it, is simple, Wells (1987) has suggested that a very young stutterer may benefit most from fluency methods, presented operantly, particularly if linguistic complexity is controlled. Psychotherapy, if needed, may be limited to environmental counseling. At older elementary school levels, Wells suggests that either fluency or symptom approaches, or a desirable mix, may be preferred. She recommends trial therapy if the decision is not clear initially, especially in working with adolescent stutterers.

What has developed is a suggestion of eclecticism, rather than depending on one theory method. By no means should the clinician go therapy shopping each time a stutterer is scheduled or each time a technique seems not to be working. Careful evaluation in selection and ongoing evaluation during use are recommended. Eclecticism creates conflicts with rigid statements such as the following:

1. Symptom therapy is acceptance of pathological behavior.
2. Operant clinicians are bean counters.
3. Children should receive fluency therapy, and adults should receive symptom therapy.
4. Use program X for clients ages three to six years, and program Y for children in the seven–ten-year age range.

Clinician maturity is required in therapy selection. Wall and Myers (1984) stress that eclectic therapy is not simple to develop. Rather, eclectic therapy requires astute observation from one who has a depth of information about stuttering. To this observation must be coupled knowledge about, and understanding of, the various therapy procedures. Of course, knowledge about the client, in normative and dysfluency terms, is also necessary. Wall and Myers also note that students tend to favor the practical side over the theoretical, and they urge the application of theory rationale to therapy planning. They summarize by stating that:

> eclecticism is governed by rationale . . . arrived at only after an examination of the stutterer's particular symptomatology and a thorough search for a match of "best fit" between symptoms and treatment. (p. 4)

THERAPY PROGRAMS

The preceding section on controversies has ended with an appeal to eclecticism, with warnings against careless or random selection. The literature, and commercial catalogs, are full of proposed or summarized programs. There actually are not many different programs dealing with stuttering therapy. Although many programs exist, their differences separate them into only a few groups. The beginning clinician, as discussed earlier, is often fearful of stuttering, or at least lacks self-confidence. In such situations it is quite natural that clinicians look for "a way" that can be applied easily. The more rigidly defined the limits of the program scope, and the more specifically procedures are detailed, the more likely some clinicians will be to use the program. As this occurs, several things may happen:

1. A program works, and the clinician goes on to apply it to the next stutterer, whether appropriate or not.
2. A program fails, and the clinician rejects future use of it, whether appropriate or not.
3. The clinician finds with repeated experience that she or he has outgrown the program and either looks for another program or begins individual planning and development.
4. Experiences are so disappointing that the clinician's attitudes of fear and avoidance are reinforced, and therapy of stuttering is avoided.

The foregoing options are not reassuring, though the third option is the one we hope for. Partly for these reasons the entire therapy portion of this book, Section III, is devoted to procedures of therapy, rather than to programs. Nevertheless, techniques in isolation are useless, or worse. They must be structured into an overall program with a beginning, a core process, and a termination that leads to transfer and response stability. For this reason the following pages are summaries of a number of therapy programs, rather than reviews of individual procedures. Some programs are available as commercially published kits or manuals, while others are presented as carefully planned and tried forms in the literature. In every section references are provided that will lead the reader to source publications or publication sources. None of the programs are recommended, or rejected, by the author. Evaluations are not provided. The author has used all of them, or used their essential forms. Some were preferred, and others were not—but on the basis of personal dynamics, and not on judgments that any particular program was good or bad. Finally, and most importantly, the following pages are not a summary of all major programs. Wells (1987), Shames and Florance (1980), and other sources are too extensive to summarize in a few paragraphs. In addition, a number of therapy programs exist in article or paper series but have not yet been collated and presented in final, single-source form.

The reader also is referred to the following sources:

- Dalton, P., *Approaches to the Treatment of Stuttering.*
- Peins, M., *Contemporary Approaches in Stuttering Therapy.*
- Speech Foundation of America, *Stuttering Therapy: Prevention and Intervention with Children*, 20.
- Wall, M.J., & Myers, F.L., *Clinical Management of Childhood Stuttering.*

- Ingham, R.J., *Stuttering and Behavior Therapy.*
- Conture, E.G., *Stuttering.*
- Leith, W.R., *Handbook of Stuttering Therapy for the School Clinician.*
- Van Riper, C., *The Treatment of Stuttering.*

Fluency Rules Therapy

Runyan and Runyan (1986) have devised a fluency rules program which they describe in general terms. The rules were applied over a period of time to nine children, about four to seven years of age. Therapy occurred in public school settings, averaging two therapy sessions per week. The seven rules are summarized below:

1. Reduced speech rate, through symbolism, modeling, and/or metronome.
2. Breath release before phonation.
3. Light articulator contacts.
4. Elimination of associated/overflow struggles.
5. Continuous movement of speech mechanism, rather than prolongation.
6. Easy onset of phonation.
7. Elimination of repetitions.

Stocker Probe

The probe therapy procedure (Stocker 1980) is based on asking questions (probes) for the client to respond to. The probes are divided into presumably increasing levels of demand, which are more likely to put stress (personal, motoric, linguistic) on the child. Therapy steps, or demand levels, are structured for operant presentation, with appropriate reinforcement schedules. Awareness, monitoring, and elimination of associated behaviors also receive attention.

Symptom Modification

Focus on symptom modification is not common among therapy procedures for young children, although many procedures borrow from it. The most symptom-oriented therapies probably are those associated with Dell (1980) and with Luper and Mulder (1964). Dell is a mixture of symptom modification, with awareness and relaxation/desensitization training. He writes for the school therapy setting and provides useful suggestions to the clinician. Luper and Mulder are classically "Van Riper" in their approaches to insight, awareness, pseudostuttering, cancellation, counseling, and other techniques of standard symptom modification. They provide a very useful section on counseling children, as well as discussing parent counseling for borderline fluency problem children.

Mowrer

Mowrer (1979) has provided a program to establish fluent speech. It requires that the client be able to read at the second-grade level. The program is made up of six subprograms, each one with an identifiable behavioral objective. In the first step (of eight) of the first program, the objective is for the client to read aloud, in five minutes, 60 two-word units with 99 percent fluency. No fluency induction modes are applied, and the stutterer is told to skip any word pair on which difficulty is experienced or anticipated. Every utterance receives a positive or negative verbal response, and error is stuttering or any "unusual behavior" (p. 14). A signal tone tape is used to key client utterances at five-second intervals. If 99 percent fluency is not obtained after 7 five-minute trials, a branch program is provided. Each subprogram has six to ten steps in it, with the final subprogram terminating in the client's participating in a five-minute conversation with the clinician, maintaining 98 percent fluency. Mowrer stresses that the program is designed only to establish fluency and would require other methods to meet needs of particular clients and to provide a maintenance structure for the acquired fluency. He developed the program initially for intensive application, utilizing up to ten student clinicians for one client. Mowrer also noted that most therapy aides could be trained to administer the program.

Gregory-Hill

The Gregory (1979, 1973) and Gregory and Hill (1984, 1980) publications have evolved a therapy program on several levels. Their evaluation procedures were discussed briefly in Chapter 3. It is intended to allow the clinician to divide children among treatment categories. The first strategy is preventive counseling with parents of rather typically disfluent children. No child therapy is involved, and emphases are on giving information to the parents and to providing suggestions that will facilitate fluency and minimize disruptions as the child matures. A follow-up check is usually scheduled.

The second strategy is for the borderline dysfluent child. Direct counseling is used, and the parents are asked to observe and chart behaviors. The parents first observe a clinician modeling good speech and interactive behaviors with their child, and then they participate on a learning basis. Follow-up procedures are scheduled to continue counseling and, if necessary, move to the third strategy.

In the third strategy, the child receives two hours of individual and 30 minutes of group therapy each week. The parents have an hour of counseling each week, plus guided observation of the therapy sessions with the child. Children are not labeled or treated as stutterers, and overt identifications are guided by the child's own labels. Play therapy and desensitization are not emphasized, and the child is taught an easy, relaxed form of speaking. This fluent speech is developed through progressive complexity levels under varying conditions. Tolerance to stress and fluency disruption, and competence in other communication areas, also is addressed. Finally, client self-confidence and self-concept acceptance are strengthened. When older, more severely stuttering children receive therapy, specific targeting of dysfluencies may occur to a limited extent.

Monterey Fluency Program

Ryan (1979, 1974, 1971) and Ryan and Van Kirk (1974, 1971) have been associated with the Monterey Program, which regards stuttering as a learned behavior and structures therapy to deal with the manner of speaking. Associated behaviors, attitudes, and emotions are presumed to be stuttering concomitants that will disappear or lose effect as fluency is established and generalized. Parent counseling and environmental manipulation are not specified in the programs. Therapy is fairly rigorous in its operant structure, with SW/M being used as the primary progress measure.

The therapy program divides into establishment, transfer, and maintenance segments. Development of fluent utterances in the establishment phase can be through a programmed variety of symptom modification procedures (see Chapter 14), through response-contingent verbal punishment strategies, through GILCU (see Chapter 7), or through the use of DAF. The last two are more commonly used, GILCU being aimed at younger and/or milder clients, and DAF at older and/or more severe clients. Transfer, which is the same for all the establishment programs, usually takes three or four months. It is structured for variation to meet individual needs. The maintenance aspect of the program, following therapy dismissal, is comprised of five steps covering nearly two years after therapy is over.

Vocal Control Therapy

Weiner's program of therapy (1984a, 1984b, 1978) combines a phonatory reconfiguration and stuttering desensitization approach. Therapy emphasis is on fluency, not on symptom modification. Although the components of the program are specified, the elements of sequence, timing, and variations are not rigidly programmed. Clinician revision and augmentation are encouraged.

The phonatory skills aspect of therapy divides into four areas of concentration: establishment of proper breathing, easy onset of speech, enhanced or optimized oral resonance, and "vowel focus." The latter target is to have the stutterer combine easy onset and enhanced resonance so that speech becomes focused on proper, easy production of a vowel in any CV (consonant-vowel) combination, with the consonant being produced without any articulator preset (preparatory set) pattern. In the development of skills, length and complexity of utterance in progressive increments is utilized.

Weiner emphasizes strongly the desensitization of the stutterer to reduce anxiety and associated tension to acceptable levels. This is seen as being necessary for the physiologic changes described in the previous paragraph to be effective, and for transfer and maintenance to occur. Systematic desensitization (Wolpe 1958) is the preferred method. However, role playing, rehearsal, assertiveness training, and controlled desensitization practice, relaxation, and fear hierarchy construction are utilized.

Transfer of therapy effects is worked with at every step of therapy progress. Emphasis is placed on establishing transfer programs, rather than just encouraging the stutterer to do develop transfer programs alone. After dismissal, maintenance involves phased-down conferences on progress and problems. This terminates with a follow-up contract that, over a period of years, can involve mail or telephone contacts and, if requested by the client, booster therapy sessions.

Systematic Fluency Training

Shine's Systematic Fluency Training for Young Children (1980a, 1980b) has been described briefly, concerning evaluation procedures, in Chapter 3. The program combines physiologic alterations in speaking patterns in teaching an "easy speaking voice," with progressive increments in the length and complexity of utterances. Different stimulus models (pictures, story books, objects) are used in rotation. The child is first taught absolute fluency, whispering if needed, so that subsequent speech activity can be manipulated within an operant framework of contingency reinforcement. Client speech is controlled and kept within the stimulus structure in order to maintain fluent responses. Intensive therapy is preferred. Verbal and token reinforcement systems are used, and the step level and overall success criterion is 0.5 or fewer SW/M.

Environment is addressed in the program, starting during the evaluation procedure. Parents are taught to observe and evaluate speech and are asked to maintain daily records of time intervals in which stuttering spasms are counted. The parents, or significant others, are asked to observe therapy sessions, then to participate in them, and then to conduct therapy procedures over steps where the pass criterion has already been met. The person learns to model a relaxed speech pattern outside the clinic and to observe the speech of the child. Shine (1980a) reported that

87 percent of 40 children did not require any out-clinic activities to effect transfer and maintenance of fluency developed during in-clinic therapy.

A Component Model

The Component Model for Treating Stuttering in Children (Riley and Riley (1986, 1984, 1979) also was discussed earlier in Chapter 3, concerning evaluation. The evaluation determines the timing, sequence, and emphasis of four areas of therapy. These four areas are environmental modification, attitude revision, therapy for neurologic components of speech, and modification of remaining dysfluencies. Environmental manipulation involves 4 to 12 one-hour parent-counseling sessions to support fluency and reduce disruptors, revise unrealistic expectations, resolve guilt, and, if needed, deal with instances of children using stuttering to manipulate family behaviors. Attitude modification deals primarily with feelings about stuttering, fluency perfectionism, and overall self-concept. Neurologic components include attending (attention span) problems, oral motor discoordination, auditory-processing difficulties, and sentence formulation problems.

In the client sample, Riley and Riley reported that 37 percent of the children did not require the final therapy step, dysfluency modification. On an age-range basis the percentage of clients needing the final step was as follows: three to four years, 20 percent; five years, 67 percent; six years, 83 percent; seven years or older, 100 percent. Therapy targets are associated struggle behaviors and avoidances, and the core stuttering spasms. The core spasms are approached either by teaching the child to substitute an easier, more normal disfluency for the abnormal one or, if needed, learning airflow and easy-onset procedures.

Double Tape Recorder Therapy

A different therapy approach was developed over the past two decades by Peins and her colleagues (Peins, McGough & Lee 1984, 1972a, 1972b; Lee, McGough & Peins 1973). It was designed to reduce clinician-client time in conventional therapy, to serve as a sole or an ancillary therapy, to facilitate maintenance, and to reduce problems in client motivation. The authors have a formal assessment protocol to establish severity, behaviors, and attitudes. The therapy goal is not fluency in the stutter-free sense, but fluency that has the speech moving easily and continuously from syllable to syllable and word to word.

The client will need two tape cassette recorders to utilize the twelve 30-minute recorded sessions. Each lesson is to be performed daily for two weeks, with the client responding and recording on the second cassette unit while playing the therapy tape on the first unit. The client erases or records over each previous practice recording, saving the last effort of the two-week cycle. In-clinic therapy occurs on a biweekly basis for 30 minutes, utilizing portions of the practice tape.

Therapy centers around the establishment of so-called legato speech, which will be discussed further in the chapters on therapy techniques. Briefly, legato speech combines rate reduction, easy onset and airflow, prolongation of continuants, and continuous phonation between sounds and words. Attention is given to speech expression, oral reading skills, and self-monitoring activities. Taped role-playing activities are used for practice. Attitude factors are not especially approached in therapy. At the termination of treatment, a maintenance reminder tape is given to the client and she or he is encouraged to return to or contact the clinic if there is a need to do so.

Preschool Fluency Development Program

The Preschool Fluency Development Program (Culp 1984), as the title implies, is directed at preschool children in individual or small-group therapy sessions. Parent-teacher training (about seven hours) is provided, and environmental observation and maintenance activities are developed on a continuing basis. (The evaluation program has been summarized previously in Chapter 3.) Therapy, in a play setting, develops in three areas: fluency of speech, cognitive abilities, and language stimulation. Emphasis is placed on establishing and developing fluency, starting at the single-word level of unison speech and moving up through conversational speech. Progressive steps increase linguistic complexity while recycling through successive levels of immediate and delayed clinician modeling and through spontaneous production by the client. These modes recur in supportive and then in disruptive situations. Cognitive capacities leading to awareness, evaluation, and internalization are developed. Suggested activities, sequences, and problem solutions are provided. The training program for parents is provided in seven sections but can be tailored and time organized to meet individual needs. Monthly observation of therapy and a bimonthly parent maintenance group is recommended. Home recording and follow-up procedures are also discussed.

Personalized Fluency Control Therapy

The Personalized Fluency Control Therapy (PFCT) program (Cooper 1984) is designed for school or clinical use and includes provision for adoption of predesigned Individual Education Program (IEP) forms and evaluation materials (Cooper & Cooper 1980, 1976). Parent and teacher interviews, the Individual Education Program (IEP) meeting, and therapy planning are described. The areas of therapy that are identified are the following:

1. **Identification and structuring.** The teacher role for the clinician is to instruct the client in the therapy program and begin developing a strong interpersonal relationship. The client is to learn to analyze/describe stuttering behaviors, feelings, and attitudes and to understand the goals and procedures of therapy.

2. **Examination and confrontation.** The clinician directs the client in eliminating behaviors associated with stuttering and identifying attitudes and behaviors that facilitate or impede fluency and attempts to strengthen the therapy relationship.

3. **Cognitive and behavioral.** The previous stage is continued with client self-evaluation and self-consequation brought in. The concept of fluency-initiating gestures, or FIGs, is introduced. Any appropriate FIG can be used. Common FIGs are slow rate, easy onset, respiratory modification, loudness and/or pitch variation, light articulation contacts, and altered syllable stress. Attitudes and personal evaluations are still stressed.

4. **Fluency control.** Transfer of FIGs to outside situations is carried out, with continued work on attitudes and feelings.

Cooper provides suggestions for materials and approaches for child or adult applications and estimated (1984, p. 33) that at least 90,000 stutterers have received therapy derived from PFCT guidelines and materials.

THE IMMUTABILITY OF METHODS?

The heading of this section is terminated with a question mark to which the answer is "no". Methods are not immutable. Neither are programs. When starting with the clinical profession, most clinicians appropriately try to duplicate what they are taught in graduate school. They learn rapidly that clients come in all sorts of different packages, and therapy has to be readjusted, revised, or substituted. Clinicians also discover that they have their own strengths, methods of approach, styles of reinforcement, and so on. This suggests that certain programs and procedures within programs will be preferred over others. It also suggests that the programs themselves, or specific procedures, can often be improved by modification to fit individual clinicians and the needs of particular clients. As a generalization, there is no technique that cannot be reshaped, and no sequence that cannot be rearranged, reduced, or augmented. If there has been a fault in our romance with behavior modification techniques of therapy, it has been in the lure to exalt the technique and rigidify it, while the practitioner fades into the background. Readers may have seen program advertisements suggesting that "anybody" can perform the activity advertised as long as they follow the step-by-step instructions, listen to the cassette, watch the videotape, and (in emergencies) use the hotline number. Some zealots have hailed the idea of therapy procedures that are "clinician proof" so that therapy can be rotated among different clinicians without loss to the client. It is almost impossible to respond to such attitudes, since they undercut the basic premise of what therapy is—an interaction between two or more persons in order to effect changes in performance or concept. The techniques are the easy part, usually learned within a short period of time. The interaction, the understanding and evaluating of behavioral parameters, and the ability to decide how and when to react, these comprise the basics of therapy. The reader is encouraged to regard every technique, every procedure, every sequence, and every packaged program as prime candidates for thoughtful, planned modification to secure the desired effects based upon the individual characteristics of each client or client group.

CHAPTER SUMMARY

In the section introduction, the author referred to an initial intention to write a few pages on factors to consider as we move into subsequent chapters on therapy. The reader is now witness to the fact that intentions and realities often fail to coincide. Some of the considerations and controversies discussed apply to every aspect of stuttering therapy, at all ages. Other aspects are quite age related, with reference to the focus of this book. It is hoped that the reader will review this chapter several times and apply its contents to what he or she thinks or knows about therapy of stuttering. We all have a tendency to let authority figures guide us in certain situations, and that is not wrong. As a student, I learned and profited from my authority figures. But ultimately I had to think and reason for myself, by myself. This chapter raises many questions and supplies only a few answers. It will help if the reader will keep these questions in mind and, over the years in this profession, acquire the experience and the new information that will help answer the questions in order to achieve the best outcomes of clinician performance and client results.

CHAPTER SIX
PLANNING THERAPY

OVERVIEW

Planning therapy has developed extensively in recent decades, mainly under impetus of modification and accountability influences. In certain situations, plans are mandated and must follow a specific format, such as with the IEP in school systems. Although lesson plans and reports sometime seem to bury clinicians in neverending paperwork, they have a value in requiring organization and accounting for therapy activities. On the negative side, forms can be restrictive in encouraging the clinician to think only along certain procedural lines that match form structures, and they make it preferable to opt for easily quantified (often trivial) measures. In this brief chapter, attention is directed toward encouraging thought and development in planning, rather than in prescribing a particular form of treatment for a certain set of behaviors. Basically, the chapter suggests certain conditions or behaviors that might be reviewed before planning therapy. These, as much as possible, are suggested in quantifiable forms to allow for baseline and progress measures—even when the quantifications are not count data but numerical-scale expressions of clinical judgments.

TERMS

Planning therapy is taught in all training programs, but terminologies differ. In this chapter use of the word *goals* is restricted to "terminal achievments of therapy," or what therapy is to achieve by the time the client is dismissed. There can be primary and secondary goals, and more than one of each, with the same client. Goals should not be confused with objectives, which are the perfomances required to achieve a goal. An example would be the following:

> GOAL: Fluency of 0.5 or less SW/M
>   Objective: wpm rate of 120, plus or minus 10
>   Objective: prolongation of continuant sounds
>   Objective: easy onset of initial sounds

Other goals can be added, such as stress resistance, language skills improvement, and environmental changes. Each goal should have objectives, and all objectives should have some criterion reference so that pretreatment baselines, therapy progress, and termination points can be marked. The criterion references can be standarized tests, data counts or time measures, percentage levels, judgments expressed against a reference scale, comparisons to a model, charting, and so on. In the example cited adequate reference points and criterion descriptions are lacking. A second example might include references:

> GOAL: Ability to control at least 90 percent of moderate or severe stuttering spasms in all situations below the 90 SUDs level (see Chapter 11).
>   Objective: Acceptable preparatory sets on 50 percent or more of moderate to severe spasms, re SUDs level.
>   Objective: Acceptable pullouts on 90 percent of stuttering spasms that lack (or were failed on) prep sets.
>   Objective: Acceptable cancellations on 95 percent of stuttering spasms on which prep sets and/or pullouts were omitted or failed, re SUDs level.

In this illustration, it is stipulated that "mild" spasms may be missed, but that 90 percent or more of the moderate to severe spasms are to be controlled. The conditions of control and stress levels are stipulated: Any situation below the client's personal SUDs rating of 90 should be characterized by 90 percent control. Objectives are described similarly, with "acceptable" depending on client/clinician definitions, since they would vary from client to client and from clinician to clinician.

Other goals can be added. In the first example, fluency therapy, one could add a goal for stress resistance and develop objectives, or a goal for self-monitoring could be included. In the symptom modification example, a goal of mild spasm control could be added. In each instance, objectives measures are needed. Depending on client characteristics and clinician orientation, one person's objectives can become major goals for another. For instance, rate control is a common objective in therapy as a step toward fluency. Some clients present a significant rate problem, stuttering aside, and rate reduction could be elevated to goal status. However, if rate is varied as a temporary expedient while fluency is established and is to be normalized subsequently, then rate is an objective and not a goal.

Each objective can be broken into steps, levels, or the like. If the objective is cancellation, for example, the possible steps might be these:

1. Ability to stop immediately after 100 percent of severe, 80 percent of moderate, and 40 percent of mild stutterings.
2. Ability to analyze and describe the location and characteristics of each stuttering with accuracy sufficient to allow replication (this can be quantified).
3. Ability to relax tense muscles, establish normal respiration, and pause at least three seconds before continuing.
4. Ability to describe (plan) what must be done in order to eliminate (cancel) the negative behaviors (also can be quantified).

For the rate reduction objective, various wpm steps and phrase-length steps, with appropriate criteria, can be established.

The value of goals-objectives-steps thinking is that it makes us look at the therapy process as a structure built of modular units. There has been (fair) criticism of some symptom and interactive therapy because it was overly wholistic in expressing goals and overly subjective in setting criteria. "Reduce stuttering severity and frequency to levels that are acceptable to the client" is not a bad goal; it is a goal badly stated. Fluency therapy has been (fairly) criticized for sometimes overparticularizing and limiting goal statements and criteria. As the next section considers preparation for therapy planning, one hopes that both extremes can be avoided.

PREPARATION FOR PLANNING

Before goals, objectives, and steps can be articulated and expanded, it is necessary to bring into focus information gathered from diagnosis and assessment activities and other sources. The decision to work on stuttering actually is a decision to provide therapy for a person who stutters. Within the week prior to writing this page, the author evaluated two stutterers: one a 16-year-old female who was about 95 percent successsful in hiding a moderate stuttering but worried about it constantly, and the other, a 9-year-old male who stuttered overtly, was quite hostile to adult authority figures, and used stuttering to manipulate parents and teachers. To say that both "need work on stuttering" is to state the obvious and miss the point. Either client could be fitted into fluency reinforcement, symptom modification, or combined therapy programs. However, placement requires that planning accompany it. The two examples cited are day-and-night comparisons, but minimal differences also require planning. On a hypothetical basis, let us posit two different 9-year-old hostile stutterers:

1. Moderate severity marked by tonoclonic spasms with frequent postponements and starters. Release efforts with timed gestures occur often, and nearly 50 percent of the spasms are marked by revision or retrial efforts.
2. Moderate severity marked by clonic spasms in which he stares fixedly at the auditor. Tends to repeat until he runs out of breath and has to start over. General speech rate seems to be extremely fast.

As an exercise, the reader might want to answer the following questions about these two stutterers:

1. What same or similar procedures might be used for both of them?
2. What would you omit or add for each?
3. In the same or similar procedures you do select, how would you need to vary your approaches?

Answering such questions is important for planning therapy, and before we do either (answer or plan), available information needs to be reviewed.

Organization of Information

In all types of therapy it is common for remediation to be planned along preset lines, ignoring much of what has been gathered during the evaluation process. This is particularly true when package programs are used. To a reasonable degree, therapy does not have to respond to every subtle variation or small datum generated during assessment. There are also the pragmatics of clinician load and time availability, in that reality imposes some constraints on the time that can be spent on planning and the areas that can be covered in therapy. Also, client time, parent availability, teacher access, and other considerations will put constraints on planning. The imperfections of the world apply to therapy as they do to all things. However, there are potential factors that should not apply—ignorance and blind habit. Ignorance involves failing to find out information that is reasonably available, and blind habit is following rigid plans of therapy when information that is present for consideration is ignored.

The information form in this section is offered, not as a form to be filled out, but as a list of key items to consider. Actually filling it out would probably be helpful, but the important idea is that the clinician consider its points before preparing a therapy plan. A decision not to plan for some factor, such as respiration, will eventually be right or wrong; but an overt decision was made, not neglected. Failure to consider the possibility of any need for attention to respiration leaves success or failure or right or wrong totally to chance, and erodes the ethical structure of the clinician. When there are time constraints or other mandates restricting therapy, it is better to make thoughtful decisions about therapy organization rather than "go with the flow" and dust off the most recently used therapy plan and apply it again. Given these considerations, the information form is reviewed here section by section.

Stuttering—specific   The first section provides for core information. *Spasms* cover frequency in SW/M, %SW, or other frequency measures. Also, spasms types and forms, locations, average durations, overt struggle, and other spasm characteristics can be reviewed. *Associated behaviors* concerns the what, when, and where of postponements, starters, substitutions, and other behaviors. The subcategory will contribute to labeling the client as covert or overt in stuttering. *Awareness* involves the client's apparent awareness of stuttering and can have been measured prior to therapy. The measure can be a data count of spasms "caught" and/or a rating scale of the client's ability to describe accurately and consistently the locations and characteristics of each stuttering spasm. *Attitude* refers to the attitude toward stuttering and also to therapy.

Communication—general   The section on general communication does not refer to the behaviors during stuttering, and they may or may not be linked to stuttering spasms. *Voice* and *articulation* refer to the standard possible problems of pitch, quality, phoneme accuracy, and the like. On a nonstandard basis, the author had an adult client who stuttered and also had a very badly repaired palatal cleft with nasality and articulation problems. Since children who stutter often present concomitant problems, this subsection requires careful consideration, particularly in view of the fact that clinicians tend to avoid working with stuttering when possible. The same comments apply to the *language* subsection; if language delays or other problems exist, fluency therapy may profitably incorporate linguistic structure in its design. For all these subsections, therapy of stuttering may result in an improvement in concomitant problems. *Rate* refers to the overall rate of speaking, measured in spm or wpm, with attention to the differences between rate in TTT terms conpared to rate when pause times are subtracted. *Prosody* might indicate problems in stereotypy of utterance, reduction/equalization of syllable stress, distortions of prosodic patterns, and so on. Again, the reference is to overall speech and not to moments of stuttering. *Awareness* in this subsection refers to general self-monitoring and to awareness of others (auditors) in communication. Similarly, *attitude* concerns attitudes toward communication in general, and self-confidence as a speaker. Measures such as the Erickson scale could be

INFORMATION FOR THERAPY PLANNING

In each category below, summarize information that might be relevant to planning therapy. Within each subcategory, when feasible, provide a description or quantification that can serve as a pretreatment baseline. Use the following items as keys to take notes, not as an outline to fill.

STUTTERING—SPECIFIC
Spasm:
Associated Behaviors:
Awareness:
Attitude:

COMMUNICATION—GENERAL
Voice:
Articulation:
Language:
Rate:
Prosody:
Awareness:
Attitude:

RELAXATION/TENSION
During stuttering:
During speech:
In general:

RESPIRATION
General:
Speech:
Stuttering:

STRESS RESPONSE
Interruption:
Correction:
Disagreement:
Situational:
Person:
Other:

ENVIRONMENT
Home:
School:
Persons:
Other:

FOUNDATION SKILLS
Attending:
Auditory Processing:
Neuromotor:
Other:

OTHER FACTORS
Availability:
Coexisting problems:
Other:

used. Motivation to improve speech can be a consideration in this subsection.

Relaxation/tension   The factor of relaxation/tension receives separate consideration because therapy can be concerned primarily with relaxation and will almost always stress it to some degree in various objectives of the steps in the therapy process. The three subsections divide tension into *stuttering, general speech,* and *overall.* Measures almost always will be subjective, although instrument ratings can be used if they are available.

Respiration   As in the previous section, respiration problems may occur in *general* when the overall pattern is deficient or abnormal. This is most likely where concomitants involve significant neuromotor problems. Speech respiration may represent abnormal autonomic function or be related to the stuttering itself. Respiration during stuttering can involve a variety of inadequacies, and the clinician may debate whether reduction of spasms will correct the problem or problems or whether separate attention is required. Measures can be quantitative in terms of volume, duration, or timing; they can also be rated subjectively.

Stress response   The category of stress response provides for consideration of the child's reaction to stress, which can come in various forms and be quite individual. *Interruption* refers to any occurrence that interrupts the child's ongoing speech, whether it is other speech, noise, or visual distraction. *Correction* is supplied as a specific subcategory, since children so often experience this type of stress. And *other* suggests that individuals have particular or unique susceptibilities to perceived stress. Measurement will typically be subjective, although count data of specific behaviors can be used as indicators of stress.

Environment   The child's environment covers areas that generally are not measurable in conventional terms. Each subcategory here would involve estimation of significance in therapy and determining whether special planning will be necessary. *Home* should cover the importance factor, need for manipulation and counseling, and the availability or accessibility of the family. *School* follows a similar pattern and can include peer, teacher, and learning problems. *Persons* can be individuals who appear to be significant contributors to fluency or dysfluency and/or can be significant contributors to the therapy process (these usually overlap with the previous areas).

Foundation skills   When working with children it is particularly important to respond to factors that may affect therapy or the child's responses to it. In the evaluation chapter, certain factors were considered and are identified here. *Attending* can be measured in seconds or in number of words or commands. Similarly, *auditory process* aspects can be expressed by test scores or in responses to selected stimuli. *Neuromotor* coordination can be measured in diadochokinetic rates or other specific counts and also described or rated in more subjective terms. These and other considerations (low frustration tolerance, hyperactivity, and so on) can be stated as separate goals that precede speech therapy or as parallel goals that are interwoven with overall therapy.

Other factors Only two other factors are suggested in the form. *Availability* will affect the intensity and frequency of therapy, time of day for scheduling, and so on. *Coexisting problems* overlaps some subcategories cited previously but actually refers to more distinct or separate problems such as retardation, special learning disabilities, and dyslexia. These problems can have their own characteristics that affect therapy, require therapy or special services from other professionals, or involve (for school children) a team approach to IEP preparation.

Summary

As stated previously, the purpose of this section is not to add to the paper load of clinicians. However, consideration of the various areas cited will help the clinician in planning therapy on an individual basis. In the next section, the planning and selection process is explored.

THERAPY PLANNING WORKSHEET

The process of planning therapy requires the mixing and adjustment of a number of factors: clinician and client time, clinician skills and resources, stuttering syndrome characteristics, relevant other conditions in the client, and factors in the environment. There can be a tendency to provide therapy by prescriptive criteria. There can also be a tendency to allow technique utilization to replace program planning, a confusion that undercuts real therapy (Conture 1982). These problems are aggravated by large caseloads, diminished availability of time, paper demands, and uncertainty about therapy needs. The previous section on client analysis will provide the clinician with an array of measures and judgments to consider. This section is intended to provide assistance to the clinician in several ways. First, a variety of clinical approaches and procedures is laid out for consideration. A STATUS column is provided so that each general approach or specific procedure can be rated in terms of its use significance in the therapy program. A *0 to 4* scale is suggested, with zero indicating nonuse and 4 indicating major use in the therapy program. Clini-

THERAPY PLANNING WORKSHEET

Client: _____ Age: ____ Sex: ____ Date: _____

For each item in the CONSIDERATION column, enter 0, 1, 2, 3, or 4 in the STATUS column. Zero indicates the approach will not be used, or at least not planned for. A 4 indicates an item would be a major focus in therapy, or at some point in therapy. Under COMMENTS, enter any explanations or special considerations.

CONSIDERATIONS	STATUS	COMMENTS
Frequency of Therapy		
Intensive		
Nonintensive		
Group/Individual		
Individual only		
Group only		
Group and Individual		
Support group		
Interactive Emphasis		
Avoidance Reduction		
Monitoring Skills		
Environment		
Parent group		
General		
Specific		
Teachers, etc.		
Rate/Duration		
Rate control		
Prolongation		
Continuous voice		
Other		
Rhythm/Timing		
Metronome		
Syllable timed		
Other		
Breathstream		
Specific errors		
Easy onset		
Airflow program		
Other		
Symptom Modification		
Assoc. behaviors		
Pseudostuttering		

CONSIDERATIONS	STATUS	COMMENTS
Cancellation		
Pullout		
Preparatory set		
Other		
General Speech		
Voice/resonance		
Articulation		
Prosody		
Other		
Motivation		
Information about stuttering		
Response Enhancement		
Attending		
Perception/processing		
Motor skills		
Self-Analysis		
General speech		
Dysfluencies		
Attitudes		
Relaxation		
Specific, focal		
General, total		
Desensitization		
To stuttering		
To situations		
To disruptors		
Language		
Improvement		
Simplification		
Transfer		
Spontaneous		
Step-by-step		
Other		
Other Factors		

cians can apply their own criteria to the five-point scale or form their own system of use indicators. The COMMENTS column provides space for the clinician to indicate variations planned in timing of initiation or termination points, special precautions or criteria, and so on. Blank spaces are provided within and at the end of the worksheet for individual considerations not covered by the outline. These added considerations might include the following:

1. Additional procedures such as breath chewing, chunking, and negative practice.
2. Preexisting or coexisting factors involving the client and/or the family. These might include child psychotherapy, marital counseling, medical regimens, or client therapy for other problems.
3. Selection of specific stutter therapy programs in commercial or published formats (see next paragraph).
4. Remeasurement dates or time intervals when progress is to be evaluated and compared against baselines.
5. Key significant others, in addition to parents, who may interact with therapy.

Other considerations can be added according to the needs of clinicians. When existing package programs are utilized, the author has an urgent recommendation: Fill out the planning worksheet, or an equivalent, and then review the intended program carefully to determine whether it fulfills the projected therapy needs. When the program omits or underemphasizes desired areas, these can be fitted appropriately into the overall program. Occasionally analysis will lead to the conclusion that a particular package program is inadequate in this particular instance, and another program (or the clinician's own planning) should be substituted.

The following comments on the therapy planning worksheet are intended to suggest how considerations might be utilized. These are suggestions, not prescriptions, and other interpretations/applications are encouraged.

Frequency: Subject to local conditions, the clinician may elect one or the other of the options or start intensive and then step down to maintenance, and so on. Nonintensive schedules can vary also.

Group/Individual: May involve stutterers only, other types of speech problems, parent-child interaction therapy, and so on. Schedule may start as individual and shift to group or to a mix. *Support group* implies that group therapy will be used only in the maintenance stage, unless Status entries indicate differently.

Interactive Emphasis: Provides clinician the opportunity to indicate how much rapport, counseling, or psychosocial factors will be stressed.

Avoidance Reduction: Can be the primary therapy goal, overlapping desensitization (see later), can be an aspect of several other therapy modes, or may not be targeted.

Monitoring Skills: Overlaps, in part, with self-analysis (see later). To what degree will self-monitoring, particularly for maintenance, be stressed?

Environment: Questions whether general parent counseling is to be used, or whether conditions require a separate but integrated plan to alter environmental conditions. For Group II children, school environment can also receive attention.

Motivation: Motivation, per se, may be a problem with Group III children; task motivation can be more frequent with children in Group I.

Information: Information about stuttering may be zero for young children but become significant as they mature.

Response Enhancement: These are more or less pretherapy factors to be corrected or compensated for, factors to be worked with as a part of overall therapy, or factors that therapy must compensate for and adjust to.

Self-Analysis: Will vary in significance from zero to 4 and may shift in value during therapy.

Relaxation: May be a total-focus program of therapy, may be limited to five minutes at each session, or may not be used at all. *Specific relaxation* refers to efforts to secure relaxation in areas of the speech mechanism, rather than total.

Desensitization: Can be aimed only at moments of stuttering, to specific disruptors, or to general situation sensitivity. Practice in reciprocal inhibition can be planned. Construction and use of a fear hierarchy ranking system can be developed.

Language: Particularly with Group I and some Group II children, there may be need to compensate for language delay or specific problems. *Simplification* refers to either a major use of procedures such as ELU or GILCU as a therapy mode or to remind the clinician to use progressive language complexity in other procedures when appropriate.

Rate/Duration: This overlaps with several other procedure areas, and they each have a "blank" category for inserted procedures. *Rate control* could be DAF, modeled speech, choral speech, shadowing, and so forth. *Prolongation* and *continuous voice* are defined in Chapter 12.

Rhythm/Timing: Overlaps with previous category. Can also include other prosody-based procedures.

Breathstream: *Specific errors* refers to, for example, strong exhalation before utterance and gasping speech. *Easy onset* is discussed in Chapter 13, and several *airflow programs* have been published. Also, a clinician can target revision of the overall postural and respiratory support system.

Symptom Modification: Motivation, self-analysis, and desensitization have been covered in other sections. *Associated behaviors* refers to reduction/elimination of specific behaviors such as postponements and starters. The other procedures are discussed in Chapter 14. As with other procedures, symptom modification can be used as a primary therapy program or, in parts, with other elements.

General Speech: Refers to improvement of coexisting problems in speech production and/ or to problems uncovered or caused (too-slow rate, prosody lacks) by therapy.

Transfer: Is transfer expected to be nearly spontaneous? Will some routine attention be required, or will careful planning be needed to secure and stabilize transfer?

Other: Considerations included by nature of the therapy program, client concomitant needs, or other special factors.

It is, of course, not necessary to fill out any worksheet. However, reviewing such a list is often valuable. The planning sheet can be expanded by putting more than one column in each category, so that blanks remain after initial planning is completed. This encourages the clinician to reevaluate therapy planning at time points in therapy and changing the therapy plan in accordance with variations among clients. It should be emphasized that to the maximum extent feasible, the clinician will want to involve the client in planning. Involvement and input at low levels of Group I may be slight and superficial but can foster a feeling of participation. As age increases, therapy planning can easily become therapy "negotiation," where client and clinician review alternatives, requirements, desired outcomes, and so forth, and the client and clinician finally agree on a mutual commitment to a particular therapy plan. We are reminded of things we otherwise might not plan for or consider, and we are cautioned against slipping into therapy automatisms at busy times. There are occasions when such a worksheet may help clinicians whose employer requires specific forms to be filled out, filed, and accounted for. The IEP is an example of such a need.

INDIVIDUAL EDUCATION PROGRAM

The IEP, according to Garbee (1985), has a variety of purposes or functions. These can include, but not be limited to, parent-school communication, resolution of differences between parent and school, formalization of resource commitment to the child, function as a management tool to cover all needs in the school setting, function as a compliance/monitoring document to determine if formal commitments are being met, and as a reference for evaluation of client progress (p.86). Garbee provides useful definitions of all IEP elements and discussion of applications. Work (1985) states that the clinician must decide what goals are to be achieved and how these goals are to be achieved. The latter involves

> the selection of objectives that specify a terminal behavior, define the conditions under which the behavior is to occur, and describe the criteria for acceptable performance of the behavior. The inclusion of procedures, content, and methods that are relevant to the objective further defines the process. (p.308)

Neidecker (1987) also provides useful discussion of the IEP and constructs a sample program to illustrate the process. Other publications have been generated through the American Speech, Language, and Hearing Association and provide additional information. It should be pointed out that IEPs and similar documents can be psychologically coercive so that the clinician swings to basic, often trivial, measures which are reflected in the goals and procedures. Accountability documents should not block statement of subjective goals or use of quantified judgments in reporting results.

CHAPTER SUMMARY

This chapter has been kept short as an expression that therapy planning is vitally important, but not to be spelled out in formulas and rigid forms. Many pages could be added to expand on possible variations in the areas suggested. The variations would be extensive, since we are considering clients ranging from the age of total dependence to those actively in the process of stepping into the adult world of independence. Adding dimensions of developmental stages, educational concerns, concomitant problems, and the like, provides the clinician with many things to consider. For these reasons the author chose to avoid a voluminous planning form and, instead, selected a reminder format. Similar variety obtains when we look at therapy options; the approach here is also to review options rather than to make recommendations. If goals and objectives are clearly articulated, information reviewed, and pretreatment measures or judgments laid out, then the structure of therapy, or the options, will tend to be self-generating and lead the clinician to the most appropriate mix of therapy choices.

In the chapters following, a number of therapy procedures and methods are reviewed. It is assumed that the clinician will not ricochet from one technique to the next but will build on this present chapter to construct a program of therapy or to modify a preexisting program. Flexibility and adaptation are frequently emphasized, but always within a frame of reference to evaluation and preplanning.

CHAPTER SEVEN
LANGUAGE
AND THERAPY
OF STUTTERING

OVERVIEW

In Chapter 2, the question of linguistic factors in fluency development and stuttering was discussed. The reader might want to review that discussion because only a brief summary is presented here.

Research has suggested that some stuttering children are significantly delayed in language (Kline & Starkweather 1979; Johnston & Schery 1976), that some may or may not be slower in reading development (Schindler 1955, affirmative; Conture & Naersson 1977, negative), and that some are more likely to present langauge and/or speech problems than are nonstutterers (Blood & Seider 1981; Conture 1982; Riley & Riley 1983). More specific suggestions have included those that stuttering children may be deficient in the use of grammatical morphemes and in areas such as word retrieval, frequency of shorter sentences, occurrence of fragmentary sentences, transpositions, word reversals, and simplification of utterances (Riley & Riley 1983, 1980, 1979).

We have also tried to investigate the factors that may be associated with language dimensions and dysfluency. Wall, Starkweather, and Cairns (1981) and Bernstein (1981) have reported that stuttering is more likely to occur at clause boundary word positions than at other locations. Stutter-

148

ing is more probable on conjunctions and pronouns than on nouns (Bloodstein and Gantwerk 1967). Danzger and Halpern (1973) found that more stuttering occurred on longer words and on words with lower frequency of use occurrence. Level of abstraction and grammatical function did not relate to stuttering frequency. Many other studies could be cited, but there is no need to overstress the point that some clincians lean strongly toward a functioning linguistic basis in stuttering.

Wall and Myers (1984) present an excellent summary of linguistic theory and knowledge, noting that before the time of Chomsky our interest was focused mainly on articulation, vocabulary, and certain linguistic areas. Chomsky, in reaction to what he felt was B.F. Skinner's too-simple view of language development, brought in the factors of affective and cognitive functions. Since then our profession has incorporated consideration of cognition, semantics, and situational pragmatics and has emphasized evaluation from a low-structure orientation with increased structure developed as our knowledge allows and needs require. Wall and Myers also discuss the significant development in psycholinguistics—that we compare disordered language (or fluency) to the developmental patterns of linguistically normal peers, rather than taking adult language as the normative model. As we have moved through these developments, we have been able to evolve therapy approaches that allow for and/or use linguistic development factors.

Not all researcher-clinicians have been positive in either the theoretical significance of language in stuttering origin and development or the necessity for or value of linguistic elements in therapy management. Hood (1973) suggests caution in drawing conclusions about disfluency and language, noting that the "potential relationships . . . are neither complete nor conclusive" (p. 545) in terms of our knowledge. Haynes and Hood (1977) investigated language and fluency in children who were four, six, and eight years of age. They reported that lingustic ability and age were positively correlated, as expected, and disfluency and age were inversely related, also as expected. They found no meaningful correlation between language and fluency variables and noted that the highest-disfluency children and the lowest-disfluency children had developmental sentence scores that differed by only 0.38 (10.9 and 10.52). Costello (1983) reviews a number of research studies wherein it is suggested that children who stutter have more trouble on longer utterances, at clause junctions, and so on. She raises the question of whether stutterers have an essential problem in planning linguistic strings or one of motoric planning for a succession of phonemic formations and transitions. In writing about language disorders and stuttering, she states that her evaluation of research "leads me to believe there exists no functional relationship between these two dimensions. Therefore, designing treatment with a language component additive would be low priority for any treatment" (p. 88). Costello has advocated that therapy should begin with emphasis on operant conditioning procedures and on bypass procedures such as relaxation, easy onset, and language simplification. Fluency should receive positive reinforcement, while dysfluency should be punished. Only if these methods fail to produce results should the clinician utilize ancillary therapy procedures, using pretherapy assessment information and in-therapy observations to determine what additional methods to use. Costello has some logic in her argument, but the author prefers to see a careful evaluation and planning procedure, as described in the previous chapter, rather than blindly starting every client with the same form of therapy.

Part of the complication in determining the significance or appropriateness of language elements in therapy has been the development of different forms of language and stuttering therapy. One of the major differences has been the contrast between low-structure and high-structure linguistic approaches to therapy. Language therapy can be administered in a high-structure or low-structure approach. In the high-structure approach, stimuli and responses are carefully controlled, reinforcements operate by schedule, and results can be measured constantly for comparison to baseline averages and/or to criterion points for success and advancement. Low-structure approaches include aspects of affect, cognitive capacity, semantic content, and situation pragmatics; they may or may not include fluency-enhancing variables. Guitar (1984) has stated that while psycholinguistic (low-structure) approaches may produce results pleasing to the "research-minded clinician," they "may be dismayed at the difficulty of knowing which variables are related to success with which children" (p. 303). He has recommended controlled comparisons, stating that the theoretical and treatment values of language variables cannot be sorted out "from the psychological counseling and motor learning treatments that are occurring concurrently" (p. 303). Wall and Myers (1984) and Riley and Riley (1983) and Nelson (1986) are notable examples of the combined linguistic approaches to stuttering therapy. Although other clinicians have established low-therapy treatments, these three present particularly thorough and clear descriptions that clinicians might find useful.

It appears that the significance of language in the development of stuttering, and the application of therapy, requires more information and further evaluation. Absolutes in either direction should be avoided. It seems feasible to suggest that some stutterers will have a significant problem in language maturity. Also, some stutterers, at least, will benefit from therapy presented in a linguistic context that simplifies both the language formulation and motoric planning requirements for communication. Many therapies deal with communication pragmatics at some stage of therapy, at least by the time maintenance steps have been reached. However, the overall rationale for, and the form of, a language-based therapy program for stuttering awaits development.

THERAPY EFFECTS

In previous discussions, reference has been made to the possibility that clinicians increased their own disfluencies as they worked with stutterers (Kimbarrow & Daly 1980). Several times references have been made to the old, and largely defunct, idea that children should not receive therapy because it might exacerbate their fluency problems. Another area of question has been whether or not therapy for language-delay problems has any relationship to the fluency of these children. Hall (1977) discusses the possibility that children receiving articulation or language therapy may show sudden increases in their disfluencies, and he describes two such cases. In another study Merits-Patterson and Reed (1981) investigated 37 preschool children, of whom 9 were normal, 9 were language delayed, and 9 were language delayed and receiving therapy. The researchers evaluated disfluencies among the three groups and reported the following:

GROUP	DISFLUENCIES PER 500 WORDS	
	RANGE	MEAN
Normal language	7–37	16.8
Delayed, nontherapy	6–43	15.43
Delayed, therapy	8–66	32.8

They also reported that the therapy-group children exhibited more PWR disfluencies than did the other two groups. One must be extremely cautious in interpreting such results. For elements of the children, the effects of therapy, the effects of the clinician, and other factors must be considered. These concerns are presented here (and the author has seen such occurrences) because one must consider what is the best therapy approach when a stuttering child is known to have a significant problem in language function. Conture (1982) suggests that with such children the priority should be language therapy (as opposed to fluency concerns), unless there are frequent prolongations combined with overt physical struggle and psychological reactions to stuttering.

The possible confusions that might arise in a therapy caseload are these:

1. Language-delayed children who were acceptably fluent but, as they progress in language therapy, find that their cognitive language formulation outstrips the motoric planning and timing capacity. Disfluencies may result.
2. Language-delayed children who also stutter may present a conflict as to which therapy should predominate, or whether a combination therapy is indicated.
3. Some stuttering children may seem to benefit particularly from linguistic simplification in therapy. Such simplification has been used for centuries but can be organized now to a high degree of structure.

There is no set answer to the confusion areas. Clinicians will need to re-spond on a case-by-case basis and avoid adopting a rigid policy in one di-rection or the other.

Age Factor

It is generally accepted that language problems are associated with childhood, although research suggests some differences or impoverish-ments among adult stutterers. Thus, relative to age, most of this chapter will be aimed at the Group I and Group II (ages three to ten) discussed in Chapter 5. However, it would be erroneous to assume that adolescents may not present residual language problems that could benefit from at-tention and possibly could reinforce the linguistic elements of fluency skills. All ages can be candidates for fluency therapy that is developed on the basis of linguistic length and complexity factors.

Concomitant Factors

Previous reference has been made to the fact that children who stut-ter also have an atypically (compared to the general population) high prevalence of language, articulation, voice, and other problems. It was suggested that where the concomitant problem was linguistic, therapy might be targeted there first—as long as the dysfluencies were not too ad-vanced in tension, struggle, and awareness reactions. Also, a caution was suggested in the possibility that language therapy might enhance linguis-tic skills for which motor sequencing and timing capabilities were weak. The writer would emphasize this particularly (imbalance between linguis-tic and motor skills) where Group I preschool children are involved. Where articulation or phonation problems are present, it is often sug-gested that they be dealt with after therapy of stuttering or phased in dur-ing the later stages of therapy. The subjective rationale for this is that fo-cusing attention on single words and sounds, or on phonation, may not be productive because it may increase the child's convictions that "things are hard to say." The result will be to exacerbate tension and struggle. These are unverified assumptions (to the author's knowledge), but they appear to have value, especially since it has been suggested that many clinicians shy away from stuttering and work with other problems first (Blood & Seider 1981). In the next section we consider several problem areas that, if present, should probably receive attention before the dysfluencies are dealt with.

Procedure versus Program

As noted before, this book does not present programs of therapy for young stutterers. However, in several places reference has been made to sources where complete programs are presented. In a later section there is a detailed presentation of a procedure involving progressive increments in utterance length and complexity. Here, and at that point also, it should be emphasized that a procedure, even a complex one, is not a program, for programs encompass a wider range of variables than do procedures, and programs require more than just following the steps or levels of a described procedure.

PRECURSORS TO THERAPY OF STUTTERING

Before one can build a house, there must be a foundation, since without a foundation the structure will sag, sink, crack, or fall. This analogy also applies to therapy: Before therapy can develop as it should, certain basic capacities, skills, or conditions must be present. It is possible to list a large number of factors, but they will be limited here to five. The first two are the following:

1. Environmental conditions that reject therapy and/or constitute a significant portion of the stuttering problem. This will be dealt with here and in the next chapter.
2. Motivation of the child to accept therapy and work on his or her fluency problems. This will be discussed in Chapter 9.

The remaining three precursors apply to other therapy procedures but receive attention here:

3. Attending capacities.
4. Auditory processing capacities.
5. Neuromotor coordination and timing capacities.

Attending Capacities

Cognitive function, and therefore linguistic development, requires sufficient attention to input stimuli. If this is lacking, then acquisition and internalization may be prevented, or be distorted, or be incomplete. It is probable that some percentage of children who stutter, especially those in the Group I age range, may present problems in attending to stimuli long enough to respond adequately and learn from them. Distractibility presumably relates to failure of the reticular activating and inhibiting systems to "tune" the appropriate sensory receptive system or systems and to sensitize or damp appropriate areas of the cerebral cortex and the associated subcortical systems. Distractible children are a clinician's bane. Wells (1987) suggests that attending disorders be worked on directly through improving eye contact, increasing attention span, and reducing occurrences of impulsive behavior. Riley and Riley (1984, 1979) also state that attending problems must be addressed before other treatment procedures can produce effective results. They provide a 13-step program, starting with a one-second attention span and increasing to eight seconds, in steps. Each step requires three correct responses before progression to the next step. Step 5 drops back to one second as a visual distraction is introduced during clinician utterance of an auditory command. Four steps take the child to eight seconds of attention (same criterion each step). In step 9 the child must perform some task for two seconds during introduction of a visual distractor. Successive steps require attention spans of eight seconds, and of one, two, and three minutes duration. Reinforcement is 100 percent during initial steps and then phased down to a ratio of 1:3. Riley and Riley suggest that where attending behavior is a major problem, the parents may need to consult their physician for medication to control the distractibility.

Clinicians can devise attending sequences of their own, working to increase both duration and resistance to distraction or disruption. Among Group I and Group II children, relaxation activities and monitoring practice efforts may also help increase attending capacities.

Auditory Processing

Research has suggested that stutterers may be less adequate than usual in auditory memory (Williams & Marks 1972) and auditory recall (Stocker & Parker 1977). They may present differences in dichotic listening preferences and in performance of dichotic listening tasks (Sommers, Brady & Moore 1975; Curry & Gregory 1969). It has also been reported that stutterers may have problems with auditory sequential memory (Wells 1987) and generally have less phonetic "sound-mindedness" (Wingate 1971a; Perozzi 1970). Riley (1980) reported that auditory memory sound blending and auditory dispersion contributed to factor discrimination of auditory perception problems among 76 children who stuttered. Earlier reference, in discussions of theory, has been made to these and other studies.

Most clinicians are familiar with procedures for improving auditory processing skills, and there have been numerous procedures published for children and for use with dysphasics. Several suggestions are offered here:

1. Allow only correct responses to questions or commands. At first permit self-correction by the child, but progress to where only one response is allowed and only correct responses receive positive reinforcement.
2. In various tasks or commands, use additional cues as needed to secure correct responses, but reduce these to minimal levels in order to force reliance on auditory systems and on their own recall and retrieval systems.
3. Practice the client learning new words, replacing incorrect labels with correct items, and so on. Be sure that words are appropriate for the child's environment and level of sophistication.

4. Give commands to the child, progressing in the number of different things commanded and/or the complexity of the command. At first allow more than one utterance of the command and provide extra cues if needed. As in 2, phase down utterances and cues.

5. Play in cumulative order word games such as "I am going on a trip and I am taking a . . ." or progressively think of words of a particular class or that start with a certain letter or are incomplete sentences for the child to finish, and so on. Older children may enjoy more sophisticated versions.

Neuromotor Function

The evaluation chapters have discussed neuromotor function and problems. That section, and part of theory discussion, has contended that a certain percentage of stutterers will present problems in the initiation, coordination, timing, and integration of motor movements. Indeed, the popular rate control, airflow, and shaping therapies today have the major effect of simplifying and slowing demands on the client's neuromotor system. Other procedures, such as some rhythm methods (Wohl 1970, 1968), also have their effects on neuromotor function. As with auditory processing problems, there is a wealth of material the clinician can use in therapy with vocal tract neuromotor functions. One can draw upon the motokinesthetic methods of Young (1965), sensorimotor therapy of McDonald (1964), aspects of Frick's (1965) motor-planning therapy techniques, chewing therapy (Froeschels 1952b), and various therapy sources that deal with dysarthric and dyspraxic speech (Brown 1985; Johns 1978; Darley, Aronson & Brown 1975).

As part of their carefully evaluated population of stuttering children, Riley and Riley (1984) identified an oral motor discoordination (OMD) subgroup and developed procedures to prepare these children for fluency therapy. They utilize their modified version of McDonald's (1964) sensory-motor approach to articulation disorders when this is needed for children who stutter. In such instances they noted that the average therapy time required was slightly over 14 hours (range 6–22 hours). They start with slow and accurate production of single syllables, working up to bisyllabic and trisyllabic productions. Production of syllable sets is controlled for five factors: number of syllables per set, number of different vowels and of different consonants, number of unvoiced consonants, and number of consonants between vowels. Four production levels are used, and the first level starts with monosyllable combinations of voiced consonants *b, d, g, m, n, v*, with the vowels *i, æ, ʌ, a, ou*, and *u*. After monosyllables, the child moves to two-syllable and then to three-syllable sets. Production starts at any rate where accuracy can be obtained and then is increased to a point where ten productions of each set occur within a certain time frame, with 90 percent accuracy in each of three consecutive efforts. The time frame is a product of Fletcher's (1972) research on diadochokinesis and the Rileys' extrapolations of his data, plus application of their own clinical experience. This table, with parameters for levels of problem severity is presented on pages 138–39 of the Rileys' chapter (Riley & Riley 1984). In a gross summary this writer would offer the following as time targets (in seconds) for ten production efforts:

> **Monosyllables**—two to three seconds, with three years at the high end and eight years at the low time figure.
> **Bisyllables**—four to six seconds, with the same age range as cited above.
> **Trisyllables**—eight to ten seconds, with no time frame for three–five years of age, ten seconds at six and seven years, and eight seconds at eight years.

The second level of the Rileys' program introduces unvoiced consonants (*p, t, k, f*), again moving through monosyllabic, bisyllabic, and trisyllabic sets. At the next level, two or three unvoiced consonants per syllable set are used in bisyllabic and then in trisyllabic sets (*t∧, t∧, t∧, b∧, p∧*). Examples could be *d∧pd∧pd∧p* at one syllable and *gupdip* at two syllables. The Rileys recommend overlearning and note that young children probably will not reach the fourth level. Frustration levels will need to be monitored, and it may be necessary to break some of the steps into substeps in order to control difficulty and reach performance targets.

The clinician will be wise to specify clearly the targets of any neuromotor therapies, establishing baseline performance levels and measuring responses consistently. Clients should have home assignment practice, usually several times daily for short periods. When parents can be involved in therapy, it is generally useful to bring them in at appropriate points, teach them the same exercises their child is practicing, and include child and parents in at least some of the outside assignments. This will aid outside transfer, improve parents' monitoring referents and skills, and possibly influence favorably the speech patterns of the parents (as well as those of the child).

Environmental Considerations

Most of the concerns about and approaches to the child's environment are discussed in Chapter 8. However, there may be specific language concerns that need attention here. Also, if therapy is emphasizing a linguistic approach, then the clinician may target or try to develop certain language behaviors in the home. It is possible that the child may have a poor language environment because the parents and the family members tend to be nontalkative, because there are few books or other sources of language stimulus, because the child is in a daycare setting with younger children, and so on. It is possible that the environment will be more actively negative in that speech rates are rapid, interruptions are frequent, language level is high, speakers are argumentative, or communication is competitive. Any of these, or others, individually or in combination may complicate therapy efforts.

As noted, although environmental manipulation is discussed in the next chapter, several suggestions relative to environmental language factors can be made at this point:

1. Adults, realistically, cannot be changed in their permanent language habits (at least, not easily). However, some "family rules" can be made and put on the refrigerator door or otherwise advocated:
   a. Speak slowly enough for the listener to comprehend.
   b. Use words the listener can understand.
   c. Notice whether the listener wants to respond.
2. Provide the child time to respond, invite responses, try not to interrupt during their pauses.
3. Adjust questions, descriptions, and commands so they match the child's capacities. If the child is receiving special therapy for auditory processing problems, work to control more thoroughly these factors.
4. Do not penalize, criticize, or correct the child's efforts, except when the clinician has established rules and procedures.
5. Be an approving, reinforcing listener in order to stimulate language activity by the child.

On some occasions the clinician will need to counsel parents about children who use stuttering for their own manipulation of the environment. Such children can become "language tyrants" if those concerned are not observant and appropriately responsive.

APPROACHES TO LINGUISTIC THERAPY

Background

There are many linguistic approaches to therapy of stuttering. General language therapy may involve vocabulary development, syntax use and comprehension, phonological skills, and pragmatic and social skills (Wells 1987). Culp (1984) describes a thorough approach to preschool fluency programs. She notes that children may need to develop listening skills. Desensitization and fluency establishment (choral speaking) are achieved. A language hierarchy is followed, moving from familiar themes to other subjects, introduction of opposites, parts of the whole concepts, associations, and sequencing. Function modes include monologue, dialogue, retelling, play, and clinician pressure. Gregory and Hill (1984) have described a complex program, including linguistic factors (they are cited again in the next subsection). The complete and complex program sources have been identified earlier, with particular mention being made of low-structure programs where a wider range of concerns and greater flexibility can be stressed. Most of these variables are addressed in the procedure chapters, so that attention here focuses on procedures that have a high-structure character and concentrate on the length of utterance and the complexity of the response.

Progressive Communication Demand

Long before linguistic research acquired its label, clinicians were aware that shorter sentences, simpler or more familiar utterances, predictable responses, and responses during conditions of lower stress were more likely to be fluent than if any of the foregoing were reversed. Such simplification or positivism reinforces fluency and facilitates the acquisition of other control methods being learned (Adams 1980). This is true whether the method is fluency enhancement or symptom modification. Such progressive developments of linguistic demand are common. Wells (1987) provides suggestions for organizing demand levels. Gregory and Hill (1984), as part of their overall complex program, describe therapy that starts with one-word responses, with a 90 percent fluency criterion over 20 trials in two consecutive sessions. Clinician models include direct, delayed, intervening, incomplete, question, and no-model forms. Home assignment practice is utilized and transfer worked on. Movement to longer client responses is developed in steps, dropping back temporarily in modes when new topics or variables suggest easing the communication load. The Stocker Probe (Stocker 1980: Stocker & Gerstman 1983) has been described previously. Designed originally as an evaluation, it was developed to provide a fluency-shaping tool. Five levels of communicative responsibility are identified: either/or questions, simple /wh/ questions, more creative /wh/ questions, "tell me about" questions, and having the child make up stories. Therapy is to start at the level below which the child displayed stuttering behaviors, dropping back whenever necessary. Appropriate reinforcement protocols are designed, and the clinician may work on parent counseling, client awareness, struggle and associated behaviors, or other factors needing attention.

A frequent mode of reference to progressive increments in linguistic demands has been extended length of utterance, or ELU. This label is somewhat misleading, since it is difficult to increase length (even in nonsense strings) without increasing complexity. Also, factors of semantic content and pragmatics tend to become involved. Nevertheless, ELU has been used frequently. Another label, similarly used, has been gradual increase in length and complexity of utterance, or GILCU, associated with Ryan's therapy writing (1974). The ELU label is more generally attributed, but it has been associated particularly with Costello (1980). In both approaches, the client begins at simple demand levels (usually single words) and progresses to conversational speech. Brundage and Ratner

(1987) have stated that morpheme, rather than syllable or word, length of an utterance is a better indicator of stuttering probabilities. Therefore, they have questioned programs such as GILCU and ELU that build primarily on word length and number.

Shames and Egolf provide an **ELU** sample (1976) of 13 steps (p. 57), starting with clinician/client utterances of single words. When five consecutive productions are fluent, the next step is solo two-word utterances, and so on. The penultimate task is 40 minutes of fluent speech, with fluency defined as no more than 1.0 SW/M. Shames and Egolf note that many would find the program "boring and repetitious." The final step is clinician observation of three outside situations (unspecified) in which no more than 1%SW occurs. If this target is met, the clinician is to "discharge the stutterer from therapy with your best wishes." In view of the authors' rejection of modification therapy because it asks the stutterer to accept stuttering and learn to live with it, and their stated goal of "speech that is free from stuttering" (p. 32), the reader may well be puzzled by this dismissal criterion and wonder where the "stutter-free" speech went, and what about the client having to accept stuttering and learning to live with it. One also might wish to speculate about the need for a maintenance program.

GILCU (Ryan 1974) involves increasing length and complexity of responses across oral reading, monologue, and conversation. The client first must establish basal fluency, with "slow and easy" speech; then he or she must move to a reading list of monosyllabic words. Progression continues, meeting the criterion fluency level at each step as word lengths are increased, up to six-word responses. Two-sentence, three-sentence, and four-sentence sequences follow; after that response is measured in time duration rather than number of words. When the eighteenth step (five minutes of reading) is reached, therapy cycles back to single-word utterances and progresses through 17 steps. At this point, recycling drops back again for progression leading to conversational activities. Ryan and Ryan (1983) reported on the use of GILCU, programmed symptom therapy, DAF, and pause therapy, with eight elementary and eight high school children. The 16 clients were divided into four groups of four, with two elementary and two high school students in each group. Each set of four was served by two clinicians, each clinician working with two clients. Each clinician was trained to administer one of the four programs cited. Criterion measures were SW/M and a rate measure in wpm. Ryan reported that GILCU produced the best overall results and the most effective transfer. However, all four programs were judged to be effective.

The ELU and GILCU programs just described, and Systematic Fluency Training for Young Children (Shine 1980a, 1980b), and a number of other programs build upon the concept of starting from minimal language demands and progressing to longer, more complex levels. Production typically begins with imitation or demand production of one-syllable words. These may or may not have been screened in advance to eliminate words on which stuttering is likely to occur or has occurred. Also, there may or may not have been preliminary activity designed to induce non-stuttered speech. Play therapy, relaxation therapy, or the easy speaking voice (Shine 1981) are among the methods used. All of the programs cited structure speech activities in an operant framework so that every response can be as follows:

1. Judged instantly as acceptable or unacceptable.
2. Responded to overtly by the clinician with a positive or a negative contingency.
3. Accumulated toward an arbitrarily set criterion of X number of correct responses (cumulative or consecutive).
4. Accumulated for tangible reinforcement (if desired).
5. Counted and charted for comparison to baseline measures.

Unlike the other two programs, Shine's program incorporates transfer into the design, whereas Costello emphasizes that her ELU design is meant only to establish fluency, and transfer must be a subsequent step if spontaneous generalization has not occurred.

An example of progressive-step language complexity is provided here. For nonreaders (clients, that is), picture cards or objects can be used, while readers can have printed words added or used as replacements. A useful step is to screen the stimuli in advance by exposing a complete sequence to the client and removing any items on which stuttering occurs (examine the rejects to see if there are any phonologic commonalities such as voiced initial sounds, stop plosives, sounds that client has trouble articulating, and so on). You might wind up with 30–50 items such as the following:

ball	car	bell	hat	one	five
sun	dog	boy	shoe	two	red
bus	cat	book	shirt	four	pear

Determine how many correct responses will be required for token reinforcement and before movement to the next step. Every response is to receive a verbal response (100%VR). It is suggested that positive responses frequently include speech references such as these:

"Right. You said that very well."
"Correct. I like your easy speech."
"Good. You were nice and slow."

All incorrect (stuttered) responses are to be stopped immediately, during utterance if possible:

"No. You stumbled that time."
"Stop. You are trying too hard."

You may model an easy, fluent utterance, but do not have the child try again on the same word. If the production is fluent but pronunciation or articulation is not adequate, deliver a positive reinforcement, model the word as it should be said, and move on. When there has been prior work on relaxation, airflow, easy onset, or other fluency enhancement modes, it is appropriate to mention good efforts in positive reinforcements and to mention and model them when negative reinforcement is required.

A typical reinforcement pattern is verbal reinforcement (VR) for every response, and token reinforcement (TR) for every 5, 10, or 15, and so on, number of correct responses. The number of correct responses may vary with age, speech characteristics, and motivation of the child. Also, whether cumulative or consecutive correct responses are required can affect criteria. Failure on an item is stuttering, or any behavior previously identified by the clinician. Reinforcement and criterion suggestions are as follows:

1. VR for every response, phase down at longer responses.
2. TR response at ratios of
    a. 5:1 (one TR for 5 VR+) for very young, severely involved, or low-motivation children.
    b. 10:1 for older or less-involved children. May be raised or made more stringent as language level advances.
3. Token conversion for rewards at a rate paralleling 2; for example, five tokens earn one minute of favorite activity or some other reward. This also can be varied.
4. Item failure can be responded to as follows:
    a. Verbal penalty (VR−) and nonearning of tokens.
    b. Loss of an earned token for every failure or for X number of item failures.
5. Pass criteria in order to progress to next step:
    a. Require X number of consecutive responses out of X number of total responses, with at least X number of the total being correct, for example, 10 consecutive correct responses out of 50 responses with at least 45 (90 percent) being correct overall.
    b. Require X number of correct responses out of the total, for example, any 45 out of 50.
6. Failure criteria and effects:
    a. Fail after X consecutive errors.
    b. More than X percent errors out of total.
    c. After failure is determined, allow earned tokens to be retained, but progress to Pass wiped out; eliminate both.
    d. After failure is determined, increase the number/time requirement for a Pass.

Many clinicians stipulate that the Pass criteria (#5) should be met twice in consecutive sessions to assure stability of fluent responses. On the same level, two consecutive failures to meet Pass criteria call for a reevaluation and restructuring of the procedure. It might be necessary to repeat, or introduce, fluency-inducing procedures such as relaxation or easy onset, or to scrutinize and simplify stimulus material. On a few occasions this author has found very young clients deliberately using stuttering to manipulate the clinician, having figured out that "boring" activities can be interrupted that way. In such cases, implementation of penalty such as time-out (TO, see Chapter 16), consultation with parents to secure stronger back-up reinforcers, and so on, usually resolve such problems.

When the monosyllabic pictures, objects, and graphemes have been performed twice up to pass criterion levels, repeat the entire step, using the same stimuli. However, this time use a printed word list read aloud for the client to imitate. This is done for several reasons:

1. Reinforcement of basic fluency and providing an almost-guaranteed success by the child.
2. Clinician modeling of easy speaking patterns, especially on stimuli failed in the previous cycle.
3. Preparation for transfer practice by the child, at home, using a different person to read the list.

In the last item listed, this initial transfer practice works best if the intended moderator can visit the therapy session, observe, participate, and be instructed. However, printed instructions can be sent home and the child instructed concerning the "rules."

> Dear Parent,
> _____ has done very well in our first step of improving speech. This progress will be aided if you will help in some home practice.
> Once each day you are to read each word aloud for the child to repeat. Say each word in your normal manner, but soften your voice and slow down a little—just as if you were a little sleepy or tired. Don't hurry!
> Your child is to repeat each word after you, without any errors. Errors are mispronunciations, repetitions, hard prolongations, or getting stuck. If there is an error, shake your head and go on to the next word. Each time they are correct, say "fine," "good," "okay," and so on, and go to the next word. At the end, compliment the child for trying hard to improve, and don't review the efforts.
> On the word list, mark each word that was an error.
> Please send this list back on _____ .

In clinical settings the foregoing can be arranged and controlled easily in most instances. In school settings it will be feasible most of the time. Check the returned sheets to see if there are too many failures. Either way query the child about the practice sessions and try to establish whether there are (or will be) problems with the attitude, pressure, modeling, or cooperation from the environment that might affect future assignments.

In the second step the child should move from monosyllabic single presentations to monosyllabic dual presentations. That is, temporarily avoid the syllabic stress variables of two-syllable words. The stimuli used previously can be reused, in paired form. Since you will want 40 or 50 trials, you will need to add new stimuli as well, starting with the familiar items. Unless you have reasons for change, the same reinforcement schedule and Pass/Fail criteria used in the first step would be applied here, and the clinician model repeat and home practice also would be used.

The third step retains two-syllable stimuli but mixes two types: two-syllable words and two monosyllabics that are syntactically connected.

father	a car	this bus
mother	my dog	that way
pizza	no sir	why not

These can shift completely to word lists or mixed pictures, objects, and modeled productions. In most instances the same reinforcement schedule and home practice applications used in prior steps would be applied in this step.

The fourth step moves to production of three syllables consecutively. For nonreaders it will be simplest to shift totally to imitative responses of the clinician (reading from printed lists). However, carrier phrases plus pictures can also be used. Anything making up three syllables can be used, but trisyllabic words within the child's vocabulary or use range are suggested. Word possibilities are *magazine, vanilla, radio, president, apartment,* and so on. The other part of the list should be syntactically related word strings:

I am home	How are you	Some pizza
Who are you	Where is it	Go quickly
May I go	Two sisters	An airplane

It is suggested that VR responses continue 100 percent, as before, but TR reinforcement requirements be doubled, unless the child is a particular problem in motivation. Pass/Fail criteria, typically, would remain unchanged. Since many of the responses can be structured to resemble ordinary verbal statements, the clinician will want to pay close attention to the child's use of syllabic stress, glottal, lingual, and labial hard attacks, rate of utterance, and other fluency parameters. However, use modeling as the therapy method unless the child twice fails the step. If this occurs, there are two options:

1. Back up and repeat the previous step.
2. Branch out to problem solving.

In the second option the clinician would want to teach, or reemphasize, some form of relaxation, breath control, easy onset, reduction of syllable stress, prolongation of vowels and continuants, continuing phonation from word termination to subsequent word initiation, and so on. The method or methods used would be practiced on the specific items failed previously. Criteria to move on should combine subjective and objective elements:

• Subjective: the clinician is satisfied that the child understands the method or methods taught.
• Objective: the child generates nine fluent utterances out of ten consecutive responses.

Then the fourth step is repeated completely. Verbal responses from the clinician should include more frequent praise and reminders of the desired fluency-enhancing behaviors.

Steps 5 and 6 each add another syllable to utterances. These will include fewer single words, since four-syllable and five-syllable words will not be common in the child's vocabulary. Mix communication and general word strings:

Step 5	Step 6
televisions	I am going home
for at he why	four some did he red
May I have some	How are you feeling
Watermelon	How do I do that

Reinforcement can be kept the same on VR and either retained or reduced at the previous TR level. In the sixth step it is suggested that fluency performance be introduced as a criterion. For example,

> In this next step, you will talk a little longer, just as in each earlier step. However, I won't just listen for you to get stuck or have trouble. I will also listen to hear if you talk too fast, too loud, make your sounds too hard, or forget to relax. I will show you what I mean.

During the sixth step, fluent utterances that fail noticeably to meet enhancement criteria are accepted, but the VR might be stated, "Good. No getting stuck there, but you forgot to . . . ," and make sure clinician speech models the desired target or targets. If this happens on more than two consecutive fluent utterances, remind the client, model the desired production mode, have the child imitate, and then remind again before the next stimulus. Remind the client again prior to the next three utterances, and then continue with the usual routine.

The seventh step is a combination of longer responses and more specific ones:

How old is your sister	Where is the swimming pool
My sister is very young	The swimming pool is over there
What is your favorite food	What is two plus two
My favorite food is pizza	Two plus two is four

These stimuli are presented for imitation, as before, and are practice in helping the child plan complete syntactic utterances. The clinician should try to use as many personally appropriate stimulus topics as possible. For instance, if the child has a dog, a younger sister, a father who is a lawyer, or enjoys TV cartoons, the following topics would be appropriate:

Do you have a sister	What work does your father do
Yes, I have a sister	My father is a lawyer
How old is your sister	What is your dog's name
My sister is two years old	My dog's name is Frank

As before, the step involves 40 or 50 child responses. Verbal reinforcement does not have to occur on each response, and TR can be scaled down further. However, any error should be stopped immediately, the stimulus remodeled, and the child expected to correct the error. Successful second tries receive a VR but do not count toward TR and do not erase the error in clinician Pass/Fail accounting. At this point, it might be useful to restate the Pass/Fail criteria:

Pass—X number of total correct responses, with the last X consecutive responses fluent. This must be accomplished twice, in separate sessions (overlap allowed). For example, 35 total correct responses out of 40 efforts, with the last consecutive 8 fluent.

Fail—errors on X consecutive responses, or more than X percent errors on the total number of responses.

In the eighth step the material from the seventh step is repeated with new items added to bring total responses up to the 40–50 range. The clinician asks a familiar question and the client, instead of imitating, answers with a complete sentence that utilizes the content of the question:

Q: Do you like to eat pizza?
A: Yes, I like to eat pizza.

Some preliminary rehearsal may be necessary, Since 50 percent of the stimuli have been co-opted by the clinician, it will be necessary to add new material. When needed, it is permissible to consult with the child concerning the form and content of the child's reply. Reinforcement and criteria continue as before. On this and the previous steps, those steps passed on an in-clinic basis can be shifted to home assignment practice.

The ninth step takes the client to originating and formulating responses on a spontaneous basis, although support material will be used. The support material can be action pictures, magazine advertisements, or other "talk about" items. The clinician may at first need to perform the tasks and then have the child respond to the same stimulus. A stopwatch, timer, or other signal system will be needed. Instructions might be as follows:

> Look at this picture. You must tell me about it or make up a story. When you start talking, I will start timing, like this, and you must keep talking until I signal you to stop, like this.

Model and practice several brief efforts, explain that prolonged pauses will increase the time demand, and remind the client of the desired fluency-enhancing behaviors. Usually it is helpful to have the child rehearse several responses, recording each one and playing it back for analysis and recommendations. When satsified with the basal capacity, proceed with the step. Stop any error immediately. Even if a response is otherwise fluent, stop for prolonged pauses, excessive rate, or other undesirable production characteristics. In general, start with a requirement of a five-second response, and target ten responses. Pass is defined as seven fluent responses, with the last three responses all being fluent. Failure will be four or more responses marred by errors *or* seven or more errors occurring in less than four responses. In the event of failure, problem solve and repeat the ten-response cycle. Provide VR to all responses and establish a tangible reinforcement for success on the ten-response cycle. After success, move to the next step.

The tenth through the fifteenth steps are the same as the ninth step except that response lengths of 10, 15, 20, 30, 45, and 60 seconds are required. The clinician will need to provide adequate stimulus material. It is useful to add "tell me about" stimuli covering favorite TV shows, movies, pets, hobbies, sports, and so on. If time requirements are met in the middle of a response, the child can pick up at that point in the next timing cycle and continue. Be sure to stop any errors at once, counsel about rate, prolongation, easy onset, and so on. Recording and playback is also often a useful teaching device in these steps, especially if the child is asked, "What is wrong?" rather than being told. If the client cannot (or will not) say, replay the tape and help them evaluate what they hear. The older the client, the more effectively this technique can be used. Criteria and reinforcement are usually the same as in the ninth step.

If home assignments are being used, this author usually suggests not using the ninth step for outside practice (it is too brief) and sending the following note home:

> Dear Parent,
>
> _____ is working on free speech, using a slower rate and an easier manner of speaking. Would you help him/her practice at home by looking below to see how long each response is to be? Pick ten pictures from the child's books or magazines and ask her/him to tell you about each. Time each response and say "stop" when the time is up. Then go to the next picture and repeat the process. If they have any trouble speaking, wave your hand for them to stop (immediately) and go to the next picture. If they have trouble on three consecutive pictures, stop the practice session, praise their effort, and let them go for now.
>
> Length of response time is _____ seconds.
>
> How many times did you signal? _____
>
> Comments: _____

Be alert for children who perform adequately on an in-clinic basis but have troubles practicing at home. Discuss any problems with the child. Possible reasons include simple change of venue, carelessness or lack of enthusiasm on the part of the child, inappropriate stimuli, apathetic parents, impatient or hypercritical parents, among other factors. Since transfer and generalization is important, this could be the time when parent counseling, parent attendance at therapy sessions, or other means could be used to improve home performance. Cooperative teachers can be used for classroom practice, whether in recitation or show-and-tell activities. With their help, classroom monologues can be rehearsed during therapy sessions.

The fifteenth step has brought the child up to a 60-second monologue. For many young children (and some older ones), this can be a demanding time factor and can be reduced for the very young. However, for children in the 8–12 year range (approximately), substeps of the fifteenth step can be implemented. These steps simply expand the monologues to two, four, and five minutes respectively. Criteria will be the same, but more attention will have to be paid to any tendencies to remain fluent while losing some or all of the fluency-enhancing behaviors. When this occurs, stop the child, correct inadequacies, and then resume the timing of the monologue.

The sixteenth step moves from monologue to dialogue, or conversational speech. This increases the linguistic load over the increments of the monologue steps. Predictability of stimulus-response drops, forward planning of language is more difficult, and monitoring includes both content and production. It also involves the responses, verbal and nonverbal, of the other participant. There should be a brief review and rehearsal with the client, with instructions and client autonomy geared to the age and maturity of the child. In this review period the clinician will want to secure several things:

1. Review and discussion of progress to date, identifying any rough spots in performance and the need for improvement.
2. Review and discussion of transfer and generalization, how well it has progressed, identification of any particular problems in performance, or trouble situations.
3. Review and reminder practice, with emphasis on self-monitoring and evaluation, and on the fluency-enhancing behaviors in use.

The targets in the preceding list can be covered with varying levels of sophistication, depending on the age of the client. With age and maturity increments the depth of coverage can be increased. At lowest levels the clinician will lead the client to organize and develop the three areas.

The performance targets in the sixteenth step should include the nonoccurrence of dysfluencies, an appropriate syllable rate, and utilization of any fluency-enhancing methods that have been applied during therapy. The client should rehearse an spm rate of 150, using reading or monologue material. With a rule of thumb of 1.5 syllables per word, this equates to approximately 100 wpm. This rate is below normal speaking rates but not too far away from a target of 120 wpm, or 180 spm. Practice should include rate procedures described in Chapter 12. Some clinicians recommend "letting fluency find itself," rather than directly instructing children. In the abstract there is a point to this view, but practicality of use and transfer is on the side of clinician assistance and direction.

When the child is able to carry the three criteria cited in the first sentence of the previous paragraph, therapy is ready for progress into the seventeenth step. This step is divided into two parts. The first part might begin with instructions such as this:

> Now we are just going to talk together, back and forth. I will time us for one minute. If you have any trouble (stutter), talk too fast, or . . . I will stop you and we will start back at zero time.

At first the clinician should guide the conversation into easy channels, starting and stopping the timing during client responses, and not timing during clinician speech. In most cases, after several rounds the clinician will find it quite feasible to estimate client time and eliminate precise timing. Clients may need to be motivated or pressured into sufficiently long responses. Clinician verbalization should be kept to the bare minimum, which differs from normal conversation. However, avoid modeling a too-clipped pattern and insert frequent nonverbal reinforcers (facial expression, nodding, eye contact), as well as interjecting social comments such as, "Umhmm . . . ," "I see . . . ," "They sure do . . . ," "That's great . . . ," and so on. Criteria and levels of the seventeenth step are as follow:

1. One minute of client speech.
2. 0%SW.
3. Rate at or below 150 spm.
4. Use of any fluency controls learned.
5. Pass: No stuttering, no more than two rate errors; no more than five fluency control lacks during the minute.

Treat the first one-minute cycle as practice, interrupting when necessary. When Pass is reached the first time, utter any comments and praise, and then repeat the step. In the second cycle, introduce the following penalties and rewards:

1. At 15-second intervals (roughly) interject a VR so that it does not interrupt unduly.
2. For each 30 seconds of fluency award 10 seconds of "therapy-free" activity at the end of the period. Mark these with tokens (TR).
3. For any stuttering wipe out accumulated time and start over. Accumulated free time is not affected.
4. For each two occurrences of fast rate or dropping of fluency control, subtract one TR. If you reach deficit TR levels, then treat the next two errors as being equal to a stuttering, and start timing over again.

Now, or later, it may be useful to introduce penalties such as time-out (Chapter 16) and/or introduce stronger and more individualized rewards.

Steps 18, 19, and 20 are continuations of step 17, with the target times changing to two, four, and six minutes respectively. Criteria will be the following:

- Step 18—two minutes time; 0%SW; rate of 150 spm or less (three errors or less); no more than three fluency control slips.
- Step 19—four minutes time; 0%SW; rate of 180 spm or less (three errors or less); no more than five fluency control slips.
- Step 20—six minutes time; 0%SW; 180 spm or less (no more than four errors); no more than six fluency control slips.

Note that in step 20, rate increases about 20 percent to 180 spm, which would approximate 120 wpm. This increase will often need a tangent for modeling and practice before continuing. Each step is to be performed twice, meeting the criteria each time.

The 21st step, the final fluency establishment, is to simulate normal conversation interaction. The characteristics of this step are the following:

- Time: five minutes
- Cycles: six times
- Criteria for each completion:
  - 0%SW

- spm rate at final target (no more than two errors)
- fluency controls with no more than three errors.

With six performance cycles, the total is 30 minutes of conversation. The last three cycles must be consecutive passes; for example, if the child stuttered in the fifth five-minute cycle, then nonstuttering sixth, seventh, and eighth cycles would be required to complete the 21st step. When the cycles have been completed, the clinician will plan further therapy on the assumption that basic fluency has been established and is relatively stable. At this point it is desirable to consider the following therapy possibilities:

1. Introducing variability and stress, desensitization, attitude alteration, and so on, as discussed in Chapters 9, 10, and 11.
2. Determining if other aspects of speech production need attention.
3. Taking progressive steps in transfer and maintenance.

Summary: Progressive Communication Development

The preceding pages have provided an example of a possible progressively developed linguistic program. It is a compilation of different structures the author has used, and is not offered as a tested and validated therapy program. The steps are offered as suggestions, not prescriptions, and clinicians are encouraged to alter and adapt it as they see fit. At the lower steps the program would be applicable to Group I children, but later steps go well past what would be expected of their levels of linguistic proficiency and motivation. Equally, the lower steps could be too simple for some Group II children, and much of the program would probably not be applicable to Group III adolescents.

PSYCHOSOCIAL CONSIDERATIONS

Other chapters of the book direct attention to pragmatic factors in communication and to psychosocial dimensions. However, it is appropriate here to stress that such considerations must be observed in the various therapy procedures. The preceding section, providing an example of progressive complexity of utterance, generally ignores pragmatic and psychosocial aspects. However, the clinician should not assume that fluency acquired through carefully graded increments in language demand will transfer automatically to other settings. Interaction of other participants, altered physical settings, distractions and disruptions, client fears and attitudes, and other factors can act to stress or break down the tentatively acquired fluency.

CHAPTER SUMMARY

There is no question that language has moved to occupy a significant place in stuttering therapy and theory research, and indeed always has been of significance in many therapies. We will not describe stuttering per se as a linguistic malfunction and assume that all children who stutter require language development or therapy of stuttering that is language based. It is appropriate that every child who stutters should receive language assessment, and a determination should made as to whether concomitant problems require specific remediation, whether language precursor or foundation skills require primary attention before fluency skills are targeted, and whether the therapy itself should emphasize language structure for the best results. Our procedures and programs, assessment and therapy, are enriched by linguistic orientations. It will certainly continue to be an area of further research and therapy experimentation and will stimulate the development of more specific procedures and programs for particular subgroups of stutterers.

CHAPTER EIGHT
ENVIRONMENTAL COUNSELING AND MANIPULATION

OVERVIEW

The title of this chapter suggests a definitional division that should be clarified. In its simplest form counseling is talking with another person (Williams, SFA #18). In more specific terms counseling might be described as therapeutic communication to identify, evaluate, introduce or eliminate, reinforce or reduce, certain attitudes on the part of one of the participants. The effects of counseling may alter attitudes and, in turn, may affect behaviors. It also is possible to target behaviors directly, and seek to alter them. On the other hand, environmental manipulation has been defined as

> therapeutic procedure which focuses on those variables operating in the child's environment which are thought to be contributing to the maintenance of the stuttering. (Shames & Florance 1982, p.204)

Although the definition is appropriate, it has certain limitations. It might be more applicable to define environmental manipulation as follows:

> Therapeutic intervention to identify and evaluate environmental factors that are most facilitating and most disruptive of fluency, and the procedures in-

volved in enhancing the facilitators and eliminating or reducing the disruptors.

As compared to counseling for attitude change, the targets here are behavioral. The word *fluency* in the preceding definition could be replaced by any other therapy target.

In the following pages, attitude and environmental therapy will mix, as will be the situation also in the next chapter. Before moving to a discussion of attitudinal and behavioral targets, it is appropriate to review briefly the background that suggests a need for these types of interventions. As we will see, in the next section and the one following, there is some controversy involved.

BACKGROUND

The family environment of stuttering children varies in importance, depending on the orientation of the clinician. Langlois, Hanrahan, and Inouye (1986) compared communication interactions between stuttering and nonstuttering children and their parents. They concluded that parents of stutterers, and the stutterers themselves, differ from the others in their communicative patterns. The stutterers' mothers made more demands, uttered more commands, and issued more requests than did the mothers of nonstutterers. With reference to the children, the authors reported that nonstutterers displayed substantially more verbal and nonverbal responses than did the stutterers. Also, the stuttering children seemed to feel obligated to reply verbally to maternal questions and did so far more often than did the nonstutterers. Moore and Nystul (1979) evaluated 27 parents of 14 stuttering children and an equal number of parents of nonstutterers. Children were matched for age, sex, and number of children in the family. Fathers of stutterers were more conventional and rigid concerning their children's behaviors, less tolerant of fighting among children, and less likely to allow expressions of curiosity about sexual matters. Stutterers' mothers also tended to repress any sexual curiosity but otherwise tended to be more democratic and protective. The stutterers' families, in general, were more rigid and stereotyped in their demands. The stuttering children displayed a positive attitude toward their mothers; whereas they were ambivalent and more frequently negative toward their fathers. Relating to attitudes and expectations, Riley (1981) found that 51 percent of the parents of the samples of stuttering children displayed unrealistic expectations of performance where "perfection" was expected. Interestingly 89 percent of the stuttering children placed perfectionistic demands upon themselves.

Family speech behaviors also have been suggested as a factor to be considered when evaluating and treating stuttering. Meyers and Freeman (1985a, 1985b, 1985c) reported that mothers of stuttering children have more rapid speech rates and that mothers in general are more likely to interrupt disfluent/dysfluent speech than fluent speech. In their review of stuttering children Riley and Riley (1983) noted that 53 percent of their population had parents who were observed to have a disruptive effect on children's speech—by use of a rapid speech rate, allowing too-brief time intervals for children to organize speech, interruptions of children as they spoke, and appearing impatient as they waited for responses from their children (p. 53).

In the diagnosis and assessment portion of this book a number of studies were commented on and summarized (Moore & Nystul 1979; Fowlie & Cooper 1978; Crowe & Cooper 1977; Allan & Williams 1974; Yairi 1973; Kasprisin-Burrelli 1972; Bloodstein 1969; Quarrington 1965; Goldman & Shames 1964; Kinstler 1961). These various studies more or less suggest a picture of the stuttering child's family in which the parents are less accepting of the stutterers than of their nonstuttering siblings, are more rigid in their own behavior and in demands on the children, are more perfectionistic in their performance expectations, and are more competitive and domineering. Fathers, in particular, may be domineering, rigid, conservative, and perfectionistic. Mothers tend to more covert rejection and less overt acceptance of stutterers and feel that their stuttering children are less well adjusted; also, the mothers may be more socially passive and more protective of their stuttering children. It was noted earlier that some studies have failed to distinguish stutterers and nonstutterers in terms of their family situations (Meyers & Freeman 1985a; Cox, Seider & Kidd 1984; Martin, Haroldson & Kuhl 1972; Bourdon & Silber 1970).

As long as flat declaratives about the adjustment and behavior of stutterers' families are avoided, the preponderance of evidence seems to suggest that it is appropriate to be concerned about the stutterer's environment. This concern may, or may not, disclose attitudes and practices in the environment that can be interpreted as having an adverse effect on speech fluency or, at the least, failing to provide maximum support for the development and transfer of fluency from therapy efforts. This question is explored further in the following section, along with the issue of whether or not clinician intervention is necessary, desirable, or proper.

CONTROVERSY

Wendell Johnson and his associates (1959) are identified particularly with the indirect therapy of environmental manipulation, since application of this approach often rejected therapy directly with the child. Although present all the time, direct therapy proponents became highly visible in the 1960s and have advanced to dominance in therapy of stuttering. In this process counseling and manipulation therapy has been questioned from various standpoints of necessity, effectiveness, and time invesment. Guitar (1984) summarizes the counseling approaches suggested by Van Riper (1973), Ainsworth and Gruss (1981), Cooper (1979), Conture (1982), and others. His conclusion is that "it is not clear how many of the children . . . would not have recovered 'spontaneously,' . . . [and] it is not even possible to state how many of the children treated with these indirect treatments recovered at all" (p. 295). On the other side, Williams (1986), while not supporting the concept that stutterers as a category form an emotional group different from nonstutterers, cautioned against hasty conclusions. He avers that this does not preclude individuals from having individual problems and feels that most of these problems relate to the family: "In fact, any time I find a child whose disfluencies [are] . . . accompanied by obvious emotional distress . . . I look for factors in the home that could account for such reactions" (p. 94). He goes on to express the idea that for the child speech is a form of reaching out to other people and other people reaching back. He continues with a superb statement:

> A child is just beginning to learn that one can hit with words, can hurt with words, can kiss with words, or caress with them . . . [and is] beginning to learn the awesome power of words. (p. 96)

When dysfluencies disrupt the words, we have a communication problem, not just a speech problem. Just as speech disruption can affect communication, communication problems (such as negative personal or environmental factors) can have effects on speech.

Costello (1983) argues strongly against environmental manipulation. She states that

> all the tenets of good parenting are invoked and the responsibility for the child's stuttering is typically placed squarely on the shoulders of the parents. Hence, the responsibility for alleviating the child's problems rests with them as well. (p. 72)

It is inappropriate for Costello forcibly to join diagnosogenesis theory of causation with practices in environmental manipulation as if performance of the latter requires agreement with the former. Such logic also suggests that environmental therapy with a dysphasic's family involves assumptions about the factors behind the stroke that caused the dysphasia. Costello correctly challenges the lack of evidence (see Ramig and Wallace, later) to support a case for environmental manipulation, as Guitar (1984) did. She states that ethics are at issue and that clinicians have no right to "ask families to rearrange their lives" (p. 72). She also questions the efficacy of indirect treatment. Costello was writing primarily to espouse direct, as opposed to indirect, treatment of stuttering. Twenty years ago, when we were escaping from the Johnsonian "no direct therapy with children" tenet, Costello's polar opposition would have been an understandable instance of gross generalization and overstatement. It is too easy to argue for or against a mode of therapy. Also, there is no doubt that fluency stimulation or shaping programs have helped many children who stutter (Costello 1980; Shine 1980a, 1980b; Ryan 1974). At the same time we have a long history of approaches to childhood stuttering where provision of information and modification of environmental behaviors have been used. It seems futile and counterproductive to champion one approach or the other as the best way. "Let us not get lost in 'either-or' thinking" (Williams, SFA 20, p. 97). There are times when the most productive, cost-effective mode of therapy will have environment as the major or sole target. In other situations speech therapy can stand alone. Certainly there will be situations where a combination of the two approaches will be most effective.

The preceding discussion did not suggest that theory and therapy should not be compatible. However, use of an environmental therapy does not require belief in environmental causation, just as use of airflow techniques does not require the clinician to subscribe to the airway dilation reflex theory. Once stuttering occurs, other factors become significant, and this significance probably increases over time as we deal with the development and maintenance of stuttering. Conture (1982) made the point succinctly when he suggested that stuttering probably occurs as a result of "a complex interaction between the stutterer's environment—and the abilities the stutterer brings to that environment" (p. 18). When a child is seen for therapy, there is no reason to assume that the complex interaction, on both sides, has terminated and that both sides will not profit from the clinician's attention.

Ramig and Wallace (1987) summarize a single-case study of indirect and combined indirect-direct therapy, concluding that the combined approach was more effective. Guitar (1984) and Shames and Florance (1982) stress the significance of parent-teacher counseling, the former beginning counseling at the time of the child's first therapy session and maintaining it on through therapy transfer activities with the child. Gregory and Hill (1984) thoroughly involve the parents in their therapy, starting with the evaluation interview and continuing as needed. Information and standard pamphlets are provided. When needed, parents are taught to chart dysfluencies by factors of person, situation, dysfluency type, child awareness, listener reaction, and dysfluency causes. The clinician may instruct the parents in speech modeling, problem solving, and other skills. General counseling in modifying expectations and resolving child behavior problems may also be used. Andronico and Blake (1971) have described a "filial therapy" process in which play therapy is used to allow the child to express feelings in a situation of acceptance and interaction. Parents observe clinician sessions for six to ten weeks and then begin similar activities in the home. (This approach will be discussed again in Chapter 10.) The overall goal of the approach is to shift family attention from speech (stuttering) to accepting and expanding interactions with the child. Riley and Riley (1984, 1979) make environmental manipulation a significant area of their multiplex therapy program, devoting from 4 to 12 one-hour counseling sessions to the area. Counseling is carried out by the child's clinician and combines continued information gathering and dispensing with counseling. Goals of therapy counseling include the following:

1. Reducing of parental guilt over occurrence and continuation of stuttering.
2. Identifying and reducing behaviors in the environment that stress the child's speech. These include, but are not limited to, difficulty in securing parental attention, interruption of child's speech, and criticism or teasing about child's speech problems.
3. Reducing unrealistic parental expectations of child, particularly in areas of speech.
4. If necessary, dealing with children who use stuttering to manipulate the family.

It is obvious that many clinicians favor the use of counseling and environmental therapy, and most of them also support the idea of direct therapy with the child. In some instances where the child is very young and severity hovers around the borderline level, it is not unusual to find indirect (counseling and environmental) therapy favored as a replacement for direct forms of intervention with the child. Williams (SFA 20) feels that where environmental pressure is high, when dysfluency occurrences can be associated with specific family situations, or when emotional factors are significant, fluency-shaping therapy is contraindicated until such time as it has been shown that environmental modification effects do not result in fluency. There seems to be no valid defense for blanket proscription against counseling and environmental therapy. When to use it, how to formulate it, skills required, problems involved, and other factors are discussed next.

VARIABLES IN COUNSELING AND ENVIRONMENTAL THERAPY

The rubrics *counseling* and *environmental manipulation* cover a wide range of meanings. At one end of the range is the clinician who summarizes the results of the diagnosis and evaluation process, utters a recommendation concerning the need (or lack of it) for direct therapy, makes a number of general suggestions to the parents, distributes one or more standard pamphlets, and encourages the parents to contact her or him if other questions develop. Also near this end of the range are package therapy programs that outline rather specifically what is to be accomplished in working with the environment. At the opposite end of the range is the practice of what some prefer to call psychotherapy. In our profession we run across instances where writers or speakers have warned speech and language clinicians against being, or trying to be, psychotherapists. Training, skills, ethics, need, value, and other considerations may be cited as arguments against practicing "psychotherapy." These arguments are a classic case of delayed closure of barn doors after the horse has bolted!

Procedures to alter the behavior of another person are psychotherapy, always. Techniques aimed at motivation, attending, cooperation, reinforcement, punishment, and other aspects of remediation—all involve psychotherapy. We are in the profession of altering the communicative behavior of human beings, and that *must* involve psychotherapy. Those who profess to ignore attitudes and anxieties of clients because amelioration of the stuttering will (supposedly) resolve these problems are practicing manipulative psychotherapy. Dalton (1983a) states that the clinician should be able to deal with stuttering in the context of the whole personality and peculiar lifestyle of the client.

> Whether this is called "work on attitudes," "counseling," or "psychotherapy," these skills need to be learned and provision for their learning should be made part of a therapist's basic training. (p. 223)

Shames and Florance (1982) do not restrict the speech and language clinician to communication disorders in counseling and note that the parents, rather than the child, can become the focus of therapy. However, they stress that interviewing and counseling skills, knowledge of child management and family dynamics, and familiarity with stuttering determine the degree of clinician involvement and whether or not problems are referred to specialists. Conture (1982) also recommends a range of capacities for the clinician, including the suggestion that they read up on baby and child care books published to help parents.

It is impossible to specify what skills a clinician will need or will have the opportunity to use (see next section). The more training experience that occurs in interpersonal and intrapersonal areas of communication, the better. However, there is no widespread agreement as to how much preparation there should be or what its form should be. The student and the new clinician need to understand that they will engage in psychotherapy, with the only question being the degree or depth of involvement. This situation requires that the clinician approach each client with several questions of his or her own:

1. What are the problems (commission and omission) in this environment that seem to affect communication behavior?
2. What standard or formalized procedures (pamphlets, audiotapes or videotapes, instructional programs, and so on) can I draw upon as a resource?
3. What personal knowledge and skills are required of me to deal with any or all of the problems in 1?
4. What constraints or mandates must I work with, in my setting, that affect my response capacity?
5. What referral sources and procedures are available?

Experience, education, continuing education opportunities, job setting, case types, and time constraints will vary the patterns of these five question areas. The important action for the clinician is to review the five questions in an ongoing pattern, for each client, and to avoid a rigid approach or philosophy to cover all situations.

LIMITATIONS AND PROBLEMS

The previous section raised questions relative to competence, but it did not answer them because there is no practicable solution except flexibility. This section may provide assistance by discussing some of the limitations that force partial answers to certain of the preceding five questions.

Although the potential limitation of *clinician competence* has just been discussed, it needs to be mentioned again. People vary in their interpersonal capacities, so some clinicians will "always" be more, or less, effective in counseling than are most of their peers. Recognising strengths, or weaknesses, and taking them into account is important in therapy planning. Clinician *time* and *rules of the workplace* are potential limitations also. Time translates either into income or caseload, or both, and some employment settings do not encourage scheduling nonclient sessions to talk with parents or other persons. The *parents,* or significant others, are another factor to consider. Leith (1984), in discussing the public school setting, has stated that parents will fall into one of four groups in terms of interest and availability: cooperative and available, cooperative and unavailable, uncooperative and available, and uncooperative and unavailable. This author identifies the environmental situation in terms of more factors, classifying availability of persons in terms of available, scheduling problems, and unavailable:

Attitude	Knowledge	Speech Behaviors	Family Situation
Overconcern	Ignorant	Facilitating	Stable
Concern	Informed	Variable	Variable
Unconcerned	Special	Disruptive	Disruptive
Hostile	Needs		

Conture (1982) has suggested that parents tend to fall into three nonexclusive groups: those expecting perfection in their child's performance, those with significant interparent disagreements over child raising, and those with a prior family history of stuttering. It is clear that parents do not fit a standard category, and each situation should be examined as a unique phenomenon and therapy planned accordingly. The clinician should be prepared for the individual responses of parents in a counseling situation. Many parents feel guilty or worry that others will label them guilty. A frequent compensation for guilt is defensiveness or reluctance to open up; this may turn into hostility if too much pressure or blame is felt. Some parents in this era feel that "cures" should be measured in terms of a few weeks, and they can be impatient or dismayed over the prospect of extended therapy. At times parents will attempt to use the clinician in an effort to assign blame to one spouse, a relative, or one side of the family. Since parents are people and people are diverse in their personality dynamics, the clinician should avoid establishing parent stereotypes. The following are statements this author has heard from parents during the past year:

- "Every time he stutters and screws his little face up, it's just more than I can bear and I have to leave the room."
- "I don't have the time to come in here after I work all day. We're paying for work with _____ , not for you to talk with us."
- "Why are you asking about his behavior at home? He's here to work on speech and you aren't psychologists."
- "I'll do what I can, but you'll have to help me out."

The last statement was included to reassure the reader that many parents are concerned and try to help as best they can.

Client responses to family intervention is a variable that many overlook. Hanley (1986) notes that the effects of environmental manipulation vary with the child. Good speech modeling by the parents may be very effective and generalizing in its effects with one child, but not with another child whose level of perceptual awareness is such that the speech changes are not noted. Similarly, children will be more, or less, responsive to attitude changes by significant others in their environment. This will also apply to directed activities by the parents, when the clinician asks them to do specific things. This area of client response will not be easy to plan for in advance, and how the child behaves (performs) with the clinician may or may not be indicative of the child's responses to similarly structured situations in the home.

GENERAL PROCEDURES

This chapter cannot teach counseling, but some suggestions can be made that are applicable across most situations. The first general procedure is to *have a plan, but be flexible.* Previous warnings have been made against rigid approaches to counseling and manipulation. However, by the time one adds the clinician's own skills and limitations, customary time and availability constraints, certain commonalities about stuttering and families, plus the input from cumulative experience, one will develop a particular plan of approach to most situations. To that, the active planning part, one must add the self-questions that bring individuality and uniqueness to every family and environment. This preplanning, subject to ongoing modifications, is necessary to avoid two of the pitfalls of counseling, formulaic coverage of rigid topics and friendly chats that, like ice cream on a hot day, leave one feeling better but do not actually solve any problems.

One thing counselors in all professions must learn is that the purpose of a session is for the *client,* not the clinician, to talk. Where the target is environmental manipulation, it is easier to instruct the auditor or auditors but it is probably better to help the client arrive at a goal by his or her own efforts. For example, the clinician could say, "I want you to slow your speech rate down around Linda's. Here, I will show you how it should sound." Another method could be this one:

C: How fast do you talk when the family is together?
P: I don't know. Like most people, I guess.
C: Well, compare to when you talk alone with your husband, or when you talk to your boss.

After the discussion, the parent decides that the family group rate is considerably faster than during other situations.

C: What do you think this faster rate does to Linda?
P: I guess it's harder for her. Gotta be!
C: Mmm-hmmm. I think so too.
P: Yes, it does. She has more trouble with us all together at one time.
C: What do you think could be done to help her out?
P: Well, slow down I suppose. That's really going to be hard, 'cause when we all get together, the words really fly back and forth.

The clinician can move directly to the issue of rate control, hold back while the parent enquires about other disruptive behaviors (interruptions, finishing words or statements, and so on), probe the client's reactions to these stresses, or just make notes for future discussion. Decisions arrived at by the counselees tend to be more acceptable to them, commit them to make an effort to change and often include more individual factors that routine advice can miss. The process is not time efficient, and sometimes must be limited, but *client talk* is generally more profitable than *clinician talk*. Most parents have little information, and possibly some misinformation, about stuttering. Counseling routinely has a goal of informing the parents about stuttering. One must be careful not to overburden the counselee with too much information, however. When a parent asks, "What causes stuttering?" the clinician can briefly explain current belief or the clinician's own theory, but without a long discourse on the different theories or the best theory. The same caution applies to giving other information. When the rare parent wants to know "everything" about stuttering, the clinician can provide the patient with, or direct him or her to, publications such as *If Your Child Stutters* (SFA 11) or Carlisle's *Tangled Tongue* (Carlisle 1985).

A routine procedure in all counseling is ongoing *observation* and *evaluation*. Previous reference has been made to the modification of counseling plans. Such modifications depend on feedback from the participants and on the clinician noting and evaluating it. Feedback can be highly specific when the client asks a question, admits a problem, or challenges a statement. One also receives feedback in client evasions, hasty changes in, or tangents to, topics, disagreements between parents, uncomfortable silences, too-hasty disclaimers or assurances, obvious halo responses, and observable changes in body language or speech production. The clinician should always review a past session by considering new information, overt or covert, that might need coverage. Also, if trying to change parental attitudes, the clinician will want to monitor the frequency and intensity of the behaviors over time in order to evaluate progress.

Finally, the clinician should always engage in self-evaluation. This is not to suggest a generalized "How did I do?" evaluation, but a specific one. Many clinicians are aided in this by drawing up a checklist such as the following:

1. Eye contact with client.
2. Clinician talking time versus client talking time.
3. Adequacy of clinician answers to questions.
4. Awareness of covert feedback from client.
5. ·Clinician response to emotional issues (if any).
6. What was accomplished, exactly, this sessions?
7. Has anything happened, or failed to happen, that would suggest a needed change in the therapy plan or approach?

The list is suggestive, not complete. Some clinicians use a bipolar checklist (warm-aloof, talkative-silent, accepting-argumentative, and so on) and mark it twice, once for the client and once for the clinician.

AREAS OF COUNSELING AND MANIPULATION

The paragraphs that follow discuss various areas with which counseling and manipulation often deal. These areas are selective and illustrative; they are not intended as a complete outline. The reader is referred to various sources already cited, with particular emphasis on Conture (1982), Ainsworth and Gruss (1981), Cooper (1979), Van Riper (1973), and the Speech Foundation of America publications 18 and 20.

The Stutterer and Individual Interactions

A child typically responds differently to various people in her or his environment, but parents may not know or observe this. The clinician wants to find out with whom the child has frequent or consistent contact. These contacts can include mother, father, siblings, other relatives, daycare personnel, other children, teachers, piano instructor, neighbors (adults and peers), and so on. This should be explored until there is a reasonably complete list of the people with whom the child interacts. The next step is to find out, in proximate terms, how much time the child spends with each of the persons identified. (Parents are often amazed, and sometimes depressed, at how little of their nonsleeping and noneating time their child actually spends with them.) After establishing the time distribution, the clinician would like to know the fluency/dysfluency pattern of the child with each of the people. At this point estimates and feelings, not hard data, are targeted. Where the parents do not know, encourage them to call or visit the people and try to secure information for a report.

Parents may need information, and reassurance, that children often stutter more with certain persons, less with others. Targeting the examples of "best" and "worst," the clinician attempts to have the parents determine the factors that might be involved. One method of doing this is to have a checklist similar to that in Table 8–1. Explain each item so they understand that 1, **Difficult to get their attention,** can, for instance, be because that person is very busy or distracted, not necessarily because he or she is unfriendly. Similarly, 5, **Responds overtly to dysfluencies,** can be either friendly efforts to help or negative criticism and scolding. Help the parents fill in all the names elicited in the procedure described earlier and talk through one or two rating procedures with them. Ask them to take the list with them but return it at the next session. It is preferable for both

TABLE 8–1. Parent Evaluation of Persons in Child's Environment

ITEM	PERSON						
1. Difficult to get their attention							
2. Difficult to hold their attention							
3. Interrupts, completes statements, etc.							
4. Shows obvious nonverbal responses to dysfluencies							
5. Responds overtly to dysfluencies							

Instructions: Identify all persons. Fill out the ratings for each person. Put a 3 if item is frequent or strong; put a 2 if item is true occasionally or mildly; put a 1 if an item is rare or absent.

parents to complete the form; if their ratings do not agree, urge them to record both judgments for comparison and discussion.

This area directs parental attention to people in the child's environment, including themselves, and how they interact communicatively. It also initiates a review of client relationships that may need explanation later. At the very least it specifies high-interaction people who may be able to provide speech modeling, behavioral changes, transfer practice opportunities, and other values in therapy. The entire process often helps the parents begin in an observation and evaluation mode that will be expanded as therapy continues. It can also aid desensitization, if needed, by subjecting the problem to the structure of analysis and charting. Table 8–1 is only an example of many different ways in which the child's environment can be evaluated. The 5 items can be rewritten, replaced, expanded to 60 items, broken down to more discreet behaviors, and the rating scale altered. The clinician profits from the information, which can aid in planning future counseling goals and in therapy with the child.

The Stutterer in Multiple Interactions

Although you are interested in the individuals in the child's environment, a certain number of the interactions take place in group situations. A first step in investigating this area is to discuss group effects with the parents and then identify the most frequent group situations met. These will tend to be family, school, or daycare, plus neighborhood peers. There may also be special groups such as scouts and church groups. Here also a sample form is provided, in Table 8–2, and the clinician again will want to

TABLE 8–2.   Parent Evaluation of Groups in the Child's Environment

ITEM	GROUP							
1. Competition in talking								
2. Competition for central role								
3. Typically one central figure								
4. Interrupting verbal behavior								
5. Nonverbal response to dysfluencies								
6. Verbal responses to dysfluencies								
7. Rapid speech rates, etc.								
8. Subjects above child's level								

Instructions: Identify all groups. Fill out ratings for each group. Put a 3 if item is very strong or frequent; put a 2 if item is true occasionally or mildly; put a 1 if item is very mild, rare, or absent.

discuss the meaning of the ratings. Item 3 suggests that the group typically has one dominant figure whose lead in attitudes and behaviors the group will usually follow. Item 7 can include vocabulary level or any other factors. With the parents identify the different groups, add any rating items that would be useful, and talk through the ratings of one group. Where parents express ignorance about a group, encourage them to observe and find out or to contact an observer who can supply information. Ask the parents to return the sheet at the next session.

Table 8–2 focuses parent attention on group situations where client needs often suffer from distraction factors due to the presence of the other persons in the group. This is also the type of situation where less desirable speech modeling, competition for talking time, interruptions, imitation, teasing and ridicule, and other stressing behaviors are likely to occur. Parents can often spend some time in this area, becoming aware of group dynamics, being encouraged to observe other group members as well, and assessing their own roles and behaviors when involved. The group category of family often means two parents and one child. However, the category may include other siblings and relatives. When this is the case, the clinician will often find it worthwhile to discuss the molecular composition of the group and its behaviors. "When your spouse isn't present, do the group ratings change?" can be queried, and the same question can be asked about other members of the usual group. Not unusually parents suddenly realize that certain group behaviors (desirable or undesirable) are strongly enhanced by one person. This is not necessarily the individual's fault. For example, grandmother may come over for lunch every Sunday for a few hours, and there is intense competition for her attention and time.

GENERAL ASPECTS OF SPEECH AND LANGUAGE

This section refers to Table 8–3 and more or less consolidates the material from the previous two sections, focusing on behaviors that might be disruptive of fluency for the child. The parents' attention is directed to general areas of home and outside environments while retaining the

TABLE 8–3. Parent Evaluation of Speech, Language, and Dysfluency Reactions in the Child's Environment

ITEM	AREAS				
	PERSON	PERSON	PERSON	HOME	OUTSIDE
1. Rapid speech rate					
2. High vocabulary rate					
3. Bilingual pressures					
4. Perfectionistic demands on pronunciation, articulation, vocabulary, etc.					
5. Quiet, nontalkative					
6. Very talkative					
7. Dysfluency reactions Interruption, stoppage					
Say things for child					
Helpful advice					
Express concern					
Criticism, comment					
Scolding					
Imitation, teasing					
Punishment					

Instruction: Identify any specific persons. Rate the behaviors. Put a 3 if behavior is frequent or strong; put a 2 if occurrence is occasional or mild; put a 1 if occurrence is rare or absent.

identification of specific persons. As before, the table is only one possible example and can be modified. Its items can provide opportunities for extended "tell me more about" questions and other expansions and variations on items. At any time prior to this or later the clinician may want to enquire about the child's reactions to different situations or behaviors. Reactions may range from none to retreats into mutism, or they may include increased dysfluency, anger, embarrassment, tears, aggression, and so on. Clinicians will not be surprised after a while at how often parents are themselves surprised to realize that the child's reactions relate to situation stress.

General Family Life

General family life is not an area of the counseling situation that can be structured in table form because its characteristics are so general. Another reason is that some parents may resist exposing their lifestyle to formal rating. Therefore topics in this section are covered best by the clinician's ability to establish good relationships, be an uncritical listener, avoid judgments, piece together scattered comments and information, encourage without pressing, and guide conversation without being obvious. Each family will present its own areas of interest or concern, and the clinician should be alert for them. In general, interest areas might be the following:

1. Spouses' marital relationship and attitudes and behaviors toward each other.
2. Availability and responsiveness of each parent in terms of work schedules and other demands.
3. Spouses' separate philosophies of child rearing and how these interact.
4. Parents' attitudes in general toward their children. Conture (1982) notes, "We never cease to be amazed at how some parents can continually and consistently selectively attend only to the negtaive aspects of their child's behavior" (p.50).
5. Disciplinary practices in the home. Who is punished for what, differences in punishment for different misbehaviors, and so on. Particular interest in child's reactions to punishment. If there are siblings, review their punishment and reactions.
6. Repeat the previous item, more or less, replacing punishment with reward, attention, love, and so on.
7. What kind of family? Closely knit or open, quiet or noisy, talkative or nontalkative, reasonable or argumentative, emotional or balanced, and so on.

Many other areas can be explored in order to fill out a picture. This picture will be useful in determining manipulation targets, areas for transfer activities, and aspects that might profit from attention in the child's therapy sessions. Halo effects can be quite strong in this section, and so less direct approaches may be most profitable.

General Client Factors

The coverage of general client factors can be as general or specific as the clinician prefers. One can go down items on a checklist, use the "tell me about" formula, or combine the two. One possible approach is to say something in the form of

> We have discussed a lot of specifics about Ernest but haven't really discussed him as a person. Suppose I am an old friend you haven't seen for years, and I ask you to tell me all about this son of yours. What would you say?

Noting what they seem to feel would be important, the clinician can maintain the "old friend" role and ask

1. How has his health been, and what is it like now?
2. What about his diet, sleep behavior, and so on?
3. How does he get along with his brothers and sisters, and with other children?
4. How does he relate to other relatives, family friends, and peers?
5. How does he like (if applicable), daycare, preschool, or school, and how does he relate to the other children there?
6. How does he relate to the workers/teachers in 5, and how do they behave toward him?
7. What are his extracurricular activities, hobbies, sports or game interests, favorite entertainments, and the like?

These questions can be expanded, and other questions can be added as needed.

Stuttering: Information for the Clinician

The diagnosis and assessment process provided extensive information about the child's fluent and dysfluent speech. However, it has been pointed out that in-clinic speech can differ materially from out-clinic behavior. Information provided by the parents at the diagnosis can be expanded or revised as they learn more informed and structured ways of looking at stuttering. A number of therapy programs assign an ongoing monitoring task to the parents, exemplified in Figure 8–1. This is a form that can be reduced to a three-by-five filecard, or enlarged. The parents are asked when they can observe the child for at least five minutes to count the stuttering occurrences. The situation may or may not actively involve the parents. Examples of times include meals, after school or work, bedtime activities, and routine play activities. The clinician writes in the times and dates on the card, with the help of the parents. It may be useful for the parents to observe a therapy session and practice noting dysfluencies. Many clinicians keep a monitoring assignment as a permanent activity, using it also to chart transfer of fluency to the out-clinic

DYSFLUENCY SUMMARY FORM			————————	through	————————		
Time	Sunday	Monday	Tuesday	Wednesday	Thursday	Friday	Saturday
Totals							

FIGURE 8–1. Example of a daily dysfluency summary for parents to use in monitoring child.

environment. After the first one or two experiences, the parents can be asked to judge spasm severities and mark them separately. Further on in therapy other behaviors can be added or changes made.

The diagnosis and assessment report covers onset, development, and present status of stuttering. Often it is not a waste of time to cover these areas again later. Situational variables and child reactions to stuttering can be followed and reviewed periodically.

Stuttering: Information to the Parents

What information to provide parents has been discussed previously, with suggested sources provided. However, it needs emphasis that professionals should not wrap disorders or problems in mystery, but should try to inform parents about stuttering. Although parents and clients cannot be told everything, they are usually able to absorb and understand a good bit of what is offered to them. Informed parents are less likely to be apathetic, argumentative, late, or create other problems for the clinician. They are more likely to work harder at transfer, be more supportive of therapy generally, and develop greater tolerance for fluency variations in their child's speech.

Alterations in the Environment

As with general family life, any alterations in the environment should be handled with diplomacy. In this section one may have to progress in small steps. The parents can be asked frequently, "Well, what do you think can be done to . . .?" where changes are needed. Their suggestions often will need reformulation and refining, but be careful not to fall into a "yes, but" pattern of rejoinders where the parents may begin to feel frustrated. If a suggestion from them does not really solve a problem but is a step forward and indicates cooperation, then accept and reinforce it while planning to elicit changes during the process of development. Areas of alteration, discussed next, are subject to individual variation and addition.

Speech modeling for parents is a traditional activity. It also tends to be futile unless it is structured. A 30+-year-old parent is not likely to change his or her speaking pattern overall for any length of time. To do so is exhausting, irritating, and boring. The author has assigned his classes to make such a change, and they uniformly report that it makes content concentration difficult, is frequently forgotten or fluctuates, and is boring. A possible sequence of speech modeling might be as follows:

1. Observe child therapy and note the clinician's speech modeling. Discuss this and practice the desired form several times during the counseling session.
2. Select situations or times in which to use speech modeling: some of the previously selected times for child-speech monitoring, every time child starts to have a fluency breakdown, when asking the child questions, when responding directly to child questions, and so on.
3. Guard against overeffort. A slightly softer voice, a 10 percent reduction in rate, a few more pauses, and so on, will be sufficient. Speech that is too dragged, slurred, or whispered may be counterproductive.
4. If only one parent is present to acquire a model speech pattern, be sure that the model is taken home to the other person, so that parents together work out 2 and 3.
5. If possible practice the pattern with each other, friends, or older family members. Solicit reactions.
6. Provide for self-monitoring, observation of child, and reporting.
7. Respond to reports, vary targets or times, praise activity, and so on. Without reinforcement most parents will become bored and slide away from modeling.

Reassure parents that although time and again they will forget and slip into their usual speech pattern, they must keep at it.

Speech opportunities involve making sure the child has the chance to talk without undue stress or interruption. Waiting out their pauses, stifling sibling interruptions, and so on, can help. Previous sections should have elicited what/where the fluency disruptors are, and these should be targeted. Establishing a few quality-time intervals is valuable—five minutes of undivided attention while the child talks about the day, a shared story at bedtime with the child asked questions about the story or asked to retell the story, are possible times. During these times the child has no stress, criticism, correction, or interruption. Later in therapy these times can be used in transfer activities. The clinician will occasionally receive reports that the child is now a "chatter box" who won't shut up! Parents might be told in such cases that the child may be making up for lost opportunities and some tolerance is in order, but that "liberty is not license." The child can be told, "David, you have had a good chance to talk while nobody interrupted. Now it's Dorothy's turn and you should wait for her and give her a chance."

Reactions to stuttering. Advice here varies with the age and awareness of the child. For all ages, preschool to adolescence, provide the following advice for the parents to follow and to communicate to others in the environment:

> When Ernest stutters, wait quietly for him or her to finish. Do not stare, but do not look away or break eye contact. Try to keep a natural expression without becoming blank in your face. Look interested and not embarrased, upset, or terribly patient. Let Ernest finish a word without interruption, finishing it for him, or offering advice. Try not to freeze, stop what you were doing, or become obviously sympathetic.

Unless therapy indications are contrary, they are not to comment afterward to young children, although this can change if the child makes a comment about difficulty just experienced. In such instances, parents can respond with, "Yes, that was a hard one, but that's why you're going to speech therapy, to learn to talk without so much trouble. We'll all help you and it will get better." Such comments by the child should be reported to the clinician and individualized responses developed for the future. When children are older and there is more overt awareness, supportive responses and willingness to listen should be obvious. However, "advice" should not be offered unless it has been preplanned with the clinician. As therapy progresses and the child develops usable fluency or symptom controls, clinicians can advise parents how to respond when stuttering occurs.

Reactions of others was mentioned earlier but needs repeating here. Parent intervention with siblings, peers, friends and relatives, teachers, and others can be important. It also tends to make parents more consistent in their own reactions, since the all are teachers and models now. In talking with school personnel the parents, or the clinicians, should stress that people should avoid "oh, you poor thing" sympathy. Emphasize that the child is working to control his or her speech and deserves courtesy and friendly support.

Overall demands and expectations of the stutterer should be examined. It is appropriate to inform parents about research indicating possible high expectations and perfectionistic demands of parents of stutterers. Note to them that children also can have high expectations of themselves. It may be necessary, starting with speech, to have the parents identify where their expectations and demands may be too high and how they can be made more realistic. Then ask the parents to identify other areas (home tasks, drawing, printing, school work, and so on) where high demands may stress the child and reinforce self-demands for fluency perfection. Acceptance of the "best you can do" may need development, for some parents will resist this suggestion, and the clinician can only do the best that can be done. On a personal note the author is not avowing a continuation of some child-rearing and educational philosophies that demands should not be made of children or expectations advanced. Simply, excesses in either direction should be avoided.

Specific stress areas operate for most children due partly to the reality of the stress and partly to the stressed person's own perceptions. Teasing, interruption, ridicule, advice, impatience, and the like, may stress any stutterer. However, what bothers one person is not necessarily noticed by another. One child may feel stress and competition any time a particular sibling is present and talking, while another child will feel stress only if the other sibling behaves competitively and/or negatively. When appropriate, parents need guidance in looking for stress points and evaluating them. They may need help to accept the idea that individual perceptions of stress differ. Occasionally, it will be necessary to move in the opposite direction and steer the parents away from overprotection of the child.

Consistency is not a strong point for most of us, except in areas of behavioral rigidity. Parents need to understand this and try for consistency where the behavior relates to the child's speech. Previous coverage areas (monitoring, speech modeling, stress reduction, and so on) will not function effectively if not employed consistently. Occasionally, clinicians will guide parents in monitoring and charting certain of their behavioral changes in order to improve consistency.

Improve life for the child by helping to raise the youngster's self-esteem and confidence. This is difficult for many parents because they cannot separate real from false praise ("That's a beautiful picture. What is it?") or differentiate reinforcement from bribery and spoiling. With the clinician's assistance parents can identify things or tasks the child can do (*not* ought to be able to do), secure their performance, and provide appropriate reinforcement or reward. Adequate quality time spent with the child may have to be planned, particularly if both parents work outside the home. Parents may need reminding to thank or praise a child for routinely putting toys or clothes away, washing properly, turning off the TV set, or other mundane things. They can be asked to "find" five things per day to praise or reinforce. Adequate nutrition, proper health care, adequate rest and sleep, balance between recreation and duties, balance between support and criticism—these and other areas can improve the life and self-perceptions of the child and provide a richer, stronger personality to support therapy progress.

Transfer of therapy activity on an out-clinic basis is a must. Spontaneous generalization can occur, especially with very young children in whom language formulation capacities have outrun motor abilities. However, the author's bias is to assume that all children need environmental support in transfer of fluency or control. The rationale for the bias is this: If not needed but used, then some effort was expended needlessly but no problems were created; if needed but not used, then the clinician and parents may have to deal with frustration, failure and feelings of failure, doubts about self-efficacy, loss of clinic program credibility, and other problems. In all subsequent chapters about therapy procedures it will be suggested that progressive levels of therapy should be transferred on an ongoing basis. Parent observation of therapy sessions facilitates transfer tasks. Parents can be trained, by observing and participating in therapy, to conduct home activities that have already met in-clinic success criteria. Assignments to monitor developed improvements can also be made, and parents and teachers can be used to support client work on self-monitoring, rate control, symptom control, or other skills.

ADOLESCENTS

The adolescent age range is mentioned separately in this chapter (it will be discussed more extensively in Chapter 9). It is appropriate to consider environmental counseling and manipulation of adolescents because an adolescent stutterer is probably the most difficult fluency problem with which to deal. Parents generally agree that adolescents are difficult to deal with, with or without stuttering! A clinician dealing with adolescent stutterers is well advised to be prepared to deal with that specific age group. Over and over again the author has seen parent-counseling sessions about adolescent stutterers shift irresistibly into parent-counseling sessions on dealing with adolescence. On the other side, adolescents often cannot separate their fluency problems and general environment problems, and the clinician often winds up as an interpreter and a buffer between alien species (adolescents and adults) and must struggle to keep therapy sessions focused on the primary dysfluency problem.

Parents can be informed about the problems and stresses of adolescents and given recommendations for responding to instances of dysfluency. Previous suggestions about individual and group speech interactions, stress producers, speech modeling, and so on, apply also to the adolescent. Direct reactions to dysfluencies and speech behaviors usually involve the assumptions that the client is overtly aware, suffers social penalties, has emotional reactions to stuttering, and engages in struggle and avoidance behaviors. These assumptions alter the way in which parents should react, and they might be expressed best in a paraphrase of what the parents of a 15-year-old stutterer reported to me:

> Don, we're real pleased you're working on your speech, and proud too, because it's not very easy. We want to help, but we don't want to bug you. What we will do is try and find the time to listen and be good listeners. If you stutter, we aren't going to look away, feel bad, or interrupt you. We'll wait until you finish. We'll be interested in what you say, not how you say it. We aren't going to give you advice, or gush over anything. If you or your teacher say we should or shouldn't do certain things, we'll try our best. If you want to talk about it, we'll listen for as long as you want—but we won't pry and we won't nag. We know you can do the job and we're here to help.

The mother was a secretary and the father an engine repair man. Neither had college educations, but their message to their son was a model for counseling goals. In therapy session the son shrugged it of with an "Aw, my folks gave me the pep talk bit," but his satisfaction was obvious. He did not experience a miracle cure, but progress was steady and stable, and three years later he was a student in my Introduction to Speech Disorders class. To qualify the happy anecdote, I must note that my ratio of family referrals to outside counselors for special therapies for adolescents is about 10 : 1, compared to other age groups.

SCHOOLS AND TEACHERS

This section on schools and teachers will be brief because the complex nature of the subject requires either brevity or extensive detail. Elsewhere entire chapters and books have been devoted to the topic of schools and teachers, but very few sources consider the classroom teacher in detail. Egland's (1970) book is devoted to speech problems and the teacher. In the chapter on stuttering he provides examples of how teachers can help or hinder therapy. He is careful to point out that "in the work of every good teacher or therapist, we find more favorable influences than unfavorable ones" (p.214). The chapter provides pages of discussions and examples of helping and hindering behaviors and suggestions for help. Leith (1984a) refers briefly to teacher significance and utilization, Wells (1987) provides several useful suggestions, and Speech Foundation of America publications provide valuable information. In general, interaction with the classroom teacher can encompass the following:

1. Information, in general, about stuttering; in particular, about the age range in which they teach.
2. Encouragement of referral. Thompson (1984) and other authors have reported that teachers are excellent referral sources.
3. Supplementing diagnosis and assessment activity by consulting teachers specifically about speech and generally about school work, attitude and behavior, and peer interactions.
4. Reports to teachers of therapy activity, goals, progress and problems, and what can be expected.

5. Working with the teacher to reduce areas of stress, facilitate communication, find areas of class performance that can be rewarded, modeling good speech patterns, and so on.

6. Monitoring child performance on the basis of clinician input as therapy progresses, cooperating in clinic and class assignments, becoming an S+ or positive reinforcer (Leith 1984a) for fluency efforts, and otherwise supporting the therapy program.

CHAPTER SUMMARY

Some will read this chapter and feel concern because it devotes pages to an area that they feel is of doubtful value to therapy or that they feel may be professionally inappropriate for the speech and language clinician. Others will read the same material and feel that too little space has been devoted to an important area of activity for the speech and language clinician. As author, I tried to stand in the middle, but personally lean to the feeling that more should be said. Although in support of the theory view of neural integrity and neurophysiological causes of stuttering, I do not downplay the significance of environment and the interactions with what the child brings to it. Parsimony or applications of Occam's razor often push the clinician to rely solely on direct therapy with the client when that is the only feasible approach. However, ignoring the environment, when necessary, is regrettable; when elective, it may be reprehensible. Commitment to the quality of therapy argues that we do our best in all areas, and this should include the environment in which the stutterer lives and interacts.

CHAPTER NINE
ATTITUDE, MOTIVATION, AND EMOTION
Concerns and Controversies

OVERVIEW

Chapter 8 focused on environment and the stutterer's interaction with the persons in it. Areas of counseling and manipulation were discussed, with the goals of reducing disruption and stress factors while enhancing those things that facilitate communication. In this chapter, and the following one, interaction continues to be emphasized, but focus now is on the client. How does he or she feel about the interactive environment? What factors need to be considered? What techniques and procedures are available for dealing with motivation, attitudes, and feelings? The author will not recommend a therapy devoted singularly to attitude therapy, just as fluency shaping or symptom control will not be advocated as complete approaches by themselves.

The first process is to review some of the information we have, and lack, concerning psychosocial aspects of stuttering in children. The agreements and disagreements among clinicians concerning the value of psychosocial concerns are also considered. It is then concluded that we lack support to mandate attitude therapy as a major part of every therapy program and have insufficient support for the general omission of psychosocial concerns in therapy. Following this conclusion, the rest of the chapter is devoted to the important topic of client motivation and factors relating to it. Chapter 10 continues the psychosocial topic and considers various approaches to and procedures for working with the stutterer's attitudes and feelings.

Points of View

Just as the significance of parents and the environment was reviewed in Chapter 2, so was the overall question of adjustment and personality factors in the stutterers. However, points of view relative to young stutterers were not emphasized. In this discussion of the points of view, some of the citations concern adult stutterers, but most deal with preschool through adolescence age groups. Moore and Nystul (1979) studied children aged 4 to 13 years and found that stutterers more often than non-stutterers had different attitudes toward their two parents. They more often were positive toward their mothers but ambivalent in feelings about their fathers. The authors commented that this split could lead to children playing off one parent against the other in order to stabilize their own environments. Such manipulative behavior could be transfered to situations outside the home. Earlier Gildston (1967) reported that junior high stutterers perceived their parents to be less accepting than did non-stutterers, and they also scored lower in self-acceptance. In a different view Yairi and Williams (1971) stated that sixth-grade and seventh-grade stutterers, compared to controls, tend to see their parents as being less hostile and controlling and as more loving and autonomous.

Stutterers have been described as more anxious, shy, and insecure, and as more hostile (Santostefano 1960), as having more anal- and oral-aggressive tendencies among adolescents (F.H. Silverman et al. 1972), and (on Rorschach plates) were more fantasy oriented, withdrawn, stimulable, and adaptable to outer reality and showed more manic trends (Meltzer 1944). It has also been reported that stutterers are less adequate in social confidence and tend more to social isolation and sensitivity (Greiner et al. 1985). High school seniors with general speech disabilities were found to be less adequate in motivation and self-image. In considering younger children, Moncur (1955) evaluated 48 stutterers, about 6.5 years of age, and reported that when compared to controls, they more often were aggressors, guarded more, had more nightmares and nocturnal enuresis (bedwetting), had more eating problems, and displayed more negativism. On the other hand, Prins (1972) failed to find a consistent relationship between stuttering and personality factors. However, the finding that the control groups scored lower in personal and social adjustment areas confused the issue and led to a recommendation of further research.

The area of stutterer attitude and anxiety has been the subject of a number of investigations. Quesal and Shank (1978), using the original

Erickson S-scale (1969) of attitudes toward speaking, evaluated stutterers, voice and articulation problems, and normal speakers. Their average scores, rounded off, were 27, 21, and 14, respectively, indicating the poorest attitudes among stutterers. Nuttall and Scheidel (1965) had stutterers and controls rate the "fear potential" of 30 speech and 24 nonspeech situations. The two groups were equivalent in rating nonspeech situations, the stutterers were significantly higher in their fear of speaking situations, and when an "if I didn't stutter" clause was introduced, they fell below the nonstutterers in their expressions of fear. Gray and Karmen (1967) investigated nonverbal anxiety among stutterers, finding differences between subgroups of stutterers and between them and nonstutterers. Peters and Hulstijn (1984) evaluated stutterers and nonstutterers on aspects of verbal anxiety and certain physiologic correlates during speech and nonspeech tasks. They found that the stutterers did not show a generally higher level of anxiety overall. However, they did differ in terms of debilitating anxiety measurement and reported higher levels of subjective anxiety. They concluded that stutterers' anxiety seems to be limited to the cognitive portion and not physiologic areas (although they suggested that their physiologic measures might have been relatively insensitive). Nevertheless, they proposed that therapy targeting cognition and attitude might be more effective than would be relaxation therapy procedures.

With the studies of attitudes and speech or nonspeech anxiety, there is a question of how aware speakers and listeners are to stuttering. Previous discussions of awareness have suggested that children, more often than many realize, are aware of their own stuttering. Thompson (1984) in her survey of 48 school-age stutterers stated that children are aware of their stuttering and often are quite knowledgeable about it. Further, she reported that nearly all children were not unwilling to talk about their stuttering, even though about 75 percent of the children had apparently received criticism, teasing, or ridicule from peers and/or siblings because of their stuttering. It seems apparent that the children are aware, and it is probable that this awareness translates into self-evaluation. F.H. Silverman and Williams (1972) evaluated the ability of 38 stutterers, grades 3 through 6, to evaluate the amounts of stuttering experienced in controlled situations. Using a seven-point scale, the children's (30 of 38) ratings were in accord with measured dysfluencies during the speaking situations. In another study Woods (1974) evaluated 24 stutterers, each, in the third and sixth grades, each class group being divided equally into mild and moderate to severe categories. Compared to nonstuttering peers, the stutterers rated themselves and were rated by their peers as being significantly poorer speakers. Yet this apparently had no effect on social position measures.

Evaluation

The foregoing paragraphs repeat what has been written previously in this text and in other sources: We do not have a typical "stuttering personality," and part of the stuttering stereotype encountered so often is not based on verified factors. Research has also failed to verify that stuttering generally has an emotional or anxiety-based etiology behind its causation. It seems, however, that stutterers do have poorer attitudes toward speaking and exhibit more anxiety and fear toward the speech act. Whether this attitude/anxiety relative to speech can be related to fluency variations is arguable (Ingham 1984), although many clinicians operate on such an assumption.

With children who stutter the psychosocial situation becomes more controversial. Studies cited in this section suggest awareness levels and accurate evaluation of stuttering by many children. Does that translate automatically into anxiety and attitude problems? Evaluative research on children, compared to that on adults, is sparse. The small amount of data available is vitiated by the situation that, for example, a 5-year-old and a 6-year-old can have many more differences (total) than two persons of 25 and 26 years of age. Grouping young children across even limited ages may blur results and render statistical significance levels (if used) meaningless. Among children below the approximate age of 8 years, research is further blurred by the possible inclusion of spontaneous remissers who seem to outgrow their stuttering and leave the population. Are they the "same thing" as stutterers who continue in the dysfluency group? If they are not, how might they affect the results of studies? Finally, the question of stutterer subgroups needs to be mentioned again. Research populations can be skewed inadvertently, especially if subgroups among children are more "pure," not having picked up any, or as many, of the psychosocial, motor, or other subgroup characteristics. Part of our problems may relate to the instruments we use. Devore, Nandur, and Manning (1984) failed to differentiate elementary school children on the A-19 attitude scale toward speaking (Guitar & Grims 1977) but found several areas of differences when projective drawings were used. They also reported that during therapy significant changes occurred in the stutterers' drawings. We may be using test instruments that are inappropriate, insensitive to subclinical problems, or subject to design and analysis problems. In looking for an anxiety disorder, we may be like the farmer who puts up fences to protect crops while tiny mites and aphids slow growth and reduce yield on the fenced-in plants. Gerstman (1983) makes two significant points about anxiety and stuttering. First, although there may not be a clinical anxiety disorder present, it is not inappropriate for a stutterer to suffer anxiety about stuttering. Second, many of the things stutterers are anx-

ious about are the same stresses that would cause anxiety for nonstutterers. In general, we have an unclear situation. Thus, in the following section we review the philosophies of various clinicians to examine attitude
and emotion in terms of therapy concerns.

THERAPY CONTROVERSIES

Background and Definitions

Sermas and Cox (1982) agree that stutterers may have excessive social sensitivity and obsessive personality trends but state that research has
failed to establish the structure of a typical stuttering personality. They
question the general efficacy of psychotherapy and suggest that physiologic, or psychophysiologic, approaches may be more appropriate in therapy. Riley and Riley (1983) reported that 83 percent of their child stutterers placed unrealistic demands upon themselves. Further, about 25
percent of the chronic-level stutterers translated emotions into specific-
word avoidance. The clinicians stated that such avoidances must be dealt
with first in therapy, a la Sheehan and Van Riper. If not, the client may
misuse various fluency-enhancing methods in order to avoid normal production of feared words.

Although the foregoing points of view about psychosocial therapy
require further discussion, first we need to consider definitions. Literally
any procedure that alters the behavior of the client is psychotherapy.
However, different clinicians use terms in various ways. Some reserve *psychotherapy* to mean the classical and innovative therapies utilized by psychi-
atrists and counseling psychologists with clients suffering from clinical
neuroses or psychoses. In such instances, other psychological treatments
are likely to be called attitude therapy, anxiety therapy, or other names.
Definitions are complicated by differing clinician practices grouped under
identical or similar labels. For instance, attitude therapy may cover only
attitudes toward stuttering, or may include attitudes in general toward
speaking, or attitudes toward self in the wholistic sense, or attitudes toward therapy, and so on. Combinations also occur. As a result, two clinicians may both reject what they term attitude therapy but define it so that
one is 100 percent pure in the rejection, while the other uses some procedures the first would call attitude therapy. Similarly, with two clinicians
who advocate and use attitude therapy, one might use certain procedures
throughout a therapy that was overwhelmingly fluency or symptom control oriented, while the other clinician's primary goal is to treat the stutterer's attitude and feelings relative to stuttering. These polychotomous
orientations need to be kept in mind as we consider therapy controversies,
especially because a person on one side may inappropriately define the
other side into the most extreme end of the definition range. The latter

technique is a convenient method of debate, but it is not useful in discussion and solution finding. With these considerations, let us review some of the questions about nonspeech emphases in therapy.

Variations in Orientation

A number of clinicians are aware of definition problems and warn against overcommitment by the clinician, especially if she or he lacks training and experience. Shames and Florance (1982) distinguish between attitude and adjustment problems, indicating that for some there is the assumption that stuttering is a surface symptom of a deeper emotional problem. They appropriately reserve such therapy to those trained in the particular specialty but question their efficacy as far as changes in speech dysfluency problems are concerned. Wingate (1984d), although arguing that client attitudes toward stuttering (and speech in general) are critical, warns that we should not get carried away over attitude except where it impinges directly on the stutterer's willingness to be objective about the problem, to accept it, and to not hide it. However, Wingate does not favor what he regards to be an overemphasis on attitude by some therapy programs. Brutten and Hegde (1984) separate classical psychotherapy and attitudinal therapy, noting that few clinicians are trained to do the former and many engage in the latter. They recognize adherents to, and critics of, attitudinal therapy and comment that since most attitude therapies also combine direct speech therapy methods as well, the validity of differing points of view is difficult to evaluate. In a similar pattern of concern, Riley and Riley (1984) caution that the speech and language clinician is not a psychotherapist involved with restructuring a child's ego, but they do maintain it is often necessary to alter a child's attitudes. Self-demands for perfection particularly are pinpointed for attention. They recommended starting with some nonspeech behavior and using this to demonstrate change possibilities. And they suggest role playing by both participants to explore behavioral alternatives. In the process the child learns to look for behavioral alternatives, to evaluate them, and to select the most viable one. Other goals include reducing any felt need for perfect speech and improving self-concept in general. We thus have two points of view stating that most of us are not qualified to perform classical psychotherapy but are equipped and should be involved in various forms of attitude therapy as long as we do not become carried away by it.

Recommendations for Psychosocial Approaches

A number of clinicians have recommended concern about attitudes, feelings, and the social interaction of stutterers (Van Riper 1973; Goraj 1974; Sheehan 1975; Shames & Florance 1982; Fiedler & Standop 1983; Guitar 1976). Some clinicians are widely encompassing in their concern, so that Dalton and Hardcastle (1977) state that all stutterers, regardless of overt symptoms, need to work on psychological aspects. Therapy may be so simple as to be limited to attitude exploration, or it may be much deeper and more extensive. Some clinicians suggest using the client as part of environmental manipulation discussed in the previous chapter. Langlois, Hanrahan, and Inouye (1986) recommend that parent-child interactions be evaluated and, when there is concern, urge the active involvement of the parents in the child's therapy sessions so that they can learn to identify and modify certain interactions. This approach is preferred over the usual parent-counseling method. Cooper (1984) objects to behavior-oriented therapy training that creates clinicians who are technicians without skills in dealing with client feelings and attitudes. Riley and Riley (1984, 1979) advocate early attention to attitude factors in children, suggesting that overall self-concept, perfectionistic fluency criteria, and dysfluency concerns often need attention. They also state that about 25 percent of their sample used stuttering to manipulate parents and the family. Murphy (1977) argued that because stutterers vary widely in their characteristics, therapy will succeed most when the entire range of the client's behaviors, not just speech, is considered. He states that the client's feelings are important and sometimes need to be the central focus of therapy.

Reservations about Psychosocial Approaches

Not all clinicians agree that feelings and attitudes are highly significant in therapy, especially among children who have not had the time/experience accumulate to favor development of problems in the area. As noted previously, some of these clinicians demur only at therapy programs that have motivation, attitude, and feelings as their major or sole focus. Others, especially in therapy with young children, question any emphasis on, or even any use of, psychosocial therapy techniques. Prins and Miller (1973) evaluated 16 adolescent stutterers on a paper-and-pencil personality scale and failed to find a relationship between test scores and therapy improvement or posttherapy regression. They suggested that in evaluating therapy, personality factors should operate as an independent variable.

Ryan (1974) has been discussed and quoted before as feeling that attitude or anxiety factors do not require attention in therapy, since they are more likely to be effects (not causes) of stuttering. If therapy achieves fluency, then anxiety and attitude problems should disappear. Webster (1979) has been identified as an opponent to therapy designed to deal with a stutterer's anxieties, attitudes, and fears. He has argued that if therapy deals appropriately with speech elements, then attitude factors "may be largely tangential to the course of treatment" (p. 227). Ryan (1979), in discussing therapy with children, expressed a similar view when he stated, "It seems far better to focus entirely on the speech act and help the child become normally fluent" (p. 150). He argued that behavior affects attitude and if we change the behavior, we change the attitude: "Is it enough to change their speech? Most of our data suggest that for many people it is enough." (p. 141). Ingham (1984) has objected to the use of counseling procedures in therapy, since they create dependency problems. He suggests that interpersonal relationships may interfere with response counting, and that the content of the client's speech is less important than its form. In discussion of therapies to reduce anxiety, he states that of the studies he reviewed, "not one has demonstrated that the treatment of speech-related or situation-related anxiety produced reduced stuttering in relevant situations" (p. 143). He was writing with reference primarily to studies where such techniques as reciprocal inhibition variations were used. Certainly some clinicians feel that research does not support the idea of attitudinal therapy needs with children. They feel that most young stutterers do not have problems in self-confidence, talkativeness, or social interaction abilities. Where these might exist to some degree, it has been suggested that therapy to secure fluency will ameliorate any possible problems as the therapy becomes effective. Planning for attitude therapy is not recommended generally and should be reserved for the specific child who overtly presents problems.

The preceding paragraphs have summarized the concerns of several clinicians about the need for, value of, and/or rationale for therapy with attitudes and feelings. The views expressed have been those of proponents and opponents and of those with reservations. Throughout this discussion the writer has been very aware of the definitions provided earlier and trusts that no clinician was placed artificially or had a philosophy overgeneralized. In the next subsection an effort is made to discuss the compatibilities or cooperations possible between the two approaches to therapy.

Amalgamation?

Most clinicians have taken the position that fluency, or symptom, therapy and attention to motivation, attitude, and feelings are not at all incompatible. They generally subscribe to the conclusions reached by Gronhovd and Zenner (1982). These authors reviewed research and therapy reports and concluded that speech situation stress tends to increase stuttering, that fluency improvements alone may not reduce anxiety about speaking, and that anxiety reduction therapy can improve fluency. All too often, research on dichotomous forms of therapy has confused results rather than clarified differences. Martin and Haroldson (1969a) evaluated two groups of stutterers (ten in each group) where one group received eight information-attitude therapy sessions and the other received eight TO conditioning treatments. The researchers reported that neither group showed pretherapy or posttherapy attitude changes. The information-attitude group showed little reduction in stuttering, and the TO group's fluency relapsed during posttreatment evaluation. With questions about subject N, group composition characteristics, content of therapy, dysfluency parameters considered, adequacy of the attitude test, appropriateness of the speaking modes used for measurement, and the validity of using eight therapy sessions to generate results, it is not surprising that final answers elude us.

A general response to therapy controversy has been to combine elements of both approaches. Cooper (1971a) was an early advocate of combining behavior modification and psychosocial methods in stuttering therapy. Ladouceur and Saint-Laurent (1986) have reported favorably on the results of combining therapy procedures to address simultaneously speech fluency, cognitive problems, and emotional areas. In a recent report Ramig and Wallace (1987) evaluated direct and combined direct-indirect therapy of dysfluency, reporting that the combined approach was more effective. Their "indirect" reference was primarily to parent counseling and environmental manipulation, but it seems likely that the same consideration would apply to combining speech production therapy and procedures dealing with feelings and attitudes.

The most appropriate conclusion seems to be that it is not safe to take a dogmatic stand about speech or about psychosocial therapy. To do so, in either direction, is to risk not meeting the needs of therapy clients. In reviewing personal experiences with 21 stuttering children, ages five years or less, the author summarized the following: Therapy was terminated for one child and referral to a child psychologist secured; three sets of parents required referral to special counselors; eight children received special attention to motivation and individual adjustments in reinforcement contingencies, behavior modification fluency therapy, and the parents participated in brief and routine counseling activities; 12 children received major attention to motivation, attitude, and emotions, along with intensified parent counseling, but all 12 children also received variations of behavior modification procedures to establish and transfer fluency.

In the next section a discussion of motivation, flexibility, and variation is emphasized.

MOTIVATION

Definition and Background

A frequent question in daily life is in some form of "What is your motivation for doing this?" It is applied by actors, business persons, sports figures—by almost everybody. Most of the time the word *motivation* translates to "reason," or "Why are you doing this?" For instance, why are you reading this book? Motivation, based on *motive,* is literally the things or conditions that move a person (motive force), or

> something that prompts a person to act in a certain way or that determines volition; incentive; the goal or object of one's actions. (Stein 1967, p. 934)

Motivation level, or strength, is an expression of how strongly we desire to achieve or perform. On a cognitive basis, motivation can be internal or external, or a combination of both. You might read a book because you are interested in it (internal motivation) or because you will be tested on its contents (external motivation). For all students perhaps there can be a combined motivation. However, on a noncognitive basis motivation is internal and is related to the functions of the reticular activating and inhibiting systems and their complex linkage with the limbic emotional and autonomic function systems. All of us have had experiences where we say, "No matter how hard I try, I can't get interested in . . . ." Assuming normalcy in other factors (health, fatigue, distraction, and so on), this is a case where cognition fails to overcome the lack of internal motivation or incentive. In therapy we deal with motivation on multiplex levels, which include, but are not limited to,

1. Motivation (awareness, concern) toward changing the speech problem.
2. Motivation (acceptance) toward entering therapy.
3. Motivation (agreement) toward the goals of a particular therapy.
4. Motivation (stimulation, liking) of specific therapy techniques and procedures.
5. Motivation (response to) toward methods used to reward and/or punish performance in therapy.
6. Motivation (belief in) toward transfering in-clinic progress to the outside world.

Without motivation, there is apathy. Persons in acute depressive states can neglect even the basic requisites of living because they lack the motivation. In the popular term *burn-out,* in the 1980s we have labeled a situation in which people appear (due to stress?) to lose the motivation they formerly had for what they were doing. The reasons may be varied, but the loss of motivation is one result. In speech and language therapy we must deal with the six (or more) aspects of motivation cited in the list. If we do not, or are not successful, then therapy suffers. When we deal with motivation, we are dealing with attitudes and emotions. They are not separable from motivation. Our motivations are reflected in our attitudes and feelings, and the latter are major factors influencing the former. Motivation is a psychophysiologic and psychosocial phenomenon, which we tend to stress as an important aspect in therapy. This is particularly true in working with child communication disorders, since the cognitive input to motivation is (usually) less than it will become as maturity occurs. Culatta and others (1985) have reviewed research and writing relative to motivation and performance in behavior modification therapy programs. Not unexpectedly the literature widely supports the importance of motivation. They link this to research suggesting that young children are not particularly concerned about their disfluencies, and they offer the implication that this lack could have a negative impact on therapy. Indeed, in considering motivation and children, there are a number of factors to evaluate.

Factors Affecting Motivation

Age of the client can affect motivation. Group I children, the youngest group, tend to be most responsive to their home environment and to follow the encouragement or mandates of their parents. Motivation and interest tend to be more transient than in older groups so the clinician needs more variation and flexibility. Cognitive factors are of less significance in this age group, so that applications of reward, pleasure, or fun, verbal and tangible, are more likely to be effective. Pressure and punishment can be effective as long as the intensity is not too high, duration too long, or frequency too great. Group II children, the elementary group, have partially exchanged their home environment for the outside world. Parents and home influences can operate strongly and be used effectively, if available. Cognitive motivation values tend to depend on the child's insight maturity, stuttering severity, and environmental penalties encountered. The clinician's authority and pressure can be powerful motivators as the child comes to accept that life seems to be made up of adults telling him or her what to do. However, this approach should not be pushed too far, and emotional motivators of reward and punishment are valuable. Group therapy, particularly in schools, can be a powerful motivator through the combined values of shared interests and problems, competition, and peer example and pressure. Group III children, those in the adolescent range, will most often pose problems in motivation. Emotional motivators can be used, but the approach often has to be cognitive in nature. The client usually must understand and accept some rationale for what she or he is doing, although rapport and emotional support may be very important. Adolescents may reject cognitive motivation simply because it originates from a suspect source (any person over 17 years of age). If they do not supply their own motivation, cognitively and emotionally, therapy rapport may be the access point for the clinician in influencing motivation.

Severity of stuttering is usually positively related to motivation. The higher the level of severity, the higher the level of motivation. In symptom therapy the ratio is almost algebraic. In fluency therapy it is less direct but may operate particularly in transfer and maintenance work when the client balances the penalties of "some stuttering" against the physical fatigue and boredom of monitoring and using fluency control methods.

Penalties felt by the stutterer usually relate to severity, but not always. Mild to moderate stuttering can receive severe penalties from some parents, teachers, and peers. In some situations this may reduce motivation to engage in any kind of speech activity, including therapy. However, in such cases, if the initial unwillingness can be pierced and reassured, the client often displays an above-average motivation.

Therapy format covers a great deal of territory. Whether or not the child likes therapy, tolerates it, or hates it is motivation all by itself. It has been stated that almost any therapy, no matter how unusual, will help some stutterers. The reverse is true in that we have no one therapy procedure that will help all stutterers. Clinicians find this out as they try to use a particular package program repetitively. Not only will children of different ages respond differently to the same program, children of exactly the same age will respond differently. Although symptom therapy is not used often with children, some (particularly adolescents) may respond well to it. Punishment, in the form of verbal feedback or TO, works very well with many children, but some respond too strongly and motivation is hurt. In the same way, certain children glow and prosper under rewards or positive reinforcement systems, while others take such systems casually and are motivated more by punishment. Therapy methods also include the clinician. E-M. Silverman and Zimmer (1982) evaluated ten male and ten female stutterers on aspects of therapy they most and least liked and similarly asked them to rate clinician attributes. Although the very small N requires interpretive caution, results indicated that attitude modification, group sharing, self-confidence building, and desensitization were among the most liked aspects of therapy. Favored clinician attributes included intelligence, competence, sincerity, and a genuine desire to help. The results do not agree with some of those who prefer a speech-shaping focus in therapy, to the exclusion of personal factors. Silverman and Zimmer maintain that success in therapy reflects how well speech behaviors and personal feelings are combined by a clinician who projects an attitude of caring, dedication, and genuine warmth. Although these data were obtained from adult subjects, there is no reason to exclude their application to children, especially the adolescents. Finally, therapy effects can be a motivating factor with certain stutterers. Nothing encourages success like success. An advantage fluency therapy has over symptom modification approaches is its near-instant creation of stutter-free speech. Children may enjoy being able to communicate without stuttering dysfluencies, and with the reinforcements they receive for fluency. However, this is not a universal. This author has had children as young as seven years reject rate control, prolongation, easy onset, and so on, because it "sounds dumb," took too much effort, and was as bad to them as stuttering was. Explaining that an early stage of therapy is not the final goal may solve the problem. Recently an adolescent stutterer reasoned thus:

> Oh, yeah, but . . . this way of talking sucks. I don't stutter, but I sound like a freak. But if I speed it up, you know, go back to the real me—then I'm gonna stutter. So where's the edge for me?

The clinician needs to probe every client in terms of responses to the particular therapy used and the component parts of it. All too often clinicians express, "That method didn't work. Now what do I do?" rather than taking a problem-solving approach to figure out why a method failed. Frequently resolution of minor problems, or slight changes in technique, will establish or restore motivation.

Perception of therapy needs to be considered in the more general sense. How does the client feel about therapy per se? Fewest problems occur in Group I, and the most occur in Group III. Adolescents, in their drives to be liberated and to be different, are often strongly opposed to anything that marks them as being different among their peers. However, the same can occur at any age (we had to include a two-year-old sibling in therapy with his four-year-old sister); usually the drive for peer acceptance and conformity is worst during the school years. Going to "speech class" is for some children like the mark of Cain, so that considerable support may be required to adjust their attitudes and motivations.

Many other factors can affect motivation. Therapy that interferes with or replaces preferred activities, time of day, "enemies" in the therapy group, and many individual factors can operate. Not all can be known, and not all known factors can be dealt with. For some children high motivation is represented by a quietly grudging willingness to work, while other children can become too motivated or excited and need quieting influences. Once in a while motivation is so lacking that therapy must be postponed, terminated, or revised drastically (Peins, McGough & Lee 1984).

ONGOING MOTIVATION

Motivation is an attitude or an emotional expression. Therefore it is a mistake to assume constancy of motivation. Boredom, disenchantment, diminished rewards, progressively more difficult tasks, altered perceptions of therapy—or of anything—can alter motivation. As this author has seen, after weeks of high motivation and hard work a child can lose most of his or her motivation because a favored peer makes a slighting remark about therapy. And so motivation must be monitored constantly. After each session the clinician should consider the following:

1. Occurrence of negative client remarks, "yes, but" responses, or other overt verbal signs.
2. Nonverbal signs in facial expressions, postural messages, slow responses, etc.
3. Late appearance for or absence from therapy sessions.
4. Backsliding in areas of previous progress, where reasons for backsliding seem to be lacking.
5. Plateauing or slowing in progress, when the therapy demands are not a probable cause.
6. Outside reports from parents, teachers, and so on.

If desired, most of the preceding listed can be translated into observable behaviors, counted, and charted as an ongoing measure of motivation.

A possible cause of motivation reduction is the therapy or the clinician, or both. Behavior modification programs are particularly susceptible to this because their multiple repetitions and carefully graduated steps can become monotonous to the child. Many programs deliberately schedule breaks to compensate for boredom and repetition fatigue. The clinician can become involved also. If one is using the same program multiple times per week with different clients, it is easy to slip into rote responses, let stereotype patterns predominate in speech, lose spontaneity, and lose that air of sincerity and genuine warmth referred to earlier.

Transfer and Maintenance Motivation

The purpose of all therapy is to alter a person's behavior or perceptions in his or her daily life. If this does not occur, then therapy has failed. Indeed, daily life, or out-clinic reality, is the final test of in-clinic achievement. A fluency rate of 0.5 or less SW/M in therapy is meaningless unless that frequency can be transferred outside the therapy setting. In-clinic ability to use pullouts or preparatory sets also is meaningless if transfer and stable use does not occur. In transfer and maintenance (both areas are discussed further in Chapter 17) motivation is a significant factor. Therapy in the clinic usually provides the clinician as a constant source of reminder and motivation. Out-clinic performance must have other motivators, however. Spontaneous transfer and stabilization can be counted on with some, but not all, Group I children. Here parents can be counseled and trained to serve as reminders and to be motivators. But the motivation problem generally increases as we go up in client age in Groups II and III, and factors that militate against motivation can be significant. Self-doubt or questions of self-efficacy, and doubts about therapy efficacy, are common problems that attack motivation. Distraction or preoccupation with more interesting things also affect motivation and incentive. However, the most universal problems are probably those relating to fatigue and boredom.

As discussed earlier, any fluency or symptom control system requires effort, and monitoring of speech also requires energy expenditure. Things that tire us over time are not likely to be high-motivation activities, especially if we are already tired or stressed for other reasons. Shames and Florance (1980) have described a nonmonitoring monitoring program, but its reality is debatable. Wingate (1984d) recommends against setting a goal of stutter-free speech, normal speech, or similar targets. He states that "some stutterers may be able to attain speech which has neither actual or incipient stutters, and many can aspire to this as an eventual goal, but it is unlikely that most stutterers will achieve it" (p. 280). When we establish a speech pattern that requires fluency planning or symptom control and monitoring, we are asking the client to engage in overt physical activity, and that can be boring and tiring. Over time, attention to minimally changing stimuli tends to reduce until it becomes nonexistent because the motivation for attention is lost. Therapy programs have included scheduling self-therapy sessions, in-clinic booster sessions, covert and overt observation, stickers with motivational phrases, posttherapy support groups, and monitoring schedules and contracts. In our fight against relapse, motivation is probably our most important tool and our most difficult challenge.

Section Summary

The issue of motivation is basic to the entire area of attitudes and emotions. At times there seems to be an effort to separate motivation from emotions and attitudes and to direct therapy activity toward it while rejecting "attitudes and emotions" as concerns as if they were not all part of one package. Such separation is not possible because one reflects the other. This section has discussed some of the factors that affect motivation and different ways in which motivation affects therapy and may be affected by it. Few specific suggestions have been offered because individual variation means that standardized approaches are not appropriate. Each client will require specific attention to his or her pattern of motivation. Indeed, a particular suggestion here is for the clinician to be careful in applying therapy procedures where motivation, reinforcement, and punishment are programmed rigidly into the process.

CHAPTER SUMMARY

As the first of two chapters dealing with nonspeech factors, attention has been focused first on issues and controversies and then on motivation in therapy. The initial review makes it clear that stutterers, as a group, do not have a particular personality profile. It is possible and probable that they may more often be overly sensitive in social interactions, have poorer self-images and higher self-expectations, and lower anxiety thresholds. ✗ There seems to be little question that attitudes toward speaking are poorer, and that stuttering or the anticipation of stuttering represents anxiety-producing factors for them. The significance of these views currently is a source of debate, with the involvement of attitudes and feelings in therapy ranging from almost none to almost total. Taking the view that reality lies somewhere between the extremes, this chapter has moved to a brief consideration of the basic psychosocial factor in therapy, motivation, to provide a bridge to the next chapter, which more directly concerns therapy procedures dealing with attitudes and emotions. Do not forget this bridge, for this chapter has acted as prologue to the next, and many of the concerns or procedures explored in the chapter that follows relate significantly to the factor of motivation.

CHAPTER TEN
ATTITUDES, MOTIVATION, AND EMOTION:
Techniques and Procedures

OVERVIEW

Background

The mature stutterer typically carries an accumulation of attitudes, fears, anxieties, and other emotions developed over the chronology of stuttering years. The focus of this accumulation may be quite narrow, targeting only speech or speaking situations, and may be limited even to the particular occasions when stuttering is most likely. Falck (1969) has commented that stutterers often tend to "think like stutterers," even when they are not talking. For others stuttering may have affected a broad range of personal feelings, attitudes, and social interactions. In the same vein, the intensity of the accumulation will vary, so that range of intensity will be from mild to extremely severe. Individual reactions will tend to vary individually in terms of their focus and intensity. We can expect, therefore, to encounter varying combinations and degrees of word fears, avoidances of various types, antiexpectancy and compensatory behaviors, disturbed evaluation and distorted self-image factors, and particularly personal modes of adjustment to stuttering. Goraj (1974), while agreeing that stutterers present no stereotyped personality profile, states that the moment of stuttering can be quite emotional. For at that moment the stutterer may feel fear, tension, frustration, impatience, embarrassment, hostility, anxiety, guilt, shame, or even panic. The variability and interaction of these possibilities, plus the variations in physical stuttering patterns, make stuttering the fascinating and challenging problem it is.

When we consider stuttering in childhood, the accumulations just described are usually quite different. The foci and intensities of attitudes and feelings may range from mild to maximum levels. In general they are assumed to be minimal for Group I levels, mild to moderate in Group II ages, and approaching or at adult levels among the Group III adolescents. However, it is never safe to generalize about stuttering, and we should anticipate only what we find, not what we are looking for. Issues relevant to adjustment, anxiety, attitudes, and other factors in the psychosocial area, reviewed in several previous chapters, are relevant here. Diagnosis and assessment can encompass all these factors if we look for them, but that is not the same as allowing for them in the therapy plan. Yet almost all therapy approaches with children, directly or indirectly, contain some degree of psychotherapy (Guitar 1984).

This chapter does not argue the pro and con of psychosocial therapy, for that debate has already been reviewed. The author takes the view, like Guitar, that psychotherapy is inherent in the therapy program. The only questions relate to how obviously it is planned, the place it has in goal structures, what form or forms it will take, and how progress will be evaluated. These questions can be rephrased as action statements to propose that therapy should do the following:

1. Have goals clearly defined to meet the client's emotional needs. These may be limited to basic motivation and reinforcement needs or extend to significant factors of attitude and social interaction.
2. Assign a value to the goals developed in 1, since goal significance will determine the organization and characteristics of therapy.
3. Be structured so that therapy meets the needs and values assigned. Behavior modification, fluency, symptom, or interaction structures (or combinations of them) should be utilized because that is what the client will respond best to. Once the basic choice is made, then the plan should consider what amendments are desirable to secure the best responses from the client.
4. Be designed so that consideration of psychosocial factors can be evaluated. If attitudes are to be changed, that change should be measured. If methods are used to secure particular responses, then occurrence of those responses should be used to measure method effectiveness. Goal statements such as "improve rapport" and evaluations such as "rapport is better" are not valid.

It must be understood that psychosocial orientations are not an excuse for passive, friendly conversation masquerading as therapy. Rather, psychosocial orientations are as accountable as a goal of reducing dysfluencies per 100 words uttered. In the following sections, measurement suggestions to facilitate accountability are offered, and the reader is encouraged to develop additional measures.

Chapter Organization

The content of this chapter relates both to the chapter preceding and the one following. In particular, relaxation and desensitization procedures in Chapter 11 overlap with procedures discussed in this chapter. For instance, the first section on self-evaluation has direct relationship to desensitization procedures, and the next section on hierarchies has a similar link to desensitization and reciprocal inhibition. However, emphases here are on methods rather than on programs. It is hoped that needful relationships will be pointed out sufficiently as we go along. Play therapy and role play receive coverage because they tie in to so many different therapy approaches, while counseling considerations pervade almost every clinical activity. Final sections on bibliotherapy and group therapy are somewhat more singular, but they also can be part of overall programs. The foregoing leads to a repeat of earlier statements: None of the sections, or procedures within sections, are advanced as total programs of therapy. They are presented as variable, changeable parts to be used, omitted, or amended in the process of planning a complete program.

SELF-EVALUATION

At one time, descriptors of childhood stuttering usually included the tag ending, "with little or no awareness." As we have seen earlier, this is a misconception, and most children who stutter know it. As they mature into school age, awareness increases. Nevertheless, awareness does not necessarily connote full understanding and descriptive capacity. There is always the possibility that the stutterer develops a "not to know" desire as covert behaviors are formulated and avoidances multiply. Many clinicians have advocated self-analysis techniques (Van Riper 1958a; Chapman 1959; Johnson 1961; Cooper 1971a; Ingham 1982; Ham 1986), while others have minimized awareness to a lesser degree of importance (Ryan 1978). Ladouceur and others (1982) evaluated awareness training as part of a regulated-breathing therapy program, concluding that such awareness training had no effect on therapy outcomes. Twelve stutterers, ages 17 to 74 years, were divided into four groups of three each. All four groups received basic awareness training in activities such as describing words stuttered on and situations causing stuttering. The "awareness group" of three received additional awareness training. One must muse over the conclusion that awareness training was not effective, considering the age range factor, the N of each group, and that each stutterer in a group had a different clinician. All of the stutterers received their basic awareness training as part of two 90-minute sessions which covered nine areas of therapy, or an average of 20 minutes per area. The "awareness group" of three also received 60 minutes of additional training, primarily in keying a counter each time they stuttered. It is quite probable that other design considerations aside, the only viable conclusion the authors should have reached was that 80 minutes of therapy, any kind of therapy, is not likely to have significant effects on the long-term fluency of a client.

Self-evaluation, or self-analysis, can run the gamut from simple counting of stuttering spasms to an evaluation of complex overt and covert behaviors and feelings. As a point of origin the author offers the following definition (Ham 1986, p. 69):

> Self-analysis encompasses the awareness of each stuttering occurrence when it happens; cognizance of the type, severity, and physical location(s) of the stuttering; descriptions of the struggle, overflow, and associated behavior patterns; understanding of attitudes concerning stuttering in particular and speech in general; and a perception of the environmental reactions to moments of stuttering, as they occur. Further, to varying degrees, self-analysis encompasses the characteristics of nonstuttered speech of the stutterer and of other speakers. These elements of self-analysis should be available as part of the stutterer's own knowledge and be functional during any situation in which he or she participates.

This definition is a no-holds-barred one, formulated with reference to mature stutterers. In working with younger children the clinician will need to modify the insight depth goal.

Group I Self-Analysis

Preschool children, Group I, usually require very little in the way of self-analysis. Yet it is not a waste of time or even counterproductive to utilize awareness procedures. Children, as they grow, learn over and over that certain of their behaviors cause trouble in daily life. Running too fast may result in a fall, talking too loudly may awaken somebody, eating too quickly may cause a mess or a stomach upset, and so on. Speech awareness can be added to that list. There usually is no need for, or value in, complex and sophisticated self-evaluation as defined in the previous paragraph. However, there are degrees of awareness available to the preschool child. Since our therapy approaches usually involve some form of direct or indirect fluency enhancement, it seems better to establish the basal fluency first, without analysis. Then, using vocabulary the child can accept, questions can be inserted during therapy:

- Did you have any trouble talking just now?
- Were you talking faster or slower than usual?
- Were you faster or slower than me?
- Were you louder or softer than last time?
- Did you use more words or less words than last time?

The answers may come easily, the child may be confused, or the child can retreat to the safety of "I donno." However, further questions, suggestions, and practice will lead the child to realize that fluent speech was slower, softer, more relaxed; it released airflow, had fewer or more words, or whatever the fluency model was. This may need to be repeated a number of times in several sessions before the child internalizes the information and adds it to the memory store. The clinician can reinforce this by stopping the child when dysfluencies occur during therapy and by going through the "What were you doing?" questions, as long as this is not done so often that the child feels badgered. Here, a tape recorder playback can be useful in teaching self-analysis.

When the child seems to have a basic understanding (and some will not), the clinician can ask additional questions:

- When you have trouble at home, do you talk fast or slow? Repeat this with other production questions.
- If you are fussing with your sister, how do you talk?
- Are you likely to have speech trouble then? Use other situation-specific questions.
- Who talks fastest, loudest, uses the biggest words, talks the most, and so on, at home?

Goals in these questions, and similar ones, are for the child to become aware of when stuttering occurs and what speech behaviors are like when it does occur. The evaluation of other family members is done mainly for practice, for awareness generalization, and to reduce any sense of pressure on the child's own speech. Also, home assignments can be structured to extend awareness. As noted children will vary widely in their capacities to develop or use awareness, and the clinician should not invest time if returns are slight. As a rule of thumb the author has considered stuttering severity, degree of at-home interruptions and speech stress, and the initial awareness responses of the child in order to decide how much effort to expend on self-analysis work.

As speech therapy continues, the self-evaluation learning can be turned more and more to self-monitoring of fluency skills and away from dysfluencies. The degree to which this is done, or the degree to which self-evaluation in general is used in therapy, should depend on the child's speech and reactions to it. Costello (1983) has recommended not explaining to a child what must be done to earn positive reinforcement, nor to explain why the child was stopped because of dysfluency. For according to her explanations tend to be confusing. While correct in saying that data to support the value of awareness training are lacking, Costello also says, "Intuitively, it seems like a good sign if a child . . . consciously understands the goals of treatment and can correctly monitor his or her own behavior" (p. 83). There is no question that some children, particularly very young ones, seem to do well in fluency therapy without awareness training. However, the time investment is small in most instances and the possible values seem worth it. On the basis of personal experience, this author feels that the need for self-evaluation training seems to increase as the child's speech shows more tension, prolongation, struggle behavior, and overt reactions to spasm occurrences. With ordinary clinical skills on the part of the clinician, there is no reason for concern that the child will become overly sensitized to dysfluency. Indeed, logic suggests that knowing what we do facilitates performance.

Group II Self-Analysis

Children at the elementary school level are generally quite capable of self-analysis in their speech behaviors. Attitudes and emotions may still be difficult for them to access and understand. However, as has been discussed earlier, school-age children have typically been exposed to teasing, imitation, and ridicule—usually from their peers. This situation greatly increases the need for, and values of, self-evaluation. Shames (1975) has emphasized that self-responsibility is an important long-term goal for the stutterer, and a powerful therapy tool. He felt that most therapists leave self-responsibility to chance or self-learning by the client. Although he favored the monitoring of fluency, rather than of dysfluency, he felt that self-monitoring is an important aspect of self-responsibility development.

Group therapy with Group II children can be particularly useful in self-evaluation development. With proper handling by the clinician, children can evaluate one another. This sharpens their own monitoring skills, builds their information base about stuttering and fluency, and also contributes to the desensitization process. In situations where performance is rotated around the group, those not performing can monitor the one who is and provide feedback about fluency performance and/or the characteristics of dysfluencies. The child focused on can be asked first to report on her or his self-evaluation, and then other group members can be allowed to correct or supplement the evaluation:

- Ernest, how did you do on your slow rate that time?
- Uh, I was too fast and . . .
- He didn't draw out his sounds or . . .
- Ann, wait until I ask you. Ernest, go on.
- Well, yeah, I didn't do that either.
- Okay, good. David, what did you notice?
- He held his breath before saying "go."
- Good, I saw that too. Okay, Ann, you pick out the next story card and try.

Rather than provide suggestions here for additional procedures, we will move on to Group III to expand the discussion there, since nearly all the Group III techniques can be scaled down and simplified for use with Group II children.

Group III Self-Analysis

In general, if many clinicians do not like to work with stutterers, they want least of all to work with adolescent stutterers. (The qualities of the adolescent stutterer are discussed further in this chapter in the section on counseling.) The complications of teen-year maturation in psychological, physical, and social areas can become almost inextricably tangled with stuttering spasms, behaviors, and attitudes. Unsorting the tangle can be complicated by the fact that although they can be penetrating and critical observers of the adult world around them, many adolescents protect their often-fragile maturation by avoiding or distorting self-insights into their own characteristics and those of the environment they identify with. The problem is often exacerbated if the adolescent perceives therapy as one more effort by "the establishment" to reject and alter his or her persona, lifestyle, behavior, music preferences, or anything else. The adolescent may resist efforts to introduce fluency therapy because alterations in rate, pauses, prolongation time, syllable stress, and so on, are perceived as being different, and the rebellious and independent adolescent is often terrified of being different if that alteration is superimposed from external sources. Symptom therapy often meets similar attitudes because of the dysfluency tolerance demands and the early-stage increments in dysfluency. Indirect therapies generally fare no better because the adolescent may doubt their efficacy and/or will not collaborate in transfer activities. Pure psychotherapy, while not necessarily a bad idea overall, usually does not have a significant effect on the fluency problem, even if otherwise feasible. This author is aware of no data one way or the other, but past experience suggests that out-and-out therapy failures (as distinguished from relapses) are highest among the adolescent group and that relapse rates are probably proportionately greater than among other age groups. Add these figures to the stutterers who either avoid or reject therapy and the stutterers who are avoided by clinicians, and the total might suggest that adolescent stuttering is the most significant, least researched, worst served fluency disorder we face.

This last paragraph is not intended to suggest that therapy is not worth the effort. Rather, it is intended to serve as a background as we look at procedures. Younger children tend to accept most procedures because of their authoritarian sources, and most adults accept procedures on a combination of cognitive evaluation and *demand characteristics* (see counseling section). But adolescents are in between, and it is wise to plan therapy slowly and use self-evaluation partially for the purpose of constructing a therapy program that best matches the "between" client's speech needs and the client's willingness to cooperate. Self-evaluation procedures can penetrate facades of protective ignorance, provide early success in skill development, and help the clinician decide the most feasible goals and the most effective procedures to teach them.

The rest of this section is divided into four subsections: general analysis, stuttering analysis, situation analysis, and evaluation of feelings and attitudes. As noted previously, most of the procedures suggested can be shortened/simplified for use with Group II and some Group I children.

General Analysis

The general analysis stage is introduced to the client as a project to find out more about speech, how people talk, and particularly to explore the disfluency situation. The client is led to the first step of analysis skills, mildly desensitized to the idea of evaluation, and given support by learning that everybody has fluency breaks. Analysis is usually preceded by a short, very short, teaching session in which the clinician discusses rate, pauses, disfluencies, and related information. The next step is to perform some analyses. A useful procedure is to prepare an audiotape cassette in advance. The first item might be a minute or so of speech by a very fluent person, such as some television network newscasters. The second item might be a talk show guest who is less fluent. Additional persons can be recorded from various broadcast and life situations. A useful system is to transfer segments of monologue from ordinary persons you have recruited. Also, the clinician can rehearse and make recordings with predetermined numbers, types, and combinations of fluency breaks (not "stutterings"). These recordings are played, analyzed, and discussed, and attention then is turned to out-clinic situations (we will return to the tapes presently).

The stutterer can be asked, in-clinic, to evaluate people in his or her environment by categories such as the following:

Fastest rate	Most talkative
Slowest rate	Least talkative
Most mispronunciations	Highest/lowest pitch
Uses longest words	Loudest/softest voice
Pauses most/longest	Physical mannerisms
Verbal automatisms	Silly verbal expressions
Lively/poker face	etc.

Outside assignments can be given to verify and expand the client's judgments, and the client can be encouraged to look for anything else that differentiates one speaker from another. Additional topics can be developed for analysis, such as evaluating the listening behaviors of auditors in varying situations, appearances of self-confidence or insecurity in speech, and so on. If desired, the client can be assigned to analyze specific persons in her or his environment (parents, siblings, teachers, peers, public figures).

Spasm Analysis

This aspect or stage of self-evaluation usually requires another short teaching insert from the clinician. The client's attention is directed to specific forms of <u>disfluency/dysfluency</u>. <u>Repetitions</u>, <u>prolongations</u>, and tense <u>pause</u> and stoppages are explained; and it will be convenient if the clinician has taped examples of these produced in rather easy, undramatic fashion, sounding as normal as possible. No effort is made to pretend that this is not zeroing in on the client's speech, so the clinician may say:

> Before we look at your stuttering, we need to know more about how break-ups in speech occur, what kinds there are, and whether or not most people have similar ones in their everyday speech.

The outside analysis procedures discussed in the previous paragraph can be recycled and then repeated again (also with taped examples) to explore the behaviors associated with normal disfluencies. These behaviors include the following, used for any reasons:

- Postponements, silent and audible
- Starters, physical or verbal
- Retrials
- Revisions
- Releases, from being "stuck" on a word

Other associated behaviors can be explored, using the information from the diagnosis and assessment chapters.

At this point, the clinician would explain how all the disfluency behaviors being evaluated are also found in the speech of stutterers. The tape recorder can be utilized with a series of short segments from real stutterers the clinician has worked with in the past (avoid familiar persons), and the clinician can record his or her own easy examples for analysis. This is a good time for the clinician to produce "live" pseudostuttering, or fakes, to provide examples for illustration and analysis (Van Riper 1973; Maxwell 1982; Ham 1986). These early fakes should be easy, slow, and uncomplicated. Useful summaries of spasm characteristics and associated behaviors can be found in a number of sources (Gottlober 1953; Van Riper 1973; Ham 1986; Wells 1987).

Spasm analysis can be transferred directly to the client's speech, with the clinician providing reinforcement for progress already made. Rather than jumping directly into self-analysis, the clinician might want to combine some in-clinic practice on simple awareness, such as the following:

1. After a brief client monologue ask, "How many times did you stutter?" or "On what words . . . ?"
2. Then play back a recording of the monologue in 1 and compare reality to the client's analysis.

#5 The client can also be asked to tap the table after each spasm, then tap during each spasm, and finally just as (or before) each spasm begins. Post-monologue counts can be compared with recordings (which will pick up the table taps). On these, and on previous exercises, performance crite-*quant.* rion levels can be set quantitatively and counted if there is a desire to *analysis* compare to baseline awareness. Similarly, reinforcement and punishment schedules can be applied. While working in the practice stage, the client can be given self-evaluation forms to complete on an out-clinic basis, with #4 the form presented in Table 10–1 serving as an example. After that more complex evaluations can be done on forms and in-clinic to establish spasm severities, combinations of behaviors used, locations of spasms, respira-tory behaviors, and so on. (The following subsection on situation analysis provides additional spasm information.) Other evaluation forms are avail-able for use or adaptation by the clinician. Severity scales have been devel-oped by Lewis and Sherman (1951), Riley (1972), and Van Riper (1972). A descriptive scale published by Johnson, Darley, and Spriestersbach (1963) has been used extensively. A variation of the descriptive scale (Ham 1986), combined with situation factors, is presented in the next sub-section.

Clinicians vary in terms of how deeply they wish to utilize the spasm analysis procedures. Fluency therapies might call mainly for spasm aware-

TABLE 10–1. Stuttering Spasm Self-Analysis

Look over the items below and for each one, under Frequency of Occurrence, check how often you stutter. For any "?" (don't know) item, try to listen to your own speech during the next five to seven days to find out the answer.

BEHAVIOR	FREQUENCY OF OCCURRENCE			
	OFTEN	SOMETIMES	NEVER	?
1. Repeat sounds, syllables, or words				
2. Prolong, stretch sounds out				
3. Stop, stuck, unable to move on				
4. Postpone, delay starting a word				
5. Starter, do something to get speech started				
6. Retrial, stop and start over				
7. Revision, change what I planned to say				
8. Substitution, one word for another				
9. Release, say or do something to get out of a stutter				
10. Distractor, say or do something to keep attention away from stuttering				

ness in self-monitoring, while symptom therapy application could utilize in-depth analysis and add client pseudostuttering (Ham 1986).

Situation Analysis

The occurrence, characteristics, and severity of stuttering is affected by situation variables. Bloodstein (1949) long ago noted a number of factors that can affect stuttering. Self-evaluation of situational factors may be particularly fruitful with adolescents, since they may have vulnerabilities greater than those of older stutterers. Such analysis also is significant in contributing to the next subsection, the discussion of attitudes and feelings, and to the hierarchies and counseling sections following. These evaluations, collectively, will be of importance in transfer and maintenance development and in therapy procedures such as desensitization, relaxation, and reciprocal inhibition.

After, or during, spasm analysis activity in self-evaluation, the clinician can bring in situational factors. This can be done thus:

> Now that we have learned a little about how you stutter, we need to look at the when-where factor. This will help us locate the best and worst spots and give us important information when we tackle the stuttering itself.

Conversation with the stutterer can begin by eliciting generalizations about when stuttering behaviors occur most and least. It may be necessary to lead the client at first by structuring a list of what situations are met on a frequent-occasional-rare basis and then tracking back through them to chart stuttering. One can prepare a list similar to that in Table 10–2 and have the client rate the probability of stuttering in each situation. This sample form provides for the addition of unique situations. It can also be reversed, as in Table 10–3, so that specific situations (those indicated in a filled-out 10–2) are targeted and stuttering behaviors in each situation analyzed.

As situations are identified and evaluated, the question of feelings and attitudes is bound to be drawn in. The factors of attitude and feeling can be integrated according to the willingness of the adolescent to expose them. The idea that different situations stimulate different reactions, and that feelings affect stuttering, is explicit in Table 10–2 and can be woven into the therapy dialogue.

Analysis of Feelings and Attitudes

The portion of self-analysis that focuses on feelings and attitude may very well be part of the counseling procedures, either functioning as the threshold of counseling or using counseling procedures to ease the adolescent into looking at feelings and attitudes. Some clients, after the preceding self-evaluation activities, will accept analysis of attitudes and feel-

TABLE 10–2. Evaluation of Situation Effects on Stuttering

Read each situation description and rate the stuttering difficulty you are likely to have in each. If the severity fluctuates a lot, check the "Varies" column and try to reason out why it varies. Leave blank any that don't apply.

SITUATION	AMOUNT OF STUTTERING				
	NONE	LITTLE	SOME	MUCH	VARIES
Telephone, talking to					
Father					
Mother					
Brother					
Sister					
Business place (pizza place)					
Employer					
Girlfriends					
Boyfriends					
Reading aloud					
By myself					
To family members					
To friends					
In class					
Before other groups					
Social conversations with					
Father					
Mother					
Brother					
Sister					
Girlfriends					
Boyfriends					
Teachers					
Strangers					
Giving verbal report to					
Class					
Employer					
Familiar group					
Unfamiliar group					
When I am					
Feeling tired					
In an argument					
Angry, upset					
Happy, amused					

TABLE 10–2.   *(cont.)*

SITUATION	AMOUNT OF STUTTERING				
	NONE	LITTLE	SOME	MUCH	VARIES
Sad, depressed					
Anxious, fearful					
Special situations					
Animals, pets					
Little children					
Acting a part					
Singing					
Doing something else while talking					
Other					

ings as a natural extension, sometimes initiating such analysis themselves. Others will not respond that way. The clinician will want to be sure of what the reaction will be and then move accordingly. The logical opener, if one is needed, could be as follows:

> You have shown me that different situations and different people can affect your stuttering. You also found out that feelings and emotions in a situation can be a factor. What I think we need to find out at this point is what your attitudes and feelings are for some of the specific situations, and for speaking in general.

Shumak (1955) produced the Stutterer's Self-Ratings of Reactions to Speech Situations. This lists 40 speech situations, and the stutterer is asked to rate each situation on four different factors, using a five-point scale. The four factors rated are *avoidance* of the situation, *feelings* about the situation, *stuttering* present in each situation, and the *frequency* with which the situation occurs. Trotter and Bergmann (1957) surveyed 50 stutterers and 100 nonstutterers with a modified version of the Shumak form. They reported that, overall, stutterers were more avoidant of speaking situations and enjoyed them less—even though the 40 situations were encountered at similar frequency rates. In general, avoidance and feelings and avoidance and fluency disruption were positively correlated. Another adaptation of this useful scale has been published by the author

TABLE 10–3.   Stutterer Failures and Successes in Communication

Read each pair of statements carefully, and circle the one that describes your behavior most of the time when stuttering occurs.

FAILURE	SUCCESS
1. Eye contact generally poor.	1. Eye contact good, especially just before stuttering.
2. Loss of eye contact while stuttering.	2. Good eye contact while stuttering.
3. Hurried or slow rate around moments of stuttering.	3. Even, normal rate before and after moments of stuttering.
4. Overly long or short pauses around stuttering.	4. Pauses appropriate to the content of the utterances.
5. Physical tension before feared words.	5. Normal tension before stuttering.
6. Behaviors used to postpone word attempts.	6. No postponements of utterances.
7. Behaviors to try to get a start on feared words.	7. No starters.
8. Facial contortions and struggle during stuttering.	8. Stutter without making faces or struggling.
9. Head jerks, shoulder movements during stuttering.	9. Normal head-shoulder postures while stuttering.
10. Retrials, stoppages during stutterings.	10. Steady completion of stuttered words.
11. Apologize, make excuses for stuttering.	11. Stutter without apology or excuse.
12. Avoid words, people, situations because of stuttering.	12. Do not allow stuttering to prevent speech.
13. Avoid speaking because of stuttering.	13. Speak any time there is something to say.
14. "Blank out" when stuttering occurs.	14. Am aware of everything and everyone when stuttering.
15. Don't know where and how stuttering occurs.	15. Am aware of where it happens and how it is formed.
16. Use tricks or devices to distract attention from stuttering.	16. Stutter openly.
17. Feel that stuttering has control.	17. Feel that stuttering is voluntary and controllable.
18. Worry about fluency and try to be fluent.	18. Try to talk without worrying about fluency or stuttering.
19. Blame other people for causing stuttering.	19. Accept the stuttering as a personal problem.
20. Show embarrassment or other reactions to stuttering.	20. Do not have strong emotional reactions to stuttering.

(Ham 1986). Another classic evaluation form has been the Iowa Scale of Attitude toward Stuttering (Ammons & Johnson 1944), which evaluates the strength of agreement or disagreement about how stutterers should behave in various communication situations. The social contexts, especially for young people, are somewhat dated on certain items now. However, the form is still in use. In a combination of stuttering behaviors and communicative attitudes, F.H. Silverman (1980) has designed the Stuttering Problem Profile. It is a mixture of statements about feelings and about behaviors. The stutterer is to circle all those statements they would like to be able to make by the time they complete therapy. There are 86 statements, and space is provided for additional, personal statements. Developing a similar list is not difficult:

- I want to feel relaxed when I talk.
- I would like never to stutter again.
- Talking on the telephone doesn't bother me.
- An occasional mild stutter is okay.
- I can be fluent when "discussing" with my father.

Please note the goal differentiation between the second and the fourth items, and the last item is an individual one. Other variations of such evaluation lists can be developed.

A popular attitude scale, toward speaking in general, was developed by Erickson (1969). In this scale the respondent answered true or false to 39 statements about their attitudes toward speaking. Although stuttering is not mentioned in the form, stutterers (with wide score ranges) averaged 26.5 and nonstutterers averaged 13.24. In spite of stutterer variability, 95 percent of them earned scores above the nonstutterer median. Andrews and Cutter (1974) modified the Erickson S-scale to 24 items (S-24), and E-M. Silverman (1980) reported that female stutterers averaged about 16, compared to the male stutterers' 19, and the nonstuttering women averaged a score of about 6 on the scale. Guitar and Bass (1978) used it in relating pretreatment attitudes to therapy outcomes. This has been questioned by Ingham (1984, 1979b) and Ulliana and Ingham (1984), so that it does not appear to be appropriate to use the S-24 as a prognostic instrument. However, it has been useful in evaluating client attitudes and changes that may occur during therapy (Ham 1986).

An indirect approach to attitudes and feelings is to utilize stuttering behaviors and relate them, in terms of successes and failures, to avoidance behaviors. Table 10–3 is based on Sheehan's philosophy about reducing avoidance behaviors (see counseling section). The stutterer reads each pair of statements and elects the one most descriptive of him or her. Another copy of the form can be filled out on the stutterer by the clinician, and if appropriate the client can ask significant others in her or his environment to fill out copies of the form. The form can be readministered during therapy as a progress measurement device.

As noted earlier, feelings and attitudes are not an isolated area of therapy, even if specific times are designated and plans made. Feelings and attitudes actually permeate every aspect of therapy and will come up repetitively as other procedures are applied. In a real sense, attitudes and feelings in addition to counseling provide the doorways to motivation and acceptance by the client. They are probably the significant determining factors in transfer, as well as in maintenance after dismissal from therapy.

HIERARCHIES

As is so often the case, different clinicians use the term *hierarchies* differently. Guitar (1984) used the term to mean finding the child's basal fluency level and then progressing hierarchically as fluency is maintained. In this chapter it is used to connote *stress hierarchy,* or

> the arrangement of stimuli (persons or situations) on an incremental basis in terms of their negative/positive effects on the feelings and speech of the stutterer.

The use of hierarchies in all types of therapies has a long history. On an informal basis hierarchies permeate therapy. Starting on sounds most likely to improve in articulation therapy is a hierarchy application. The ELU and GILCU approaches discussed in another chapter are linguistic hierarchies. Rapport development in counseling therapy follows a feelings hierarchy. Even the training of clinicians follows a number of hierarchies.

In stuttering therapy "establishing a hierarchy" (without the addition of modifiers) refers to the identification of a fear, or stress, hierarchy. Symptom therapy has for many years involved the use of stress hierarchies. Gronhovd and Zenner (1982) recommend the development of fear hierarchies and brief sketches of each item so that they can be used in role-playing, visualization, and desensitization activities. Hierarchies are used extensively in transfer and maintenance activities, and they have major significance in desensitization, reciprocal inhibition, flooding or implosion therapy, personal construct therapy, assertiveness training, and many other therapy procedures. Some specific values of hierarchy development include the following:

1. Awareness, insight, evaluation skills of the client.
2. Determination of covert characteristics and avoidance predominance in the client's behavior.
3. Selection, timing, pressure of procedures used in therapy.
4. Information needed for specific therapy procedures.
5. Progressive escalation of outside assignments.
6. Transfer, maintenance, and self-therapy activities.

Preparation of hierarchies is not complex as far as structure is concerned. The clinician and the client together establish the kinds of situations the stutterer meets. The list is then ranked according to the communication disruption that is likely to occur, or is feared to occur by the stutterer. The structural simplicity is complicated by any tendencies the client has to avoid potentially embarrassing honesty. Also, the client may not list certain appropriate situations because they are avoided routinely and, hence, are not considered. The author had an adolescent assure him that he never had any trouble on the telephone—only to find out later that there was no trouble because the client flatly refused to use the telephone.

The example in Table 10–4 illustrates how a hierarchy can be developed. The Basic list groups a range of situations under gross categories and provides some information about general *types* of situations. These general categories can be ranked or not, but it is necessary to progress to the Complex column of Table 10–4. Only two categories, *using the telephone,* and *talking to groups,* are illustrated. Note that there is a mix of situation and person factors. For instance, any stranger (general) may be difficult to talk to on the telephone, and talking to G-Mom may be easier than talking to Carol Ann (specific). (Further breakdowns and variations are discussed in the Group III subsection that follows later.) Nearly all clinicians use such hierarchies, with or without formal structure.

Group I Hierarchies

The use of hierarchies with children is not new in clinical work (Brutten & Shoemaker 1967), and it is suggested that every therapy program should have its equivalent, even if use is delayed until transfer-

TABLE 10–4.   Preliminary Fear Hierarchy Development

BASIC	COMPLEX

1. Talking on the telephone
2. Talking with family members
3. Talking with friends
4. Talking with strangers
5. Talking in front of groups
	1. Talking on the telephone to
	   Mother
	   Father
	   Carol Ann (sister)
	   G-Mom (grandmother)
	   Close friends
	   Strangers, when they call
	   My boss at the restaurant
	   Sell tickets for Rainbow Girls
	2. Talking in front of groups
	   Asking questions in class
	   Answering questions in class
	   Giving class reports
	   Reading aloud at church
	   Treasurer's report at Girl Scouts
	   Telling a joke

maintenance stages. Children do not have to be able to read or write in order to participate in hierarchy construction. The clinician can describe different situations or use pictures to simulate them. Labeled cards, or pictures, can be arranged physically on the table in a hierarchy. A possible approach might be this one:

> Sometimes people or things make us get all tight and nervous. Sometimes we may get scared, or even get mad. When that happens, we may get stuck or have trouble getting some words out. Can you think of some times when that happens?

It may be necessary to lead the child, cite examples, and as a model build a parallel hierarchy for the clinician. Attention is directed to other situations, neutral or easy ones are brought up, and the clinician probes as needed to bring in situations the child has not mentioned. After a number of situations have been identified (perhaps 20–30), it is necessary to rank them. This can be done grossly by grouped rankings of "awful," "hard," "okay," "easy." Parents can be consulted for their perception of stress hierarchies and assigned to monitor and evaluate them for details the clinician can use in therapy. Emphasis on hierarchy use will depend on the child's severity and reactions to stuttering and on what is revealed in early development of hierarchy lists.

Group II Hierarchies

Construction of hierarchies in the first and second grades will be quite similar to that described for Group I children. However, methodology and depth rapidly change as the child learns literacy skills, develops nonhome interaction situations, improves insight skills, and probably experiences an increase in social penalties for stuttering. Most of the procedural discussion is reserved for Group III coverage, since it is essentially the same, but two new factors can be commented on at this age level: the school environment and the use of group therapy.

The school environment creates a new world for the child, generally fraught with potentially negative factors. The stutterer faces uncertain parameters, emphasis on speed of response, depersonalized institutional treatment of children, and loss of old, familiar cues. Almost certainly the child will receive negative attention from peers because of stuttering. This attention can vary from obvious surprise and embarrassment to laughter, ridicule, and rejection. Teachers are usually supportive and accepting, but the reaction of some may be traumatic! Of those who are supportive, some may be too sympathetic and obvious in their sympathy for and protection of the child.

In hierarchy construction, the clinician will want to include school-related situations, such as:

Waiting for school bus	Volunteering in class
Riding school bus	Answering questions in class
Playground activity	Show-and-tell
Lunchroom situations	Classroom teacher
Lunch table peers	Specialty teachers

As the children are older, more situations occur and feelings are more likely to focus around certain ones. It may also be useful to add specific persons to the hierarchy list with older children.

Group therapy offers particular advantages and disadvantages in hierarchy construction. The advantages stem from clients realizing that they are not alone in having anxiety about particular situations and/or persons and from cross-prompts to bring them up. It also tends to be helpful for one child to see that although many factors are held in common, each child tends to have a different arrangement in his or her own hierarchy. On the minus side, the clinician may not hear of some situations or problem persons if the child feels other group members might be amused or scornful were they revealed.

Group III Hierarchies

The older preteen and the adolescent can approach hierarchy construction on a full cognitive, as well as emotional, level. The material presented in Table 10–4 can be expanded and used as the basis for a wide range of therapy approaches. Yet another way of approaching hierarchy development is illustrated in Table 10–5. Five different hierarchies are presented, with the client asked to fill in items under each category and rate the stress values. Only one Other is shown in each category, but as many as needed can be used. Additional categories can be used, or existing categories subdivided. In order to have a true hierarchy the clinician will want easy or neutral items, as well as including those likely to cause speech disruption. Although a five-point stress scale is illustrated, many methods can be used. Wolpe (1973) suggested the client use "subjective units of disturbance," or SUDs, to describe anxiety level. The client is asked to identify what they would evaluate as the most anxiety-producing experiences they ever had (one also could construct an imaginary situation). This worst-case situation is a value of 100 SUDs. Next the client is asked to identify a neutral, no-fear situation, and this is given a value of zero SUDs. With the two reference points, all situations and persons on a hierarchy can be assigned a SUDs value. The client is supposed to use the SUDs system in desensitization work, but this system can also be applied in initial hierarchy construction. For children too young to encompass the cognitive aspects of a 0–100 scale, simpler systems can be used.

TABLE 10–5. Ways to Develop Stress Hierarchies

FACTOR	STRESS
For each of the categories below, list factors in terms of how much stress they put on your speech. In the column labeled stress, put a 1, 2, 3, 4, or 5. A 1 means little or no stress and a 5 indicates maximum stress. Each category has two examples. Rate them if they apply, and add other factors of your own.	
People	
Members of the opposite sex _____	_____
Talking with my mother _____	_____
Other _____	_____
Situations	
Answering questions in class _____	_____
Talking at the lunch table _____	_____
Other _____	_____
Emotions	
Talking when I feel good, relaxed _____	_____
Arguing when I'm angry _____	_____
Other _____	_____
Speech Production	
When I try to speed up _____	_____
When I talk more softly _____	_____
Language	
When I use unfamiliar words _____	_____
When I use words that have been trouble before _____	_____

PLAY AND ROLE PLAY

When the author entered the speech and language pathology profession, most children who stuttered were not enrolled for therapy. Those who were enrolled often received play therapy. In many instances this was no more than scheduled indoor recreation activity, under the explanation that the child needed opportunities to relax and enjoy a nonpressured communication situation. At times this explanation also covered the fact that the clinician either had no idea of what to do or was reluctant to try anything for fear the child would explode into advanced secondary stuttering behaviors. Today we have a far different situation, not only in terms of therapy with children but also with reference to play therapy and its use. In this section we will look at some uses of play therapy, as well as consider role play and its applications.

Play therapy and role play are, in many instances, separable techniques, particularly in psychotherapy. However, in our field and at the lower end of the age range covered, distinction can become blurred between the approaches. Further, clinician management procedures for the two approaches have many points in common. Riley & Riley (1984), in writing of the game type of play, defined it as "an activity between two or more independent decision makers, seeking to achieve their objectives in some limiting context" (p. 36). A rather grand label for hop scotch, but valid when one analyzes play characteristics. Sapora and Mitchell (1961) provide a prolonged view of about 40 years of work with and evaluation of play uses. Although social contexts have changed extensively during those eras, the same basic values were found in play. Refinements and organization in play therapy have been extensive. In the following group discussions play therapy and role play separate as age progression continues.

Group I Play

At this early stage, separation of play and role play is not as easy as it is for older children. The concept of play and of games is easier to establish as we grow older. However, at early ages the following demarcations might be observed: random sensorimotor play, imitative sensorimotor and/or symbolic play, organized and diversified play forms. In the latter, playing hopscotch and "playing house" follow different rules and serve different purposes. Marzollo and Lloyd (1972) developed an extensive resource of play activities for young children. Each section (language development, problem solving, self-esteem, and so on) has a series of play activities that can be used with preschool children. Specific rules, instructions, and needed supplies or equipment for every activity are listed. Manning and Sharp (1977) provide both preschool and early school play activities, presenting dialogues and evaluations of possible results and effects.

In general play therapy with Group I children will be needed more in situations where the primary focus is parent counseling rather than fluency therapy for the child. Gregory and Hill (1984) question the value of traditional play therapy, "together with desensitization therapy, in facilitating and generalizing fluency" (p. 87). They feel this is particularly true if there are any special problems such as attending, hyperactivity, or delays in speech and/or language development. However, it is possible to take special problems and make them (not fluency) the focus of play therapy. Thus play therapy can be used if there are particular reasons to strengthen the child's abilities or willingness to engage in interactive relationships, increase verbal output, improve attending skills, and so on. Play therapy can be used to prepare the child for more sophisticated forms of role-play activity and to learn about behavioral alternatives. Van Riper (1973) has recommended the use of play therapy in two possible forms.

One approach is *unstructured play therapy,* used as a relaxation and rapport builder, into which progressively structured speech therapy is insinuated. The other approach is a *play psychotherapy* designed to allow the child to express feelings and release emotions. Speech therapy in the direct sense is not involved. Since most young child stutterers may exhibit language delays or deficits, the research by Roth and Clark (1987) on language-impaired children's capacities in symbolic play and social participation may be applicable to some stutterers. The researchers reported that language-impaired children displayed more nonplay, more solitary play, and more parallel play activities. Correspondingly, they displayed significant inadequacies in integrative, adaptive, and symbolic play behaviors.

Another aspect of play therapy is "filial therapy," described by Andronico and Blake (1971) and based on Guerney's (1964) work in general psychotherapy with children. Over a period of six to ten weeks parents are introduced gradually into their child's play therapy sessions. They learn how to express empathy, accept expression of feelings, and otherwise act supportively to the child. After this time period phased transfer activities, for outside generalization, are developed. Curry (1974) emphasized strongly the values she perceived in play therapy, utilizing dramatic play. She contrasted the abbreviated, imitative, repetitive dramatic play of three-year-old children with the much longer, varied, and complex "plays" children of four years of age would develop on the same topic. Curry argued that such role play prepares children to think in abstract symbols, develop problem-solving capacities, begin complex (but flexible) learning strategies, and move away from strongly egocentric orientations. Familiar occurrences are useful material to work with, and *sensorimotor* play can be used to develop into *symbolic* play. For instance, giving a child tools and having him or her pretend to do something can slide easily into being someone else and acting out a role. When the child can sustain a role, the clinician will be needed as "a facilitator, a referee, a representation of reality, and for cognitive and sensory input" (p. 70). Curry draws upon Smilansky's work and lists the following elements comprising a child's role-play behavior:

1. Imitation of a role.
2. Make-believe concerning objects.
3. Make-believe concerning actions and situations.
4. Persistence.
5. Interaction with one or more other players.
6. Verbal communication.

Group II Play

The young school child has less need for generalized play therapy and can profit from development of role play, although the back-and-forth overlap between Group I and Group II can be extensive. In both groups parents and home situations are often resources for role-play activity.

Lemert and Van Riper (1958) discussed the value of psychodrama in treating speech disorders. They stated that having the client play other roles can help insight and favor emotional release. Letting the client help in the development, scripting, and directing of a role-play situation can also aid in catharsis and insight. The authors noted that it can be useful to the clinician to have the stutterer recreate the people she or he deals with on a daily basis. They warn that negative reactions can develop if the client falls too quickly into certain insights or releases too much emotion too early. Riley and Riley (1984, 1979) utilize role play to help the child resolve frustrations and learn to select alternative behaviors that will eliminate or reduce the frustration problem. Moore and Nystul (1979) have stated that research indicates that young child stutterers are more likely to be more positive toward their mothers and ambivalent toward their fathers. The stress of sibling rivalry was also noted in their discussion. Without going into in-depth psychotherapy, the speech and language clinician can structure play and role-play activities so that father characters have opportunities to be loving, approving, problem solving, and flexible. Female characters are not to be cast in a negative light by comparison. Simultaneously, in parent counseling the father can be aided in altering certain behaviors and becoming more available and open to the child.

Shames and Egolf (1976) experimented with parent-child and clinician-child interaction dyads in terms of the effects of different parent behaviors on the child's speech. The clinician works to replicate parent behaviors to the opposite degree (Shames & Florance 1982) until desired fluency is obtained. Parents can then be inserted into therapy sessions for experience in the types of social verbal interactions that will favor fluency. Guitar (1984) reported a single-case study of therapy similar to the interaction dyad described by Shames and Egolf (1976) and by others (Kasprisin-Burelli, Egolf & Shames 1972). He indicated positive and stable results. Riley and Riley (1984) describe the use of role play, usually starting with nonspeech areas, and the clinician enacting the child's role. The clinician, before reaching expressions of frustration or hurt, reviews alternative changes that would resolve the situation satisfactorily. The child then reenacts the situation. Other situations are practiced until the child sees that there is more than one way to behave in a situation. Speech frustration situations are brought in and developed. As real situations of frustration occur in therapy, the child can be stopped, alternatives reviewed and acted out, and the child asked to select the most appropriate alternative.

The preceding paragraphs seem to indicate a wider interest and use of play and role play in therapy than one might expect. Indeed, a number of clinicians report effective use of role and role play (Dalali & Sheets 1974; Luper 1974). In the Group III discussion, more specific comments about applications and use of play therapy are provided.

Group III Play

Role play, not play therapy, with adolescents presents unique challenges and opportunities. On the one hand, adolescents can be extremely wary of exposing themselves, as they see it, embarrassingly. On the other hand, many of them will delight in examining and recreating the behaviors of other people. Honig (1947), writing about younger children, made suggestions that are applicable to Group III stutterers as well. She recommended a warm-up to role playing, rather than jumping into simulated real situations. She also suggested acting out a variety of roles and situations—mother, father, teacher, sibling, and so on. This variation will develop the overall context of the various favorable and unfavorable factors involved in the client's social interactions. Subsequently Honig moved to dramatization of prospective stress situations in real life, exploring feelings and ways in which the situations could be improved. After the real situation had occurred, the stutterer reported back, and dialogue and further role play were used in evaluation and revision. Maxwell (1982) recommends the use of role play in group situations. Chapman (1959), in her group therapy manual, followed in Bryngelson's pattern in a heavy use of role play with adolescents. Although needing updates in some of the social interaction contexts, both sources have worthwhile ideas for using role play.

Role play has been described and recommended for adolescents by Rustin (1978) in the context of interactive group therapy. Its use is suggested for the rapid integration of group members, to explore alternate modes of behavior, and to rehearse for difficult real situations. Rustin notes that role play validates fluency in a variety of situations and often provides insight into how stuttering is used in social interactions. Harris (1977), as part of a counseling approach to therapy, recommended behavioral rehearsal, or role playing with role reversal experience, to prepare the client for outside situations. A particular use of role play has been in assertiveness training, an approach discussed in the following section on counseling. Higgins, Frisch, and Smith (1983) reported that assertiveness practice in role play was reflected in the behavior of the participants, compared to those who did not receive assertive emphasis. As noted before, problem solving, tolerance, insight into others' behavior, and many other factors can be explored, rehearsed, or altered in role play.

Role play is not a "Let's do it!" type of undisciplined activity; rather, it functions best with structure and a script (not necessarily written). Before initiating a scene several points need to be covered with the participants:

1. What is the situation and its characteristics?
2. Who are the characters, what are they doing, and how do they interact?
3. What is the purpose of the enactment?
4. Who plays what characters?

For instance, the purpose of a scene might be to explore different ways that auditors react to stuttering. The situation will be one in which the stutterer takes a job in a fast-food restaurant. Characters will include the manager and two customers (number of characters can be adjusted to group size, or individuals can play more than one role). The behaviors and attitudes expressed by the characters should be outlined generally, and the sequence of the situation decided. It is possible to be very specific, up to planning script lines, or to be as general as, "You be a person calling a girl for a date, and you be the father who's a real squidge about stutterers." The purpose of the enactment affects the postscene activity. Purposes can include exploration of feelings, desensitization, practice in reciprocal inhibition relaxation, analysis of stuttering behaviors, practice in various fluency or symptom control methods, use of pseudostuttering, role rehearsal for behavioral change, rehearsal for real situations that are going to occur, and analysis of real situations that have occurred.

Very often role scenes are repeated a number of times. Reasons for repetition can include, but are not limited to, the following:

1. One of the scene purposes (cancellation, prolongation, experiencing rejection, and so on) was not met, was inappropriate in degree, or was performed incorrectly.
2. A decision is made to repeat the scene on a "what if" basis, altering one or more of the characters or behaviors.
3. It is desirable for participants to experience enacting different characters in the same scene.
4. Similar to 2, but aimed at determining what needs to be changed so the scene can have a satisfactory, rewarding result.

In group therapy, critiques are not difficult to elicit, and the "actors" can be very discerning and demanding with each other. Group situations also allow the clinician to step back, or fade, from scenes and become an observer, commentator, and moderator to guide the activities of the role players.

Role playing can become quite complex, with scripts and properties and amateur directors. The clinician will need to guard therapy time so that it is not spent on writing and preparation activities that the clients can do on their own, outside of sessions. Occasionally, the clinician needs to interfere if scenes begin to stretch out to unprofitable length. Once in a rare while actors can become too involved in the pseudoreality of the situation, so that the clinician will need to relax tensions and direct discussion in order to reestablish a balance. Yet role play can be used with any type of therapy program, for its depth can be controlled so that it stops at a level of simple simulation for practice of various behaviors, or it can dig deeply into psychosocial feelings and interactions. The training and experience of the clinician will guide the way in which it is used. With Group III adolescents the clinician should be aware of daily increased role playing by the stutterers. Therapy role playing can provide opportunities for stutterers to examine the falsely structured roles from real life and so discuss and possibly alter them. Carlisle (1985), in his stutterer's autobiography, described a large number of roles he learned to play deliberately, depending on the group or person he was with. He noted that clinicians might not approve of false role playing in real life to support fluency, but that he had been willing to adopt any role if it would help him.

Before possibly rejecting play therapy or role therapy, the clinician should remember that therapy is an artificial, nonreal environment. Whatever program we structure, we want the client to transfer its effects to outside life. Whereas spontaneous generalization may be feasible with some young children, it will not occur with all of them, and will decrease rapidly with age. Role play, aside from other possible uses that have been discussed, is one of several useful techniques for promoting transfer and practicing behavioral changes.

COUNSELING

The dictionary (Stein 1967) defines counseling as

> advice; opinions or instructions given in directing the judgment or conduct of another. (p. 332)

On the basis of this definition, there can be no doubt that every clinician, in every therapy session, engages in counseling. Additional considerations of client motivation, stimulus presentation, and response reinforcement increase the counseling component of therapy. In spite of this there are clinicians who argue against "counseling-oriented" therapy, because they perceive a demarcation between speech therapy and counseling therapy. Literally, there is no demarcation and the difference is only one of degree. However, in practical terms it is possible, although difficult, to categorize into one hegemony overt speech behaviors, covert speech behaviors, and feelings and attitudes about speech. The other grouping on categories involves the behaviors, feelings, and attitudes that supposedly are not involved in communication and, therefore, are not appropriate for address by the speech and language clinician. Wingate (1976) states that "we must acknowledge stuttering to be basically a speech problem" (p. 326). He disagrees with Sheehan in saying that observable occurrences

in stuttering are "something that *happens*. It is not meaningfully understood as essentially something one *does*" (p. 326). Wingate continues and
states that stumbling, yawning, trembling, hiccoughing, and so on also are
things that *happen*. Unfortunately, Wingate's analogy is seriously flawed.
If a yawn routinely elicited the personal and social reactions that stuttering does, then we would record the development of yawn avoidances,
yawn struggles, yawn fear and anxiety, and we certainly would have
"yawn therapy." Stuttering, postulating a neurophysiological origin, probably does 'happen' in most instances. However, its development and evolution into advanced stages most certainly is a result of what the speaker
does in an effort not to have the stuttering happen. Wingate does not reject the presence of attitude and emotion in stuttering and therapy;
rather, he places them in a position of secondary importance to the
speech problem itself. This is probably appropriate in most instances.
However, the therapy that ignores feelings and attitudes among older
children and adults is likely to produce a relapsed client for some future
clinician to struggle with. Sheehan (1978) speaks quite strongly to this issue:

> Until operant conditioners and others have really demonstrated that they
> can stretch laboratory fluency into real life, until they stop pretending there
> is no such thing as anxiety, and until they give stutterers tools for dealing
> with future fear, they will continue to help themselves more than they ever
> help the stutterers. (p. 185)

The foregoing represent opposite, but not irreconcilable, points of view,
attitudes which have been explored several times previously in this book.
Conture (1982) has suggested that some have scrambled so hard to develop quantitative and accountable procedures, and to count or measure
various behaviors, that they may have lost sight of the content of behavior. He argues that charting behaviors over time does not explain the behaviors, either to ourselves or to others (p. 82).

Part of the disagreement relates to how different persons define
counseling. Some limit counseling to a quality one might call the therapy
relationship. Brutten and Shoemaker (1967) support a learning theory
and conditioning approach to therapy, but they do not negate the importance of psychological factors. They stress the significance of client motivation and state that "the therapeutic relationship should also serve as a
stimulus situation that will inhibit negative emotion" and go on to say,
"Success in therapy is highly dependent on the relationship between the
patient and the therapist" (p. 91). Attitudes and feelings have been discussed already, and motivation has been stressed in this text as well as by
other authors (Van Riper 1973; Conture 1982; Wells 1987). Hood (1973)
has expressed an orientation based upon Rogers's theory of client-
centered therapy, particularly with the later stages of therapy. He cited

clinician genuineness and sincerity, warmth for and acceptance of the client, and a sensitivity that would allow the clinician to view the client's world as the client perceives it.

A more comprehensive orientation to counseling has been expressed by R.D. Harris (1977). He discussed the speech and language clinician as a counselor and made the initial point that therapy is affected by two conditions, *demand characteristics* and the *clinician-client relationship*. Demand characteristics is a somewhat nebulous concept that covers the client's expectations of therapy, the attitudes of clinical support staff, and the aura of the clinician. The more positive the demand characteristics, the more trust and reliance the client will have in the clinician. Factors or occurrences that create negative demand characteristics would include the following:

"You're the first stutterer I have worked with."
"This is my supervisor, who will keep an eye on things."
Supervisor comments, corrections, interruptions during therapy.
"Mr. Jones, your case number is X5012Z."
"If you work hard and do what we say, your problem should get better."

Included among negative demand characteristics are any factors that reduce impressions of clinician competence or caring, institutional impersonality and routine procedures, attitudes or expressions of boredom, and behaviors that reduce the autonomy and maturity of the client. These and many other possibilities tend to reduce clinician effectiveness, predetermine the atmosphere and relationship in therapy, and predispose the client to behave in particular ways. The clinician should consider that the opening preliminaries of therapy may create demand characteristics that will color all of therapy. For instance, starting with a sheaf of forms and reports to fill in may persuade the client that he or she is a nonhuman set of data responses and the clinician does not see the client as a person. Similarly, a prolonged "rapport discussion" of parking, traffic, the weather, and other chit-chat may cause the client to think that her or his problem is being avoided and/or the clinician really does not have a therapy plan.

Harris also makes an important distinction between interpersonal and noninterpersonal communication. The latter is any type of communication which is not centered on the auditor-client but deals with categories, stereotypes, or external references. Whenever we say or think, "The stutterer typically . . . ," follow a set routine, or use automatic questions and responses, we are using noninterpersonal communication. Such behaviors have positive values in time saving, efficiency, output, measurement activity, and protecting the psyche of the clinician from erosion by the emotions of a series of clients. However, such behaviors promote stereotypy, reduce communication, and foster client perceptions that "I, as a person, am not very important here." Operant procedures are particularly conducive to noninterpersonal communication. Harris states that counseling involves interpersonal communication and that this is required for mutual understanding and trust to develop, for information to be exchanged, and for action to be planned and carried out under the supervision of the clinician. The first essential step is understanding; until this happens, effective action cannot occur.

Understanding involves information about, and empathy for, what the client's situation is at the present time. Harris states that failure to achieve the status of understanding will minimize treatment success because

1. Client confidence and trust has not been established.
2. The clinician has not become a figure of positive social reinforcement and client motivation to "please the clinician" is undeveloped.
3. The clinician lacks information about what realistically can be expected from the client.
4. Therapy goals are likely to be clinician based rather than client based.

In order to achieve understanding of the client, the clinician needs to function in a variety of ways, some of which are summarized in Table 10–6. All of the suggestions are standard in counseling situations, but the clinician might periodically review the table or its equivalent. On the ac-

TABLE 10–6. Clinician Behaviors Contributing to Understanding of Client

Attending—to the client with a listening posture, good eye contact, interested expression, and generally positive nonverbal signals. Relaxed and confident attitude should be projected.

Nonverbal Behavior—actively monitoring the client's postures, facial expressions, inflections, tension signs, etc. Harris suggests that over 90% of meaning is conveyed nonverbally.

Verbal Behavior—active listening to and monitoring of verbal behavior, both for what is said and how it is expressed. Be a good listener with clinician-uttered sounds or words indicating interest, and give appropriate restatements or summaries of things the client has said.

Empathy—is easier to do than define. Feeling what the client feels without becoming involved (accurate empathy) is required. Check on it by trying to describe how you think the client feels about a subject that has been discussed, and see if the client agrees with you.

Concreteness—in both directions. The client often needs to have vague and rambling statements rephrased into the first person and related to the present time. Through example and questioning help the client to be more organized and explicit. The clinician should communicate similarly.

Goal Setting—press early for the client to articulate what his or her goals are. It is permissible to try to revise the client's goals, but therapy should start with them, not with the clinician's goals. By all means avoid allowing a nongoal situation where stuttering is talked about and worked on, but without articulated targets.

Source: Adapted from R.D. Harris, The speech pathologist as counselor, *Australian Journal of Human Communication Disorders* 5(1977):72–78.

tion side Harris favors role playing to rehearse behaviors, outside assignments to transfer in-clinic successes, and behavior shaping by breaking changes into small steps and moving progressively through them. If necessary, the speech and language clinician always has the option of referral to or consultation with psychological counselors in various areas.

In the following subsections, various approaches or procedures will be suggested, but there will be no recommendation for various forms of in-depth counseling or psychotherapy. Doll play, puppetry, clay therapy, structured psychodrama, nondirective therapy, rational emotive therapy, and other techniques have been raised to levels of complexity that make them inappropriate or ethically suspect for use by the untrained person. However, all of the procedures just listed contain basic elements used in general therapies. For example, puppets have been used frequently in various speech and language therapies, and rational emotive therapy (RET) principles are involved any time the clinician guides the client to take a rational look at emotional feelings about stuttering or speech. What will be emphasized are basic techniques rather than program approaches. As a final reminder of care over procedures, and consideration of the client, it would not be inappropriate for the clinician to gain insight into what is involved in behavioral change. Lay (1982) has suggested that during training clinicians should experience what is involved in altering an aspect of personal behavior. He structured such an assignment for his graduate class in fluency disorders and concluded it was a worthwhile experience for the students. They learned to appreciate the complexities of identifying and selecting targets, determining *what* to modify, and deciding *how* to go about it. The process of change, some failures, and the effects of change afterward were valuable to the student clinicians' understanding of the client's point of view. It is never a bad idea to ask clinicians to experience what they ask the client to go through!

Group I Counseling

Counseling, in the traditional sense of the term, occurs rarely and minimally among preschool children. Sheehan (1978) favored working with the parents and, if direct child therapy was necessary, using permissive response to stuttering with rewards for "openness and courage, not for achieved fluency" (p. 186). Costello (1983) has stressed that explanations of therapy to children may not be understood and can waste time in therapy. However, Wells (1987) has stated that young children may not understand their problem and, therefore, may not be cooperative. This is accentuated if the child perceives no relationship between the therapy and their own stuttering.

On the basis of personal experience and bias, this author prefers counseling the child as to why he or she is in therapy, and keeping the child informed of reasons as therapy progresses. Explanations need to be short and simple, and vocabulary can be adjusted to the child's level of comprehension. If there are specific reasons not to counsel the child, then it is appropriate to stop counseling; but this author prefers to provide counseling unless it is contraindicated, rather than not to begin counseling at all.

More complex problems and needs of the client, such as behavioral rigidity, perfectionism, social isolation, stress from the environment, loss of communication motivation, fear of failure, and so on, can require attention. These are better approached through environmental counseling and manipulation, or indirectly with the child through play, role play, puppetry, and other procedures discussed previously.

Group II Counseling

Depending on the maturity and insight of the child, the preceding approach may also apply best here. Because school children have, or rapidly acquire, a respect for therapy (usually), this approach can be used for a while in dealing with some of the problems discussed under Group I. Young children can often be motivated out of a desire to please an adult, the clinician. And the clinician should not fail to exploit this and should value rapport-building time with the client. Authority has its values with the young, but this is not to recommend an authoritarian, impersonal role for the clinician. Rather, positive attitudes, clear planning and organization, and a confident manner project an authoritative aura to the child. With older children, however, too much authority may boomerang and stimulate client resistance.

In Group II it is usually wise to probe for areas that may need counseling support. As Carlisle (1985) noted in his autobiography, his external appearances and behavior (except when speaking) gave no indication of the frustration, embarrassment, rage, and bitterly unhappy feelings he had. Previous research cited has suggested that stuttering children are perceived as being inferior in communication by their peers and tend to be stereotyped by parents, teachers, and clinicians. Problems in this area should be open to discussion, and efforts should be made to help the client arrive at solutions or, where this is the only option, at a better understanding of and tolerance for them. Several approaches are discussed next in the Group III section following.

Group III Counseling

Background   Adolescence has been described by many authors in the literature, and these descriptions tend to focus on traumatic and negative factors. Over the years, in university classes, this author has queried students about their adolescent years (just past or in final stages), and they have overwhelmingly rejected any hypothetical opportunity to relive those years. Adolescent change, upheaval, and trauma usually strike at about age 14, but may occur at 11 or 12 years of age, and occasionally earlier. Many books, professional and otherwise, have been written about adolescence. Most clinicians benefit from coursework in adolescent psychology and from reading among the books available. When stuttering and adolescence combine, therapy can become particularly complex and counseling approaches are emphasized with this group because there may be resistance to the very concept of therapy, not just to aspects of it. Questioning of and rebellion against adult authority occur frequently and therapy may be viewed as just another establishment trick to single the adolescent out and make life difficult. This is likely to be reinforced if the adolescent has experienced therapy in previous years. The rebellion against entrenched adults is often accompanied by a drive to establish a "difference" from the perceived establishment, usually through overconformity with the current beliefs, behaviors, and fashions of their peer adolescent society. As a parent, this author has watched bemusedly as his assertively different children would disappear into a peer group that dressed, ate, talked, and behaved indistinguishably from one another— with one of the conformities being a uniform insistence upon their individuality. Adolescents often do not want to differ, or seem to differ, from their peers.

Stuttering, of course, creates a difference. However, that can become an accepted difference, a familiar stigmata if you will, and therapy can become threatening. Therapy alters school schedules, calls attention to the "accepted" problem, changes speech patterns, and calls up personal attention. Indeed, adolescents may regard therapy changes as being worse than stuttering, which they have more or less learned to live with. As a result therapy can become a classic approach-avoidance conflict for the client or, as indicated in Figure 10-1, a double approach-avoidance problem. If there is no motivation for fluency, or if the motivations in various directions are seriously in conflict, then the clinician must secure changes in the motivations, or not attempt therapy. Similarly, in initial goal setting and during various therapy procedures, counseling may be needed to effect agreement and cooperation.

The basic relationship in therapy determines how well the therapy

FIGURE 10-1.

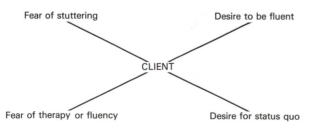

itself progresses. As it evolves, the success of transfer and maintenance will be affected by the stutterer's capacities to convert mechanical skills into social interactions. Simple modification of spasms, or acquisition of fluency modes, will not usually be enough. As an example of this, Cohen and others (1974) expressed the feeling that relapses after successful therapy were often due to a lack of self-confidence in interpersonal communication situations. This deficit erodes the stutterer's self-confidence and slides her or him back toward dysfluency as anxieties and tensions return. Their suggested solution is assertiveness training, which they feel restructures the client's interaction capacities. On the same idea Schloss and others (1987) have described a program of assertiveness training used with stutterers. They reported a substantial increase in the occurrence of desired behaviors and a noticeable decrease in stuttering. While not making definitive claims, the authors recommended its further development and exploration. Assertiveness therapy, discussed further under group therapy, is just one possible approach. Suggestions are made in the next few paragraphs to help the clinician clear the line between authoritarian or impersonal therapy techniques and trying to become a "groovy buddy" of the Group III client (Conture 1982) while trying to separate adolescent problems from stuttering problems. The approaches include *thematic content, avoidance reduction,* and *personal constructs*—all offered as auxiliary procedures or methods to blend into therapy, and not as total programs. In each approach references are provided for those who wish to study them more extensively.

Thematic content   Communication is controlled to a surprising extent by the auditor. Any teacher who stands before a class experiences this repeatedly. In conversation simple behaviors such as retaining or shifting eye contact by the auditor can cause the speaker to stumble, alter the speech pattern, and even to lose speaking place to interruption from a previously silent person to whom the auditor has shifted eye contact. All of us have experienced modifying, emphasizing, or qualifying behaviors because of the inflection of an "Oh" from our listener, shifts in (or lack of) facial expression from listeners, and so on. Clinicians have used this in interview and therapy activities also. How we respond as listeners can influence what people say and the ways in which they say it.

Shames and Egolf (1976) reported on the use of *thematic response* (TR) therapy, in which positive (TR+) statements are reinforced and negative (TR−) statements are ignored or punished. Examples of the two forms are the following:

TR+	TR−
I can improve my speech.	Stuttering runs my life.
	You must cure my problem.

TR+	TR−
I feel more confident.	I never succeed at anything.
	You have to come with me.
I must not avoid situations.	People don't like stutterers.
	I look for easy people to talk to.

Reinforcement can be the understanding behaviors cited by Harris (1977) earlier in this chapter, as well as more overt approvals. Clinician punishment can range from nonresponses to nonaccepting facial expressions or gestures, or to overt statements disagreeing with or not accepting TR− verbalizations. Shames and Egolf stated that over time clients usually become more positive in their statements and that TR+ increments are usually accompanied by stuttering decrements. However, they agree that changes in stuttering can occur "quite independently of changes in beliefs" (p. 142) and that changing observable content of utterances does not mean automatically that there has been a change in feelings.

Egolf, Shames, and Blind (1971) describe a three-stage program combining operant procedures and psychosocial therapy measures. Four establishment sessions used eye contact as a criterion measure (eye contact loss on one percent or less of the total words) while developing a clinical relationship and maintaining verbal output. The second step used the Thematic Content Modification Program (Shames, Egolf & Rhodes 1969) described earlier. To meet criterion levels 24 therapy sessions were required. The final stage, 15 sessions, involved Sheehan avoidance-reduction therapy, mixed with elements of semantogenic orientation. The authors reported satisfactory results that were maintained during the follow-up period. Thematic content therapy in the Speech Foundation of America publication (Shames 1978), and the positive and negative response categories from that source, are presented in Table 10–7. Responses, scored TR+ and TR−, can be counted and accumulated for operant structuring and for measurement against baseline scores.

For a number of years the author has used variations of the thematic content concept. One arrangement or variation is presented in Table 10–8. In this form, positive and negative utterance categories are contrasted. The number of categories used has varied from two to ten and can be altered for individual clients. The F1 and F2 categories are cumulative totals of positive and negative statements. Category G would be the sum of F1 + F2, plus all statements irrelevant to therapy (talk about the weather, purchase of a new record, and so on). This category allows the clinician to plot how much time (by utterance frequency) the client spends in trying to discuss nontherapy topics. Also, shifts in positive/negative statements can be plotted by taking F1 and dividing it by the sum F1 + F2. The clinician can be covert in using the procedure, or it is possible to explain things to the client and identify undesirable types of statements (attitudes), count their occurrences openly, and discuss results with the client. Such direct-discussion possibilities lead us to avoidance-reduction therapy, discussed in the next section.

TABLE 10–7. Positive and Negative Thematic Content Response Categories

RESPONSE CATEGORY	DEFINITION	EXAMPLE
1. Concurrent Variables	Statements which reflect client's awareness or growing awareness of events or situations which accompany his stuttering or fluency.	"I stutter when I'm talking on the phone," or "I don't stutter much around home."
2. Controlling Variables	Statements which reflect client's awareness or growing awareness of events which control or cause his stuttering behavior or fluency.	"Maybe I stutter because I think about how I'm going to talk before I say anything."
3. Description of Struggle Behavior	Statements which describe a client's overt motor struggle behavior when speaking.	"I blink my eyes when I stutter."
4. Description of Avoidance Behavior	Statements which describe or report a client's avoidance behavior at word, situation, and interpersonal levels.	"I sometimes change words when I think I'm going to stutter."
5. Positive Affect	Statements which describe or evaluate a client's feelings or emotional state in a positive manner.	"It makes me feel good not to stutter."
6. Negative Affect	Statements which describe or evaluate a client's feelings or emotional state in a negative manner.	"I sometimes hate everybody in the world."
7. Contemplated Action	Statements which report the contemplation of engaging in activities or meeting situations which involve speaking.	"I think I'll call him on the phone tonight."
8. Completed Action	Statements which report the completion of action involving speaking.	"I finally talked to my boss today about the raise."
9. Ambiguous Amorphous Entities	Statements referring to speech or stuttering which are imprecise, vague, or nondescriptive. Must contain the key words *it, this, or this thing.*	"It occurs when I start to talk." Or, "I just don't know what to do about this thing."
10. Helplessness Victimization	Statements reflecting client's perceptions of stuttering as an event which renders him helpless, incapable of acting, or as being the victim of outside events over which he has no control.	"I can't get the word out." "I'm just not able to say it." "When this stuttering happens, the word gets caught and I can't get it out."

Source: Reprinted from G. H. Shames, Operant conditioning and therapy for stuttering, In *Conditioning in Stuttering Therapy,* 7. Memphis: Speech Foundation of America, 1973, 7, p. 31.

TABLE 10–8. Client Attitude Content and Utterance

STATEMENTS RELEVANT TO STUTTERING THERAPY

Positive	Negative
A1 _____ Personal responsibility for stuttering	A2 _____ External factors that "make" me stutter
B1 _____ Personal responsibility for stuttering	B2 _____ Stuttering is an entity that "does things" to me
C1 _____ Approach comments about talking	C2 _____ Avoidance comments about talking
D1 _____ Other positive, optimistic statements about speech	D2 _____ Other negative, self-derogatory statements about speech
E1 _____ Clear, precise statements in first person use	E2 _____ Vague, rambling, ambiguous, or third person statements
F1 _____ TOTAL POSITIVE STATEMENTS	F2 _____ TOTAL NEGATIVE STATEMENTS

G _____ Total statements uttered (including ones irrelevant to therapy)

Percentage of positive statements:

$$\frac{F1}{F1 + F2} \times 100 = \underline{\hspace{2cm}} \%$$

Percentage of statements relevant to therapy:

$$\frac{F1 + F2}{G} \times 100 = \underline{\hspace{2cm}} \%$$

AVOIDANCE-REDUCTION THERAPY

For many clinicians avoidance is the core of stuttering and an application of what Wendell Johnson used to describe when he said that stuttering was what the person did when he or she tried to avoid stuttering. Symptom modification therapies deal with avoidances to varying degrees. However, some clinicians have targeted avoidances as the main area of concern and structured therapy accordingly. Sheehan (1970) has been noted for his approach-avoidance theory of stuttering, in which stuttering is a "false-role disorder." That is, the stutterer attempts to behave as a fluent person and in this process exacerbates negative feelings and dysfluencies. In role therapy, or avoidance-reduction therapy, Sheehan stresses a number of concepts that the stutterer must come to accept and internalize:

1. Behaviors to hide or postpone stuttering must be eliminated. Until this happens, conflict over speaking will occur, and conflict generates stuttering. As long as a person pretends not to be a stutterer, he or she cannot break the stutterer role.

2. Most stutterers, whatever the therapy, will probably retain some residual stuttering for the rest of their lives.

3. Most of what is called stuttering are the avoidance and camouflage behaviors engaged in to prevent the occurrence of dysfluency. The hidden portion, and hiding efforts, will prevent improvement of fluency.

4. Stuttering, or not, is not the question. How evenly, and in what form, is open to amelioration.

5. The stutterer is not a "victim" of stuttering. Stuttering is a behavior, not a condition.

6. The stutterer should learn to abolish avoidances and other tricks and to stutter openly and honestly. By accepting the stuttering self it will become possible to relax in speaking and to stutter more smoothly without the excess baggage of other behaviors.

In avoidance-reduction therapy Sheehan recommends a number of procedures or goals that are associated classically with symptom modification therapy. However, Sheehan did not agree with what he called "shotgun therapy" (1979), since avoidance-reduction therapy "has tended to be an incidental aspect" of the programs (p. 145). Although not comprising the overall role therapy program advocated by Sheehan, the following goals or assignments are part of the therapy he recommended. They are summarized briefly here, and the reader is directed to the original sources (1970, 1979) for more information and examples:

1. **Eye contact.** Learn to look at persons while speaking, preferring to overdo it rather than back away. By all means let every stuttering be a signal to establish and hold eye contact. Later on, when eye contact is not stressful, the stutterer can modify the eye contact.

2. **Openness.** The stutterer must be able and willing to discuss his or her stuttering with others. Assignments start with family or friends and then expand to include strangers.

3. **Stuttering analysis.** Study the stuttering pattern to isolate and identify all behaviors used to try to hide or avoid stuttering. These would include eye contact avoidance, substitution, postponement devices, starters, releases, and so on.

4. **Responsibility.** Monitor your own language for acceptance of, and responsibility for, stuttering. Failures are phrases such as "my head jerks" rather than "I jerk my head" or "my foot taps" or other phrases in which stuttering is doing something to the speaker rather than the speaker performing the behaviors.

5. **Monitoring.** Learn to observe the behaviors that occur during stuttering. Start monitoring a single avoidance behavior in easy and then in progressively more difficult situations. Add more behaviors until near-total awareness in any situation is possible.

6. **Desensitization.** The stutterer, on a progressive basis, is deliberately to use feared words and engage in behaviors usually avoided because of speech fears.

7. **Evaluate successes and failure in speaking.** Sheehan provides a list of 15 failures and 10 successes, as well as a charting form to use in keep-

ing track of various successes. A variation of this is provided later on in this section.

8. **Exposure.** Sheehan compares stuttering to an iceberg, with the avoidances, fears, guilt, covert behaviors, and so on, as the hidden portion. The aspects of acceptance, eye contact, stuttering openly, and so on, are the visible portion. The stutterer is directed to draw her or his "iceberg," and then to redraw it as the overall size changes and the above-water and below-water ratios change.

9. **Open stuttering.** The stutterer is asked to stutter, without preambles, without struggles, and without covering behaviors. Progressive assignments are recommended.

10. **Pressure resistance.** Learn to resist pressure to respond quickly, rush utterances, and so on. These pressures may be external or self-induced.

11. **Phrasing.** The stutterer is to evaluate his or her breathing, phrasing, and pause patterns in order to control resistance to pressure and establish a self-regulated time sequence.

12. **Struggle reduction.** Efforts are to be made to relax while stuttering, to identify what the stutterer has been trying to hide, and to relax and stop struggling to hide it.

13. **Voluntary stuttering.** This is to occur on nonfeared words and to be performed so that none of the avoidance behaviors or failure behaviors are utilized. Sheehan divides this area into three subtargets and suggests progressive levels.

14. **Tolerance.** Rather than straining and guarding to be fluent, the stutterer is to stutter voluntarily in order to reduce fears of losing fluency. Sheehan states that increased fluency will result from this behavior.

All of the foregoing items go well beyond consideration of basic counseling procedures. However, they were not eliminated here because they provided one of the opportunities, discussed earlier in the text, to take separate procedures and show them sequenced into an overall therapy program.

PERSONAL CONSTRUCT THERAPY

The counseling approach discussed in this section is not so much a recommendation of a specific therapy technique as an example of the type. The focus is on the stutterer and how he or she perceives self in relation to other people, to different situations, and to communication. The clinician guides the client in evaluating several question areas:

1. How do you compare yourself to other people in your environment?
2. What positive and negative factors in peoples' behaviors affect you?
3. What are the positive and negative factors in your behaviors that affect communication?

4. What situation factors have positive or negative effects on you, and how do these effects operate?
5. Specifically, what communication behaviors of others have positive or negative effects on you?

Group distinctions are not discussed here, since the cognitive capacities and insight levels of the client will determine the extent to which these areas can be evaluated and discussed directly. As an example of an approach procedure, the personal construct orientation is used.

In counseling therapy with children, usually adolescents, the clinician may apply some of the elements of Kelly's (1955) *personal construct therapy.* This psychotherapy is built around Kelly's view that people find their place in life and define their roles by using personal constructs. A construct is a discrimination made between contrasting characteristics or qualities, and it tends to be bipolar. For instance, good-bad, attractive-unattractive, successful-unsuccessful, fluent-stuttering, are bipolar constructs. In broad categories of comparison, the construct is *superordinal.* These superordinal constructs can have *subordinate* constructs contained within them. Examples of this might be the following:

SUPERORDINATE	SUBORDINATE
Attractive-Unattractive	short-tall, slender-fat, nice smile–silly grin, brown eyes–blue eyes, and so on
Confident-Unconfident	introduces self–stands around; seeks people–avoids people, says words–avoids words, good eye contact–poor eye contact
Fluent-Unfluent	smooth speech–jerky speech, hesitate–steady, broken words–finishes words, relaxed–struggles, and so on.

The subordinate constructs can have varying personal values so that, for one person, *fat-slender* might have more discriminative value than *smile-grin,* and so on. Constructs can be placed on a grid with various combinations decided by the client and the clinician. For example, a simple grid might include fluent-unfluent and confident-unconfident as displayed in Figure 10-2a. Onto this grid the client places *elements*—those things or persons that have characteristics associated with the constructs displayed. In our example people are used as the elements and the client places self and various persons on the grid, as shown in Figure 10-2b. In this figure Don is seen as being very confident and fluent; Frank is not very fluent but fairly confident; Carol Ann is fairly confident and fluent; Linda is fairly fluent but not very confident; the client sees self as very lacking in both fluency and confidence. On these bases the client described his or her place and role by comparisons to other persons. The grid could be

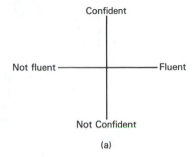

FIGURE 10-2a. A basic construct grid with only two categories.

(a)

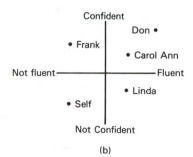

FIGURE 10-2b. A two-category construct grid with people elements entered on it.

(b)

reused, changing the elements to "situations that affect fluency and affect confidence." Then the client would disclose the situations that have positive and that have negative factors, a form of hierarchy in more than one dimension.

Fransella (1981, 1975, 1974a, 1974b, 1974c, 1972, 1970) has published extensively on the use of personal construct therapy with stutterers. Personal qualities, fluency desires, stuttering fears, situation anxieties, and other factors can be developed into personal construct grids. In the therapy process the client concentrates on the changes that will lead to fluency, rather than trying to learn to tolerate or accept the role of being a stutterer. Dalton (1983c) and Hayhow (1983), in Dalton's (1983b) book on therapy methods, provide an extensive explanation, summary, and examples of personal construct therapy with stutterers.

As a formal therapy, personal construct approaches require study, training, and supervised experience. However, as a concept the approach offers useful suggestions to the clinician for methods to help the client gain insight into self. Also, it can be applied in the client's efforts to evaluate people in her or his environment and how interaction with them facilitates or disrupts fluency. Similarly, situation categorization, communication fears, therapy goals, and other factors can be explored through this method.

GROUP THERAPY

In speech and language areas there are three forms of group therapy. First there is therapy with more than one person at the same time. This occurs typically because budget and time constraints require it. Clients receive clinician attention in rotation, and involvement outside the clients "turn" varies from nil to extensive. When it is extensive we have the second type of group therapy. In the second type, therapy can be organized in three ways:

1. Focus on production and perception skills so that when a client is not producing speech he or she has to monitor, evaluate, time, and so on, the production of some other member of the group.
2. Focus is on the psychosocial interactions of group members, using these to foster reductions in undesirable attitudes and behaviors and to promote increments in desired ones. This focus may be a primary target at the time of therapy initiation, may appear progressively as transfer becomes more significant, or may function in a support group after the termination of formal therapy.
3. Combinations of the first two.

The third approach to group therapy covers a variety of psychotherapy techniques that use group therapy formats. This format is used widely in mainstream psychotherapy and includes therapy with psychiatric disorders, phobic anxieties, grief therapy, substance abuse control, weight control, marital counseling, vocational rehabilitation, and so on. As with other psychotherapy approaches, special training and experience is required for clinicians. However, also as before, a number of principles can be and are utilized in more generalized group therapies.

Economics aside, group therapy has advantages and disadvantages in what is required and what can be gained. Slocum (1987) noted that psychotherapy clients are less motivated to join group therapy (preferring individual therapy) and are more likely to drop out of group therapy than the other. Slocum surveyed 96 college students seeking counseling for personal or vocational reasons and compared their pretreatment attitudes toward group therapy with the attitudes of 110 controls. Three unfavorable expectations or attitudes were found: (1) Group therapy is unpredictable, (2) it is not as effective as individual therapy, and (3) it may even be detrimental to the interests of the individual client. These expectations or concerns can be applied equally to Group III and some Group II clients—and have some validity. Indeed, if one reviews the three concerns, they are not inappropriate. The third concern, possible detriment, functions in any kind of group situation where self-perceived individual needs may be ignored and self-preferred individual behaviors may be discouraged or submitted to change pressures from the group.

Clinician planning for and manipulation of a group is a complex skill, and many do not do it well. Each member of the group must be planned for, observed, and reacted to as an individual—even as the *gestalt* of the group operates as an example of the whole being greater than the sum of its parts. Ordinarily this gestalt is a prime rationale for organizing group therapy in the first place, to utilize the group personality in therapy. Nevertheless, it must be recognized that some groups will be set up because, and only because, of time and cost factors and the intent to practice therapy parsimony in explanations, demonstrations, practice, and evaluation. While the foregoing reality cannot be ignored, and one can recognize the useful aspects of group therapy from the managerial view (see the list that follows), it is regrettable if certain values of group therapy remain untapped. In summary, some of the values of group therapy can be stated as follows:

1. Reduction of time spent in scheduling (usually) three to five individuals. This saving can range from one hour up to five or six hours per week.
2. Possibly scheduling longer and/or more frequent sessions because of the overall time saving.
3. Mixing individual and group sessions to garner the best values of both.
4. Desensitization through the exposure of each client to other persons who stutter. Tolerance and acceptance tend to be reinforced.
5. Cognitive values in becoming aware of the different forms fluency disruptions can take.
6. Encouragement to share feelings and experiences from the past, during therapy, and to anticipate future experiences and problems. Exposure to the idea that there is more than one way to view experiences and problems.
7. Practice in monitoring skills by evaluating others and by having self-monitoring efforts compared to others' evaluations.
8. Group interactions in activities such as role play and behavior rehearsal.
9. Opportunities for shared assignments, practice efforts, evaluation and mutual support on activities, outside of therapy sessions.
10. Peer pressure in motivation and standards of performance.

Group I Groups

Very young children are worked with individually. However, group activity can be used easily in several areas. Play therapy and desensitization to fluency disruption can be performed usefully in group therapy. To this author it would seem that fluency establishment and progress through early fluency criterion steps are accomplished best during individual therapy—but no absolutes are stated. As a child reaches the advanced stages of fluency stabilization, I usually try to find opportunities for group interaction in order to foster transfer practice while the clinician can be in control and monitor events.

Group II Groups

Therapy in a group form with Group II very likely will be structured for reasons of time economy, as well as therapy effects, particularly in the schools. One clinician commented to me, "Three separate children in a two-session, 20-minute schedule take two hours of time a week. I can see them in a group twice a week for 30–35 minutes, and still save time." Any form of therapy can be utilized with groups, such as the Shames and Florance program (1980), which provides specific adaptations for group use. Role play, at simple levels, can be utilized, as can behavior rehearsal activities.

Group III Groups

Group therapy seems particularly useful in this age range. It appears that adolescents respond well to having others to identify with, and group therapy may lessen the problem of communication between client and clinician. There is a caveat to be observed, however. At times an adolescent group can develop an "us-you" attitude toward the clinician and frustrate everything attempted. In my first day of student teaching I was given a group of six adolescent stutterers, and left alone. To this day I have sympathy for the mouse trapped in a corner by the playful cat! For weeks my only therapy planning was developed from the base, "What are they going to do to me *this* session?" In most cases group failures are the fault of an inexperienced clinician. But it is also possible for one or more adolescents to resist or even sabotage deliberately their group sessions, and the skill and experience of the clinician often cannot overcome this problem. Fortunately, this does not occur frequently.

If options on membership are open, the clinician may want to consider candidates. It usually helps if severity ranges are not sharply separated, particularly if only one member would be severe and the others mild. Age discrepancy can be a problem because of possible attitudes from other members, the practicalities of school class schedules, extracurricular activities, employment variables, and social interactions. Intelligence, at the extremes, can be both a cognitive and a potential attitude problem. A major factor in selection will be the individual's attitude toward group therapy. Finally, and possibly related to the prior concern, is the consideration of the overall adjustment and personality of individuals. In different situations, for a variety of reasons, the clinician may decide that a period of individual therapy may be required before a child can make the transition to group therapy. In arranging groups the clinician will also have specific considerations based on the individuals who are group candidates: A and B are brothers, A and C used to date but broke up, D has to leave early for band practice, and so on.

In adolescent group therapy this author has found it useful to set some ground rules or guidelines at the outset. This may be done during the first session or established after therapy preliminaries. For example,

> Okay, you all know who the others are now. This term we will be working together on your stuttering to understand what goes on and to work on bringing it under control. First, though, we need to know a little bit about each other. I want each of you to tell the rest of us about your stuttering history—when did it start, how has it developed, and what has to be done to help it. _____, why don't you start the histories?

If responses are open, this activity can take several sessions, especially if the clinician probes for further information and encourages other group members to ask questions. After this initial commitment, or some equivalent, then the clinician might lay down ground rules. These could originate totally from the clinician, from group discussion, or a mixture of both. Possible ground rules might include the following:

1. No cuts, and be on time.
2. Never laugh at a member's problems. We all have them.
3. Don't put down another's suggestion, but you are encouraged to suggest alternatives.
4. When you stutter, look at all of us. Never look away!
5. When somebody else stutters, establish and keep eye contact with them.
6. Become able to describe exactly what each person does when he or she stutters.

Other rules can be added or developed as the group takes on its own characteristics. One clinician's group added a rule, later, that at the end of each session, they would identify the person who had contributed most and best that day.

The form of group therapy is open to any kind of approach, or combination thereof. As discussed earlier, behavior modification and personal interaction can be stressed separately or mixed together. Similarly, fluency and symptom modification methods can be separated or mixed. Whatever the final program design is, a nonchanging principle should be that *every activity must be of value to the entire group.* If client A is practicing some skills, then B, C, and D should be interacting or have some assignment to monitor, evaluate, or consequate performance. If there is a discussion mode, the clinician must assure that all members participate. Constant monitoring of individual reactions and group interactions are needed, and the clinician should be ready to improvise, alter conditions, relieve stress, support varying efforts, and foster group strength. Role play and behavior rehearsal are particularly applicable in group therapy with adolescents, and the clinician can retire to the role of executive producer, supporting and observing as the clients conduct most of the activity among themselves. (Group therapy has particular values in maintenance, and this aspect is discussed in Chapter 17.)

BIBLIOTHERAPY

"And, of course, you can use bibliotherapy." This throwaway phrase is heard in many lectures but rarely explained. As a matter of fact, bibliotherapy can be very useful and we have some excellent sources for it. There has already been discussion of resources for use with parents in counseling and environmental manipulation. However, older Group II and the Group III children can profit from bibliotherapy. It provides organized information in readable form, saves time for the clinician, and can be used as background for in-clinic discussions and/or for expansion of in-clinic introductions.

Sources for bibliotherapy can be limited. However, the limitation can be dealt with in part by judicious photocopying of relevant sections of various books, with proper observation of copyright regulations. Such copies can be used, filed, and used again. If the clinician feels confident in doing so, he or she can use text sources, notes, and experiences to write material for personal use. In several in-service programs, this author noticed the groups had divided up self-assignments to write about, and collect materials on, various communication problems. Clinicians prepared material in areas they felt more strength in, and the results were copied and shared among the group. Also, over time clinicians tend to develop files that can be used in bibliotherapy—and it is never too early to start. One school district this author visited had a "rule" that at their monthly staff meeting clinicians would bring copies of all printed materials they had developed and used in the past month (form letters, word lists, information pages, and so on) and share them.

Specific bibliotherapy material should be used with several considerations in mind. Is the material relevant and appropriate to the situation? Is it written at a vocabulary and semantic level that is not too much above or below the clients' levels? Has the clinician read the material, and is it understood? Years ago, after reading a pamphlet a client asked me, "What does it mean here, 'When you want to call a spade a spatula . . . ?'" It took me some time to formulate a reply about the semantic concept of labeling. On practical terms the clinician should keep more than one copy of useful materials, or have the client buy them. Materials can quickly become torn, stained, crumpled, and lost. This year a college-age stutterer was loaned my personal copy of Murray's (1980) *A Stutterer's Story*, and the client chewed the binding off the back! All of the items from the Speech Foundation of America can be ordered at very reasonable rates. Suggested items, and comments, are as follows:

DIRECT MATERIAL

BARBARA, D. A., *A Practical Self-Help Guide for Stutterers*. Springfield, Ill.: Charles C. Thomas, 1983. Somewhat casual in style, but easy to read; particularly good coverage on feelings and attitudes.

CARLISLE, J. A., *Tangled Tongue: Living with a Stutter*. Toronto: University of Toronto Press, 1985. Autobiography. Excellent overviews of theories and therapies of stuttering, as well as the author's personal experiences.

MURRAY, F. P., *A Stutterer's Story*. Danville, Ill.: The Interstate, 1980. Autobiography. Similar to Carlisle, but more therapy oriented. Author became a speech and language pathologist.

Speech Foundation of America. P.O. Box 11749, Memphis, Tennessee, 38111.
Do You Stutter: A Guide for Teens, 21 (1987). "Writes down" somewhat, and the cartoons are rather cutesy, but it has useful information about stuttering and therapy. Might be particularly useful with young adolescents.
Self-Therapy for Stutterers (revised), 12 (1987). Written as if stutterer will be own clinician, but also useful in clinician therapy. Valuable mainly in symptom modification, avoidance-reduction, and desensitization therapies.
To The Stutterer, 9 (1972). A series of short chapters by 25 clinicians who work with stutterers, and many also are stutterers. Useful overall, or through selection of specific areas.

BOOK CHAPTERS

BLOODSTEIN, O., *Speech Pathology: An Introduction*. Boston: Houghton Mifflin, 1979. Chapter 4 provides a thorough, readable discussion of stuttering for the adolescent and the young adult.

CONTURE, E. G., Introduction. In E.G. Conture, *Stuttering*. Englewood Cliffs, N.J.: Prentice Hall, 1982. Most of book is clinician oriented, but the first chapter provides a clear description of stuttering, along with therapy implications.

CURLEE, R. F., Disorders of fluency. In P.H. Skinner and R.L. Shelton (eds.), *Speech, Language, and Hearing: Normal Processes and Disorders*. 2d ed. New York: John Wiley, 1985. An excellent overview chapter. More detailed and technical than some, but very readable. Best for older child, or for clinician to extract specific parts.

EGLAND, G. O., *Speech and Language Problems: A Guide for the Classroom Teacher*. Englewood Cliffs, N.J.: Prentice Hall, 1970. May have to find in a library. Chapter 8 on fluency disorders provides about 70 pages of material that can be used or adapted for use with teachers.

FLORANCE, C. L., and Shames, G.H., Stuttering treatment: Issues in transfer and maintenance. In W.H. Perkins (ed.), *Strategies in Stuttering Therapy*. Seminars in Speech, Language, and Hearing. New York: Thieme-Stratton, 1980. Will require some editing to remove technical summaries, but other summaries and text discuss transfer and maintenance issues very clearly.

SHAMES, G. H., Disorders of fluency. In G.H. Shames and E.H. Wiig (eds.), *Human Communication Disorders*. 2d ed., Columbus, Ohio: Charles E. Merrill, 1986. A very basic, easy-to-read overview of stuttering in general.

REFERENCE TEXTS

SILVERMAN, F. H., *Speech-Language Pathology and Audiology: An Introduction*. Columbus, Ohio: Charles E. Merrill, 1984. This book is written differently than most, and stuttering topics are scattered across various chapters. However, the table of contents tracks topics well, and usable material can be retrieved easily.

St. Louis, K. O. (ed.), *The Atypical Stutterer*. New York: Academic Press, 1986. A series of chapters by different authors, each considering "different stutterers." Areas of particular interest include cultural factors, female stutterers, extreme severity, clutterers, and neurogenic stuttering. Selection and revision may be needed.

Stuttering Therapy: Transfer and Maintenance. Memphis, Tenn.: Speech Foundation of America, 19, n.d. A series of chapters by various clinicians, touching upon issues and information concerning transfer and maintenance.

Van Riper, C., *The Treatment of Stuttering*. Englewood Cliffs, N.J.: Prentice Hall, 1973. Wide-ranging coverage of many different therapies and aspects of stuttering. Selection required.

Van Riper, C., *The Nature of Stuttering*. Englewood Cliffs, N.J.: Prentice Hall, 1982. Wide-ranging coverage of origins, development, and characteristics of stuttering. Selection and revision required.

Wingate, M. E., *Stuttering Theory and Treatment*. New York: John Wiley, 1976. May have to find in library. Excellent at pulling areas together, synthesizing material in easily understood terms, and telling reader "what things mean."

CHAPTER SUMMARY

This chapter cut across the wide range of motivation, attitudes, and emotions of stutterers, discussing their significance to therapy and indicating several procedures that can be used. Some of the procedures, such as self-analysis, relate strongly to the central theme of the chapter, and hierarchy development and use also relate to the central theme. However, both self-analysis and hierarchies have significant values for other areas of therapy focus, such as relaxation-desensitization therapy, out-clinic assignments in symptom therapy, and for any therapy mode in the maintenance stage. Group therapy and bibliotherapy were presented more as general therapy methods, but their potential impacts on attitudes and feelings should be clear. Counseling activities, the core of therapy, pervade in every type of therapy approach. Even the most formal of behavior modification therapies, cast in an operant structure, possess a counseling dynamism based, at least, on therapy presence and authority of the clinician. Something is being "said" to the client in any mode of therapy. Perhaps that is the epigram of this chapter. Therapy is communication on a psychosocial basis, and it is most appropriate for us to consider and plan for the most effective modes of communication as we give significance to the motivation, attitudes, and feelings of the client.

CHAPTER ELEVEN
RELAXATION AND DESENSITIZATION

OVERVIEW

Anxiety and tension have received attention a number of times already in this book. Clinicians tend to separate into three groups, according to their views on anxiety and tension and their significance. Some (Sheehan 1975) appear to feel that anxiety can be a causative agent and should receive major attention in therapy. Other clinicians (Van Riper 1973) regard anxiety as an important factor to be dealt with in therapy, but not necessarily as a major factor. The third group (Ryan 1974) seem to feel that anxiety is an antecedent response to stuttering and that therapy to relieve or remove the dysfluency eliminates a need to deal with the anxiety and tension as specific phenomena. These points of view tend to merge or overlap with many clinicians as they deal with different stutterers over time. Some stutterers, particularly the very young (and perhaps the elderly), may present very little in the way of state or trait anxiety, and therapy that removes or significantly reduces dysfluency frequency and severity may be sufficient unto itself. There will be other stutterers, especially in Group III and young adult categories, where state anxiety (Spielberger 1966) occurs prior to and during dysfluency events. Therapy to enhance fluency or control symptoms may not resolve a lifetime of emo-

259

tional abrasion and trauma, and successful transfer and maintenance requires dealing with significant residual anxiety and tension. A few stutterers, as in the fluent population, will be characterized by trait anxiety
(Spielberger 1966), in which the person perceives and feels stress and
anxiety where none ordinarily exists and/or feels at a much higher intensity than most other people would.

A problem in anxiety and stuttering has been contradictory views
and reports on the condition. Boland (1953) argued for the existence of
higher state and trait anxiety levels in stutterers, while Andrews (1974)
failed to find a relationship, and Ingham (1984) felt the hunt for the relationship had not been successful (p. 133). Anxiety during the act of stuttering has generated equally contradictory views (Brutten 1963; Gray &
Brutten 1965; Sherrard 1975; Ragsdale 1976). Research has indicated
that stutterers' avoidance reactions to speech situations is greater than the
avoidances by nonstutterers (Johnson, Darley & Spriestersbach 1963).
The stutterer's perception of a situation (audience) also seems to relate to
the speech difficulty experienced (Porter 1939; Berwick 1955; Sheehan,
Hadley & Gould 1967). The simple factor of audience size also seems to
relate to stuttering difficulty, being positively related (Shulman 1955;
Siegel & Haugen 1964). However, at least with reference to the number
of listeners, Young (1965) found that adolescent stutterers were not affected in their speech by groups of one to four listeners. The possibly
significant factor in this study is that the speaker-subjects were not told
beforehand how many listeners would be present. Stutterers seem to have
anxieties about the same types of speaking situations as do nonstutterers
(except that the telephone usually ranks higher on the stutterers' anxiety
lists), but their avoidance of such situations seems to range widely from
maximal to minimal. State anxiety seems to be a frequent, but variable,
concomitant of stuttering, and research does suggest that situation-
specific, or state, anxiety problems occur with some stutterers (Moore,
Soderberg & Powell 1952; Goss 1952, 1956; Forte & Schlesinger 1972).

How anxiety affects the speaker is complex but significant. Aside
from certain instinctive fears, anxiety must start at the neurological level
where sensory stimuli are interpreted and associated with stored memories. The association process extends to include the *limbic system,* a complex of neurological centers and pathways that provide for emotional
tone, attitudes, feelings, and so on, involved in our responses. The limbic
system, through interaction with the *reticular* and *autonomic* systems, produces effects on awareness, stimulus sensitivity, motivation, and physiological responses of the body to emotion. Depending on the emotion and
its strength, physiological responses can include such effects as tears, tension of muscles, adrenalin release, and altered vascular states. For example, Ickes and Pierce (1973) reported that stutterers, compared to nonstutterers, had significantly greater vasoconstriction prior to speaking and
had even higher vasoconstriction levels prior to stuttering spasms.

To a certain degree, an emotion and its typical physiological concomitants become reflexive and reciprocal—one can trigger the other. Most of the time, through corticothalamic connections, the limbic system is guided and restrained so that excessive emotional responses do not occur or, if they do, are quickly brought under control. However, limbic reactions are more difficult to access and control when they affect behaviors that have "slipped" from high levels of cortical control to the semiautomatic control systems in the cerebellar-midbrain-basal ganglia circuits. Limbic reactions are also more difficult to control if they are stronger than usual and if the person cognitively concludes that the fear, anxiety, embarrassment, or whatever, is "justified." That is, if you know you may stutter and the stuttering will be unpleasant and produce negative reactions from auditors, you may conclude that anxiety is appropriate—and this will weaken control of limbic activity and facilitate avoidance behaviors as the best antidote for anxiety.

The subsequent sections of this chapter concentrate on three separate approaches to relaxation and desensitization: (1) the cognitive (cortical) factors in anxiety reduction or control, (2) the reduction of emotional (limbic) responses directly, or (3) the suppression or redirection of the physiological (autonomic) concomitants associated with emotions. In some procedures the three aspects are mixed or combined. This results in some overlap between the topic areas of desensitization and relaxation. However, these areas are first discussed as separate issues before combinations are considered.

RELAXATION

Background

Tension is the normal state of the organism, and muscle tonus is a requisite of normal muscle function. The concept of tonus refers to a low-level of constant muscle contraction for maintenance of posture, circulation of blood, and support of general body functions (Friel 1965). A muscle without tension is a lifeless muscle. However, the general use of the words *tense* and *tension* usually occurs in the sense of hypertense, that is, excessive levels of tension. Van Riper (1973) has indicated that relaxation historically occupied a place in stuttering therapy. Many years ago Boome and Richardson (1939) observed that "the basis of all treatment for stammerers—whether individually or in a group—should be relaxation" (p. 101). But reviews of relaxation as a primary therapy (Bloodstein 1969; Van Riper 1973; Ingham 1984) have not reported particularly impressive, or supportable, results. During the author's student days, formal relaxation therapy was regarded as quackery unless it was presented in a psychotherapy context. However, in the past 20 years or so there has grown a recognition that relaxation is, or can be, involved in many different therapy procedures. Also, there has been a renewed interest in relaxation from the desensitization standpoint and from therapists applying biofeedback procedures.

Many clinicians today would agree with Dalton and Hardcastle (1977) who observed that relaxation therapy alone is not very successful. They feel, though, that it seems to be essential for relaxation to be integrated into whatever modification therapy is being used and that relaxation should be practiced progressively, starting with in-clinic steps (Gregory 1968; Bloodstein 1969; Wingate 1976; Crystal 1980; Fiedler & Standop 1983).

Presumably relaxation is antagonistic to feelings of anxiety and tension. It favors reductions in rate and increases in the frequency and duration of pause time; it also facilitates elongation of vowels and continuant consonants. Articulatory contacts are likely to be made with less pressure (and precision), and respiratory patterns typically become more stable and uniform against the cardiac pulse rate of the individual. Under such conditions stuttering behaviors are less likely to occur, or to occur with less intensity and with fewer associated behaviors.

The following subsections consider relaxation procedures from the aspects of general or whole-body relaxation, specific applications, and special procedures that can be used.

Deep Relaxation

Deep, whole-body, or progressive relaxation has been used for many years in therapies and has been associated mainly with Jacobson (1938). A number of clinicians, particularly Overstake (1979), Wohl (1970), and Gronhovd (1977) have published versions of Jacobson-type relaxation procedures. In most cases the intense practice of relaxation (anywhere from 4 to 12 sessions) is preliminary to other therapy—desensitization, airflow retraining, easy onset speech, and so on. The author has published a version of Jacobson-style relaxation therapy (Ham 1986, pp. 127–30) (an abbreviated form is presented in Table 11–1). More extended sequences can be used, different parts of the body involved, or different tensing methods applied than those suggested in Table 11–1. In each activity, the particular muscle group or area is to be tensed strongly and then relaxed thoroughly. The client is to feel the difference between the two tension levels and begin to learn to judge degree of tension. Two complete cycles in one therapy session are probably sufficient. As soon as the client has demonstrated an ability to perform the full cycle successfully, she or he should be assigned to practice the relaxation sequence at home. One or two out-clinic sessions per day are usually adequate; these can be set at convenient times, such as lunch, midafternoon, after school, or bedtime. If available and feasible, a cassette recorder can be used to

TABLE 11–1. Short Sequence for Progressive Relaxation

1. Explain relaxation, tension, purposes, and procedures.
2. Environment: dim or redirect lights, have client lie supine on pad or mattress.
3. Suggestion: clinician use relaxed speech pattern; use background sound or music if desired; direct client to clear mind or concentrate on relaxing thoughts or visualizations; reinforce feelings of quiet and relaxation.
4. Instructions to client: tell client what he or she is to do, what signals will be used, what procedures followed (clinician maintains relaxed speech pattern).
5. Elevate each leg in turn for five seconds, relax and let fall, repeat; verbally stress and reinforce difference between relaxation and tension.
6. Strongly contract abdominal muscles as if resisting weight, hold for five seconds, release; repeat (clinician reinforces relaxation).
7. Clench fists, tighten shoulders and shrug them toward ears, hold for five seconds and relax; repeat (clinician reinforces relaxation).
8. In sequence, holding each for five seconds and then relaxing, form an exaggerated and tensed version of each of the following: forehead frown, eyes squinted shut, nose-lip wrinkle, smile or grin, tongue pressure against hard palate, jaw clench; repeat entire cycle (clinician reinforces relaxation).
9. Between each of steps 5 through 8, and also before the repeat cycles of each step, clinician may want client to concentrate on breathing evenly and deeply, clearing the mind, while clinician verbally reinforces relaxation.

tape a successful in-clinic session, for the client to use during out-clinic practice.

The clinician should keep in mind that Group I children do not usually require, and do not respond well to, progressive relaxation therapy. This also is true of many Group II children, especially in group therapy situations. However, relaxation can be used profitably with any age—it is just that younger children do not seem to respond as well to the "exercise" aspect of progressive relaxation therapy. In contrast, Group III children may have some initial shyness and resistance behavior but often respond well, ultimately, to whole-body relaxation therapy, especially with the hectic pace at which so many adolescents seem to live.

Specific Applications

There are several specific applications of deep-relaxation therapy. Wells (1987) supplies an outline of specific differential exercises for hands and arms, stomach and breathing, eyes, jaw, lips, tongue, and larynx. For each area she provides tension activities and progressive levels of increasing tension. Wells states that weeks or months of twice-daily exercises are needed to accrue full benefits of relaxation. Conture (1982) has recommended relaxation in order to reduce speech rate and dysfluency severity in children. An illustrative model he cites is that of comparing the scarecrow (relaxation) to the tin woodsman (tension). The author has paired statue with rag doll, lazy dog and crazy cat, and other combinations for children to imitate. Mental imagery has been suggested as a method of achieving relaxation. Breathing exercises to deepen, regulate, and retime respiratory patterns tend to have a relaxing effect (Fiedler & Standop 1983; Azrin & Nunn 1974) and are often an extra benefit in fluency or symptom therapy where respiration or an easy onset of phonation receives attention. Other therapy instructions may involve, require, or promote relaxation as part of their procedures. An example of this is Runyan and Runyan's (1986) listing of "rules" for young school-age stutterers. The rules include practice in reducing oral tension, relaxing muscle groups not involved actively in speech production, eliminating rigid articulatory postures, and relaxing the laryngeal area through breathstream release and gentle phonatory onsets.

Falck (1969) follows the pattern set by many clinicians, particularly those working with symptom modification procedures, in suggesting a limited and specific use of relaxation. Overall, general body relaxation is not favored, but specific relaxation of speech mechanism muscle groups is. The training sequence might be summarized as follows:

1. Imitate a stuttering spasm; then increase its tension and push hard with the articulators. If the fake becomes real, that does not interrupt.
2. Stop the production effort, relax all tension, and return articulators to the rest position.
3. Feel the difference between tension and relaxation; analyze it for each area or muscle group.
4. Repeat the previous three steps until tension differences can be quickly identified and evaluated.

Falck notes that the benefits of relaxation differ for different stutterers. Gottlober (1953) approached relaxation from the systematic and differential view, combining it with psychotherapy. Alone, it is only a symptomatic treatment and will have, at best, "only limited benefits and temporary effect" (p. 230). Relaxation is regarded as a balance between desirable and unnecessary levels of tension. The client first must have quiet and relaxation-conducive surroundings to achieve mental "quiet" relaxation. Gottlober then identifies twenty muscle group areas to be highly tensed, separately, for about 20 seconds each, and then relaxed. When this can be done, the client is to carry the exercise through twice daily, preferably at noon and at 4:00 P.M. After two or three weeks of practice the client should try to achieve the same degree of relaxation without the exercises and try to extend the duration of time the relaxation can be held. Mental calmness or relaxation is a requisite. Differential relaxation follows, in which the client surveys daily activities (reading, writing, walking, and so on) and tries to slightly relax the active muscle groups and more thoroughly relax the muscle groups not directly involved. Speech is the final target, involving respiration, phonation, and articulation.

Special Applications

Relaxation can be induced or supported by other methods. Audio-tape recordings of environmental sounds or soothing music can be used, and the author has used a tape that is silent except for a quiet, high-pitched ring of a chime sounding at five-second intervals. The client was to clear the mind, float in the silence, and listen for the chime, letting it "fill your mind." Commercial audiotapes of relaxation exercises are available, and videotapes can be used to project scenes that are conducive to relaxation. Postures and behaviors borrowed from yoga and transcendental meditation (McIntyre, Silverman & Trotter 1974) have been used, and the author has found them to be quite effective. Also reported has been the use of carbon dioxide inhalation as an anxiety inhibitor (Meduna 1958; Kent 1961; Wells & Malcolm 1971). And hypnosis and biofeedback applications have been used in order to promote or train relaxation methods.

There will be no discussion of CO_2 and the psychopharmacologicals because the reports of their effects have been quite mixed, more so than usual. Also, their use requires medical administration and/or supervision and monitoring. Immediate and long-term side effects can be a question, especially since some drugs appear to create a neurogenic fluency problem or, at worst, result in major neuromotor problems such as tardive dyskinesia. In past contacts with stutterers who, individually and apart from therapy, were on medical regimens of tranquilizing drugs, the author observed reductions in anxiety and in dysfluency levels. However, there frequently was a reduction in the motivation toward, and the willingness to work in, therapy.

Neither will hypnosis be discussed extensively, although some have supported its use (Falck 1969). Ingham (1984) reviews hypnosis use, finding "woefully inadequate" (p. 412) evidence either to support or to decry its value. However, Ingham suggests the possibility that it may be of value and have a very useful place in therapy. While this may be possible, there again is the problem of training the clinician and integrating hypnosis into an overall therapy plan. Also, and especially with young children, potential problems with parents, school boards, and interest groups can become a critical issue. Since for many decades media entertainment has portrayed hypnotism as the fiendish tool of that madman, evil Dr. X, many persons in the lay public may bristle at the thought of children being hypnotized.

Biofeedback has been adopted by the communication disorders field and applied in many different ways. In general terms biofeedback is a system by which some biological activity of the organism is detected, transmitted back to the organism emitting the activity, and used by the organism as a signal to alter the activity. Often the returned signal acts as a scale against which the organism can measure the change in activity that has occurred. Usually, but not always, the biological signal is amplified or otherwise modified, and it may be used to trigger an intervening signal or scale that will be more noticeable, and useful, to the organism. For instance, having the client tactilely monitor her or his carotid pulse is direct, unaltered biofeedback. Electronic monitoring of blood pressure, temperatures of body surfaces or orifices, brain-wave activity, and other complex functions have also been utilized. The most common approaches in communication disorders have been through galvanic skin response (GSR) and electromyography (EMG) procedures. A GSR involves placing contact electrodes (usually on hand palmar surfaces or finger thenar surfaces) where electrodermal conductivity changes are detected, amplified, and displayed on meters or graph paper. The EMG techniques use surface electrodes or invasive (needle) microelectrodes to detect and amplify the chemoelectric action of final motor pathways as alpha motoneurons deliver impulses to the motor endplates of striated muscle groups. As before, detected signals are displayed on meters or on paper. Both GSR and EMG signals, with the EMG being used more frequently, can be used to drive auxiliary signaling systems. Strength of the detected signals can also be displayed—the number of lights illuminated on a panel or board, or the brightness of lumen, or changes in color, for example. Specially labeled meters, digital-readout counters, rising and falling forms, and other signals can be used. Auditory signals have included tone emission when an arbitrary level is reached, discrete tones or clicks where speed of production is proportional to activity strength, and signal loudness or pitch that is related to activity level. Other signal methods have been used, being limited only by ingenuity and budget. In all instances the person generating the activity can be trained to associate the signals with designated activity states and to alter those states by working to change the signal or its characteristics. In many instances, how the person achieves this change is not understood, and success varies with different individuals.

In relaxation therapy, biofeedback has been used in some of the ways described previously. Client participation can be *active* or *passive*. In passive biofeedback the client practices keeping the measurement signal at some desirable level, with progressive stress or stimulation increments occurring as the stabilization ability improves. In active biofeedback the client is practiced in deliberately altering tension levels in order to change the output of the measurement signal. Hanna, Wilfing, and McNeil (1975), in a single-case study, attempted to evaluate biofeedback and relaxation using EMG laryngeal signals to trigger a variable-pitch auditory signal. Pitch level was dependent on degree of laryngeal muscle tension. Results were confused, adaptation may have blurred results, and few conclusions can be drawn from the stuttering decrements measured in two sessions. Guitar (1975) found that several stutterers could learn passive muscle relaxation using analog EMG feedback from various muscle groups. The clients then were trained to transfer the relaxation to speech activity. Results indicated that relaxation and stuttering decrements occurred, but individual stutterers varied in the relationship between stuttering decrements and the muscle area or areas showing the most relaxation. It appears that we cannot assume for any one stutterer what muscle groups contribute most to spasm activity or whether one or more muscle groups is involved significantly. Yonovitz, Shepherd, and Garrett (1977) used biofeedback (GSR) signals to trigger a variable pitch generator as the client practiced relaxation. When relaxation was established, visualization of aversive stimuli was introduced in progressive steps. St. Louis and others (1982) reported successful, although difficult, efforts to use EMG biofeedback in training a preschool stutterer to secure relaxation in the laryngeal area and so reduce stuttering. Shames and Egolf (1976) suggest that clinicians can learn to teach the stutterer how to recognize and regulate internal excitement levels. The goal of such therapy would not be to teach relaxation in the presence of stress and stimuli, but "how to cope with excitement, how to participate in and experience the emotional situations that are available in society, with the same relative fluency that the nonstutterer emits during states of emotional excitement" (p. 144). Exactly how this differs from "relaxation in the presence of stress" is never explained by the authors. Ingham (1984) provides an excellent review of biofeedback studies in stuttering in terms of describing stuttering and in therapy uses. He is impressed by the potential of biofeedback but depressed by the lack of creativity in its use. Ingham feels that its use in relaxation training does not appear to be any more effective than relaxation therapy itself, yet he does note that biofeedback is highly suited for use in behavior therapy. When more appropriate applications have been developed, "biofeedback methodology will become an essential feature of much stuttering therapy" (p. 408). This author feels that adequate training of student clinicians needs to be planned, the expense of multiple EMG unit acquisitions and maintenance dealt with, the expense of equipping clinicians in the workplace budgeted, and the probable wide variations in EMG responsiveness compensated for. Until that time biofeedback will continue to be found most in laboratory research, in training programs, and in a few practice sites.

In summary, relaxation in stuttering therapy has a long history, a high level of present use, and a promising future. In today's therapies clinicians tend to use it as an adjunct to facilitate other therapy procedures or to make it an integral part of certain fluency or symptom modification techniques. At present more or less traditional relaxation methods are the primary approaches in such therapy. Drug therapy has not been sufficiently rewarding, and the valuable tool of hypnosis has a number of constraints. While agreeing with Ingham about the potential value of biofeedback, this author is doubtful about its wide implementation in the near future.

DESENSITIZATION

Background

To desensitize means to eliminate or reduce the occurrence of a response to stimuli of a particular form or type. Altering the stimulus is not desensitization. Desensitization can occur if a stimulus is presented repeatedly across appropriate time intervals so that response adaptation occurs, temporarily or permanently. The folk cliché of returning to a traumatic experience "or you never will again" is founded partially on this concept. Therapy assignments that have the client make many telephone calls consecutively is another example. Desensitization may occur if the stimulus is raised to extremely high levels so that responses reduce as a result of overstimulation (unless the result is response exaggeration to match the stimulus increment). *Implosive,* or *emotional flooding,* therapy is an application of the overstimulation concept. Another desensitization procedure is to begin stimulation at infrathreshold levels and intensify the stimulus in small increments, stopping short of response threshold, and then starting over again. *Basal fluency* therapy applies this process. Situation fears may be dealt with in this fashion when working with mature stutterers: Start with situations that can be handled and slowly progress along the fear hierarchy. Desensitization can also be approached on the cognitive level to foster cortical inhibition of limbic activity. "Fear of the unknown," another cliché, is handled by this approach, based on the idea that information and logic bring understanding, and understanding can reduce fear. Of course, understanding can also increase fear and tension because the person no longer fears the unknown. Instead, he or she now fears a specific thing! Finally, desensitization can be fostered by interposing a second, competing response to the stimulus, so that the first or primary response cannot occur or is reduced in strength. Telling a person to "first, count slowly to 10" is a common application of this approach. If one is slowly, quietly counting, it is difficult to express or feel anger. So-called systematic desensitization, or reciprocal inhibition therapy, is a clinical example of this desensitization principle.

Types of Desensitization

There are two general types of desensitization, implicit and explicit. *Implicit desensitization* involves procedures in which emotional reduction is not a direct goal, although it occurs. The clinician is a desensitizing agent because she or he is a friendly, concerned, interactive listener and projects confidence in self-efficacy and the therapy program. "Tell me about your stuttering" and "let's analyze each stuttering spasm" and many other therapy activities tend to be desensitizing. Even the process of constructing a fear hierarchy can reduce anxiety and tension in some clients. Further, implicit desensitization can occur when the activity of the moment prevents or reduces anxiety responses (reciprocal inhibition). Thus, if the client is concentrating on a 120-wpm rate, syllable prolongation, self-monitoring, and so on, anxiety is less easily stimulated because of the blocking activity. In contrast, *explicit desensitization* involves the direct goal of identifying sensitivity or anxiety and making overt attempts to control it. Many of the implicit activities that have been cited previously can be applied in explicit desensitization. The differentiation is not vital except where clinicians who question the use of desensitization therapy fail to realize just how much of the implicit form they use daily in therapy. Actually, the only questions are how much will it be emphasized, and what format will be followed. In the following paragraphs, explicit desensitization is reviewed in several forms as a primary therapy and as an adjunct in composite therapy programs.

Transfer of Desensitization

Adams (1982) notes that the most persistent problem faced by clinicians is that in-clinic speech fluency of stutterers tends to fall apart when it is carried over into daily life. He states that this problem is particularly significant in situations where the client encounters anxiety or emotional stress. Many clinicians have expressed the attitude that significant desensitization should precede therapy in which intensive fluency shaping is planned. The impact of stutter desensitization on the listener was investigated by Tatchell, van den Berg, and Lerman (1983), who applied previous research and therapy concerns about eye contact to audience ratings of four videotapes in which low or high eye contact and fluent or disfluent speech were paired. Findings were quite clear that low eye contact plus disfluent speech resulted in uniformly low auditor perceptions of speaker competence, credibility, and dynamism. Particularly interesting was the result that good eye contact plus disfluent speech was rated better than low eye contact with fluent speech. Frequency of eye contact was, at least in this situation, more important than was fluency (the disfluency enacted was not stuttering).

Desensitization and Inhibition

The popular combination of systematic desensitization and reciprocal inhibition has received considerable attention, and a number of favorable reports about it have been issued (Lanyon 1969; Webster 1970; Adams 1972; Gray & England 1972; Tyre, Maisto & Companik 1973).

Most of the studies just cited, plus others, are reviewed by Gronhovd and Zenner (1982), who concluded that systematic desensitization and reciprocal inhibition are generally effective in reducing anxiety related to speech and may help improve fluency. Gronhovd and Zenner also support the idea of learning and overlearning of fluency methods through behavior modification but object to any program that then leaves the stutterer to "go it alone." They insist that such intervention must be followed by anxiety-reduction therapy, or we are in the position of only partially preparing the stutterer for the stress that may occur in out-clinic communication. Ingham (1984) criticized the research done in this area of anxiety reduction, suggesting that the research may not be focused appropriately because it is arguable whether or not tension states are necessarily negative in their effects and they "must" increase stuttering.

Applications of Desensitization

As indicated, desensitization therapy has been applied in a variety of ways, and reports of effects have varied. Adams (1972) reported that 75 percent of 12 stutterers showed some favorable fluency responses as a result of ten weeks of reciprocal inhibition therapy. In the same vein, Boudreau and Jeffrey (1973) described a trial of systematic desensitization therapy, starting with relaxation, hierarchy construction, and systematic desensitization. After 13 therapy sessions, five clients showed "marked improvement" and three had relatively little change. It was noted that the least improvement was shown by the mildest stutterers, and those who were rated most severe (pretreatment) showed the greatest reductions in stuttering. In comparison to more standard speech therapy approaches, desensitization and inhibition received a favorable evaluation. Walton and Mather (1963) described two stutterers where evaluation indicated significant emotional problems and for whom direct speech therapy procedures (shadowing) failed to provide adequate speech outside the clinic. But utilizing desensitization and stimulus generalization procedures, they reported satisfactory results. This study might emphasize simultaneously the points that some stutterers require major attention to out-clinic desensitization and that not all stutterers require intensive desensitization. Berecz (1973) describes cognitive arousal and cognitive conditioning therapy in which the stutterer is taught to imagine vividly re-creations of scenes (cognitive arousal) from a hierarchy list. When the re-creation is at its most vivid, the client is to self-administer the precision punishment of an electrical shock (cognitive conditioning). Yet systematic desensitization has also received unfavorable reviews. Moleski and Tosi (1976) compared systematic desensitization to RET, rational emotive therapy (see Chapter 10), and to no therapy during eight sessions, with five stutterers in each group. The authors concluded that RET was more effective in reducing stuttering behaviors and anxieties but that systematic desensitization was better than no therapy. They also reported that controlled real-life assignment practice was helpful in improving client attitudes toward speech. Conture (1982) stated that desensitization should develop tolerance for, not dysfluency, but fluency disruptors. These disruptors can be subtle, such as the auditor losing eye contact, or more direct, as when a stutterer is interrupted or "helped." Particular topics and types of situations can also function as disruptors.

Controversy over Desensitization

The previous paragraph summarized a mixed, and somewhat confusing, series of reports and comments about desensitization—focusing on it as a major therapy. There also is the question of how well desensitization is used in terms of integration and appropriateness in a more generalized program of therapy. Wohl (1966) criticized most applications of desensitization therapy because they fail to prepare the stutterer for the transfer to real-life situations. Wohl describes a Wolpe-type system (without hypnosis), which is followed by a fluency reinforcement therapy (for example, using a metronome) that is felt to be appropriate for the client. But the issue of appropriateness has been raised about desensitization itself. Adams (1983), making the point that stutterers are a diverse group of persons, stated that a therapy can fail because clinicians do not consider client individuality. This occurs particularly where stereotypes of stutterers are held. Using anxiety deconditioning (desensitization) as one example of therapies that can be applied inappropriately, Adams pointed out that many stutterers are anxious, some are extremely anxious, and some show quite low levels of anxiety; and so to utilize desensitization or any other anxiety-reduction procedures with all stutterers, or to the same degree, or in the same form, is as inappropriate as not considering or applying such procedures with any stutterer.

Thus, in addition to separations between implicit and explicit desensitization, to joining reciprocal inhibition with it, and to applying various combinations of either or both, there are cautions about how well the methods are used and questions about how appropriate they are for use with all clients. In the following subsections various approaches to desensitization are described so that the reader can gain some sense of various possibilities and then consider how they might be used.

Classical Desensitization and Reciprocal Inhibition

Although desensitization has been utilized for centuries both formally and informally, the present-day concept of *systematic desensitization* is associated most often with Wolpe (1973). In laboratory settings, Wolpe had conditioned a cat to an eating neurosis by pairing food presentation with severe electrical shocks (Pavlov's dog was more fortunate!). Once the anxiety neurosis was established, Wolpe worked to decondition the cat by presenting the food in low-anxiety settings. The results were promising but incomplete, and Wolpe continued to work to refine and establish his procedures. With the use of the personal imagination of humans to create feelings of anxiety at graded levels, systematic desensitization finally evolved. In brief, the process included the following:

1. Progressive, deep muscle relaxation in the Jacobson (1938) mode.
2. With the client, definition and establishment of a scale to quantify feelings of subjective anxiety.
3. Development and refinement of a hierarchy of anxiety-provoking situations.
4. Opposition use of relaxation and recall visualization of scenes from the hierarchy, starting with those lowest on the scale.

In Wolpe's design the deep muscle relaxation sequence of therapy sets up a reversal of the limbic-autonomic sequence described earlier. By putting the body into all the physical characteristics associated with a nonanxiety state, the "backflow" supposedly blunts limbic effects and alters reticular sensitization patterns. At this point, cognitive recall and visualization of anxiety-producing events occurs without the limbic effects and autonomic nervous system (ANS) reactions associated with anxiety. The patient is able to contemplate anxiety stimuli without becoming anxious. Wolpe did not claim that systematic desensitization was universally effective: "Human variations are so complex and subtle that even the most extensive experience can provide no absolute insurance against disappointments" (1973, p. 132).

Gronhovd and Zenner (1982) use Wolpe's principles and provide a thorough description of an anxiety-reduction program. The program, as described, would be applicable to Group III children. Their sequence divides into *visualization* and *reality* stages. In the visualization process the first step is a thorough development of an anxiety or stress hierarchy. Each item is developed as a little "scene" that lasts from 20 to 30 seconds (as opposed to Wolpe's 5 to 7 seconds) and includes some normal disfluencies as well as occasional stuttering dysfluencies. Relaxation training is used to provide a secure base in which visualization can occur, to focus awareness on the scenes visualized, and to help the client ignore other distractions. Before actually starting desensitization visualization, Gronhovd and Zenner may have the client perform simple behaviors that take 30–40 sec and then, afterward, visualize them again step by step. In this practice, the clinician's questions to make the client recall every small aspect of the behavior. The client should need no more than about 5 sec to visualize a complete scene, although this is not the actual duration of the original situation, and the client should be practiced until this frequency of recall occurs consistently. In scene presentation the authors use Wolpe's (1973) *subjective units of disturbance* SUDs scale described in Chapter 10. Starting at the low end of the hierarchy scale, the first scene is visualized. If the client reports very low (below 20) or no SUDs, that is, no anxiety, the scene is visualized five times again and then dropped; then the next scene is taken up. If the client feels anxiety, he or she is directed to take several deep breaths and shift visualization to a neutral scene before trying again. When a scene has to be stopped several times, and the reported SUDs level stays above 20, the process stops. The trouble scene is then shifted to a higher point on the hierarchy, and a new scene is selected for visualization. Scenes visualized successfully are repeated as home assignments. Gronhovd and Zenner describe a number of ingenious variations of scene presentation, including the use of out-loud speech by the client, audio and video material, and GSR feedback.

Real-life experiences, according to Gronhovd and Zenner, are absolutely essential as part of the desensitization process. This writer strongly agrees. Without controlled transfer, this type of desensitization is not likely to generalize spontaneously. Gronhovd and Zenner recommend transfer initiation when the client, on an in-clinic basis, is about one-third through the hierarchy list. Starting with the easiest items, reality situations should resemble the visualizations as much as possible—and the client *always* must preplan alternatives in the event that anxiety should become unmanageable. The alternatives may include escape or starting over. The researchers recognize a recurrent problem, where a high-SUDs item is met frequently, such as a stutterer hating to answer questions in class but being required to do so on a daily basis. They suggest the clinician do everything possible to secure a temporary removal or amelioration of the demand until the stutterer is ready to meet it. Indeed, they are quite emphatic about this suggestion and discuss its various aspects as well as the responsibilities of the clinician. Other transfer methods are also discussed.

Systematic desensitization, in the classical form, does not appear to have sufficient support to justify its use as a sole therapy of stuttering. Aside from that, few speech and language clinicians have received adequate training in psychotherapy, which is needed to implement its complexities. However, there is frequent use of systematic desensitization concepts as an identifiable stage or phase in a number of stuttering therapies covering both fluency reinforcement and symptom modification. Yet there are variations in desensitization that depart from the applications of reciprocal inhibition applications as discussed previously, and these are considered next.

Implosive Therapy

Reciprocal inhibition in desensitization sets up a competing, incompatible physiological state (relaxation) during visualization or recall of scenes that typically create the opposite state (tension). In implosive therapy, or emotional flooding, the principle of *supersaturation* is applied. *In sensu* or *in situ,* overstimulation of the limbic system without the reinforcement of real consequences will result in the lowering of response strength. It is an application of the old principle, "If you are afraid to do something, imagine the very worst that could happen, and then what actually happens won't be nearly as bad." Emotional flooding, or implosive therapy, as a formal procedure stems from work done in psychotherapy (Stampfl & Levis 1967). However, the author was taught a variant of the approach in 1953 by Van Riper, who also described it later (1973). The basic premise is that repeated exposure to high levels of emotional stimulus, especially if no consequences occur, will result in reduction or extinction of the person's response. Adams (1982) describes a single-case study where flooding was used with success, noting that as repeated floodings lowered emotional responses, the client was able to engage in behavioral rehearsals and thus experience and practice success in advance.

Implosive therapy requires significant insight and maturity on the part of the client. In the author's opinion, it can be a useful method for many (but not all) Group III adolescents and, as a variation, can be used in a group setting through role play. Clients enact worst-case scenarios and so discharge much anxiety. Also, stimuli can be exaggerated to burlesque so that clients begin to "laugh at our fears," and that tends to reduce the anxiety valence of reality. This author does not recommend implosive therapy for children in Groups I and II. All too often they lack maturity and insight, and they cannot adequately internalize unreal levels of hyperstimulation as not actually representing reality. Bedtime ghost stories to the young are classic examples of this! Where desensitization is desired for younger children, basal fluency expansion may be more productive.

Basal Fluency Expansion

Many years ago the author faced the emotional crisis—that childhood rite of passage—of the public piano recital. Appetite disappeared, sleep was disrupted, and seriously considered were the advantages of the faraway foreign legion, where savage desert tribesmen would be less frightening an adversary than a public piano recital audience. My mother took charge and tied me (figuratively) to the piano for extra hours of practice. Then she had me "perform" for her. Next, I played before the assembled family and an enlarging group of friends and relatives. In this progression I increased the adequacy of my motor performance, learned to correct or compensate for errors, and reduced my fears of audience pressure. In short my mother had successfully applied the principles of *basal fluency expansion.* This same procedure used in stuttering therapy combines support and reinforcement of fluency while manipulating the factors that disrupt fluency.

Desensitization therapy with children, according to Shames and Florance (1982), was developed earlier to help the child cope with the normal stresses of the everyday environment, and the idea has been utilized for generations. The clinician determines what fluency disruptors exist *for the child* in the child's environment. The italicized phrase in the preceding sentence is important. We might assume appropriately that "Shut up if you can't talk right!" is disruptive to a child and plan to use environmental manipulation to deal with it. But some stuttering children find any questions, or requests to repeat an utterance, or other mild stimuli, to be disruptors. And some children are stressed by the auditor's loss of facial mobility or eye contact. It may take time, effort, and close observation, but various disruptors can be identified and described. When the disruptors have been identified, therapy focuses around eliminating them until fluency is established and stable. Such an environment might involve the following:

1. Quiet play with art materials.
2. No questions, interruptions, criticisms.
3. Quiet, parallel activity and monologue by clinician.
4. Nonintrusive reinforcement of child's activity.

When client fluency is stable, the clinician might start to elicit more verbalization through friendly questions such as "That's a great airplane. Where is it going?" As the child becomes more verbal and remains fluent, the clinician begins to increase pressure on this *basal fluency*. Pressures might include more demanding or less-favored activities, faster work pace, more frequent activity changes, less familiar activities, clinician speech that is less facilitating (faster, louder, more complex, and so on), less cooperative or more competitive play activities, interruption, criticism, more demanding or critical questions, and so on. These are not loosed in a sudden barrage, and approaches differ. Some clinicians escalate one factor progressively while keeping others stable. Some prefer to escalate several factors at a time, in small increments. At any rate, the target is to approach, but not actuate, fluency disruption. The clinician is to watch for behaviors typical of the client that presage fluency breakdown. These might be increments or decrements in body movements, speech production changes, speech output changes, altered facial expressions, or changes in play performance. When the presumed stress peak is reached, the clinician is to drop quickly back to basal fluency levels, stabilize for a while, and then start the cycle again. The goal is to raise the disruption threshold progressively. Cycle lengths vary, but usually no more than two or three cycles per session are feasible. This form of desensitization therapy can be a total program, combined with parent counseling, used with filial therapy, or integrated with more direct therapies such as fluency reinforcement. Client manipulation and social interaction skills are paramount requirements of the clinician.

TABLE 11–2.   Integration of BFE into Therapy Programs at Different Age Levels

---

GROUP I

Mild or Inconsistent Dysfluency
   Parent counseling to reduce home disruptors and support fluency;
   Play therapy for fluency enhancement, parent observation, and filial interaction therapy;
   Relaxation games to slow speech rate, reduce production tension, and increase fluency;
   BFE to increase disruptor tolerance.
More Severe or Consistent Dysfluency
   Parent counseling, as above, plus more specific in-home procedures;
   Language facilitation, if needed, and/or work on attending, auditory processing, etc.;
   Fluency reinforcement, organized, such as Shine's (1980) program;
   BFE during latter stages of, or after, fluency stabilization, bringing in parent observation and
   interaction.

GROUP II

Mild Dysfluency, Minimal Struggle
   Teacher planning to reduce class stress, monitor speech, build ego, control peers;
   Parent conferences to inform, counsel, secure monitoring;
   Fluency therapy, such as ELU, particularly if there are language weaknesses;
   BFE before, during, and after fluency reinforcement.
More Severe plus Avoidance Behaviors
   Teacher planning, as before;
   Parent conferences, as before;
   Relaxation therapy in game or exercise form to reduce tension and struggle;
   Breathstream management to reinforce relaxation and focus it on the speech mechanism;
   BFE, probably in overt form where client and clinician talk about disruptors and practice
   with them. May lead to role play or to more formal desensitization procedures.

GROUP III

BFE unlikely except when clinician varies in-clinic pressures on the client to observe effects,
or as the client increases abilities to tolerate pressure;
Desensitization will be through role play, fear hierarchy formulation, reciprocal inhibition
(relaxation), implosive therapy, or specific desensitization of identified fears;
Therapy will focus on, or combine, counseling, symptom modification, and fluency
reinforcement.

Conture (1982) suggested that the older child (nine to adolescence) who has a low awareness of stuttering may benefit from desensitization activities to help the client develop more tolerance for fluency disruptors. Emphasis is situational and not fluency or dysfluency oriented. The clinician identifies situation factors that facilitate fluency and develops them to establish a basal fluency level. Identifying the characteristics associated with basal fluency is necessary because the therapy procedures will require many returns to that level. When basal fluency is established, the clinician introduces fluency disruptors, or "barbs." Barbs are to be inventoried and selected from the child's experience, not specially designed. However, barbs can involve abrupt topic change, eye-contact shift, interruption, requesting repeats, etc. Conture's basal fluency process is an example of the many that have been used over past decades. In Table 11–2 the author has provided an example of how basal fluency expansion (BFE) can be integrated into an overall therapy program at different age levels. The plan is flexible, and many other combinations can be used.

Specific Desensitization

Although many clinicians utilize the BFE procedures described in the previous section, use of the total relaxation and reciprocal inhibition therapies is less extensive. This is due, in part, to the skills and experience required of the clinician. Also, many clinicians have not supported use of these programs, claiming that they are too generalized, too difficult to transfer effectively, and fail to deal specifically with particular fears and avoidances of stutterers. In his avoidance-reduction therapy, Sheehan (1980, 1975, 1970) focused on facing the stuttering and learning to accept the role of stutterers. Fears must be faced over and over again, as discussed in Chapter 10. Van Riper (1973, 1971a) long has been identified with desensitization as a part of his MIDVAS (1963) therapy, in which desensitization (the D of MIDVAS) was to follow and build on the identification stage of therapy. The goal of therapy is to toughen the stutterer "to those factors which normally increase the frequency and severity of his stuttering" (1963, p. 396). Prior stages of therapy have targeted desensitization as a secondary, or indirect, byproduct of work on motivation and identification. At the D stage the stutterer is challenged to "consciously endure stress" (p. 396), seek it out deliberately, and hold on to feelings and speech during stress. Van Riper emphasizes clinician skill and empathy requirements, as well as motivation/manipulation of the client to participate actively in planning desensitization assignments. Difficulty should be phased in, should be in the out-clinic world, and should involve the clinician modeling and pseuodstuttering while the client observes and evaluates. Suggested areas include the following:

- **Penalties.** Solicit penalties, either for stuttering or for other behaviors.
- **Frustration.** Perform behaviors that are frustrating.
- **Feelings.** Design assignments where feelings are expressed by the behavior or by actual verbal identification.
- **Stress Resistance.** Deliberately plan or spontaneously enter situations that create high stress levels.
- **Situation Fears.** Target feared situations and enter as many as you can.
- **Word Fears.** Take usually feared words and set goals for their use, especially in situations likely to cause stuttering.

Van Riper (1973) rejected the use of generalized relaxation techniques and the development of hierarchies. He replaced imagination and recall of scenes with direct participation in the actual scenes, often while practicing assertive or positive behaviors. The author was trained in this system and has used it for many years, in various ways. Comparisons between this form of desensitization and those discussed earlier show some similarities and differences:

1. In-clinic cognitive analysis of stuttering behaviors, situation characteristics, and client feelings are used to reduce limbic (emotional) effects of stuttering.
2. In-clinic practice of target behaviors is used to semihabituate them, increase cognitive acceptance of them, and increase feelings of self-efficacy.
3. Whether or not a formal hierarchy is constructed, the client is led through a series of situations of graduated difficulty levels. Often the clinician models and pseudostutters for the client.
4. The client usually has some assigned task (maintaining eye contact, counting stuttering spasms, and so on) during situations. This elevates cognitive function and, therefore, further reduces limbic effects.
5. Repeated, controlled exposures are used to stabilize results.

As the reader can see, the differences among the methods become less clear when such comparisons are made. One might also mention another difference. Periodically, and without warning, Van Riper would declare "role reversal" day, and clinicians would have to perform all the assignments they had prepared for their individual stutterers to do. They did these as "stutterers," and the clients functioned as observing and evaluating clinicians. This helped the clients both cognitively and emotionally, kept the clinicians empathetic in their assignment planning, and also contributed to an important therapy area—desensitizing clinicians! Finally, clients were given extensive assignments to perform on their own between each clinic session.

In a variation of the Van Riper type of stuttering desensitization, Gendelman (1977) used "confrontation therapy" in working with adolescent stutterers. Gendelman felt that practicing only in-clinic was less productive than out-clinic experience. The clinician and client engage in a prolonged analysis of stuttering, factors that affect it, thoughts and feelings surrounding stuttering situations, and a very detailed analysis of each situation. Feared figures are ranked in stress order, and then either they are brought to the clinic or the client is taken to them. Gendelman reported that of 40 adolescents involved, 23 were dismissed as fluent, 13 were rated as improved, and 4 were not helped. In follow-up, averaging about six months after dismissal, 22 had retained their dismissal speech fluency ratings, and 5 had suffered "slight relapses." The intense, focused desensitization therapy discussed here is not appropriate for Group I, and most Group II, clients. It can be utilized extensively with most Group III clients, however, if such procedures can be integrated into the overall therapy program.

Mention was made earlier of the clinician modeling desired behaviors, and pseudostuttering, in real situations—making telephone calls, going to shopping malls, and so on. In these situations the clinician is to be a stutterer and the client is to have assignments as if she or he were the observing and evaluating clinician. Even during early stages of therapy the clinician will usually pseudostutter in a forthright, matter-of-fact manner, keeping eye contact and minimizing associated behaviors (unless demonstrating types). In symptom therapy, the clinician can model preparatory sets, pullouts, and cancellations. Fallback methods when preferred control methods fail can also be demonstrated. For fluency therapy, the clinician can demonstrate the method being used and show how to regain fluency if it is temporarily disrupted by a "real" stuttering spasm. *In situ* relaxation methods, avoidance-reduction, and other behaviors can also be demonstrated through reality modeling by the clinician.

Whatever the method, the client benefits from modeling and pseudostuttering by the clinician by observing another person survive such experiences without noticeable trauma. It also helps for the client to play the clinician role with its requirements of monitoring, evaluation, and objectivity. Where symptom or fluency techniques are involved, desensitization is facilitated as the stutterer develops greater confidence in the particular techniques because he or she sees another person use it in real life. Pairing stutterers to work together on assignments can have similar effects, but the participation of the clinician should not be omitted. Pseudostuttering has been supported for clinician use by this author before (Ham 1986). In a study of the effects of pseudostuttering on normal speakers, Klinger (1987) concluded that it was a viable method for student clinicians to use in experiencing and feeling the negative emotions that stutterers have. Whether the feelings of real stutterers and pseudostutterers are exactly the same is not important; the experience for clinicians, and clients, is useful.

CHAPTER SUMMARY

Ingham (1984) raised the question of whether or not certain tension levels might be desirable in communication and whether overrelaxation might not act against speech control. The same concept might be applied to desensitization—too much, and the client will not care if stuttering occurs. However, communication is two-way, and auditors may care very much if there is stuttering. At any rate the question posed by Ingham does not stipulate how much is enough for either tension or relaxation, just as we have not established what percentage, or form, or intensity of residual stuttering is required for fluency and how this should be differentiated from the residual dysfluency of symptom modification therapy. Nevertheless, relaxation is almost a universal factor in every form of therapy, and desensitization procedures are not far behind. Many clinicians who disavow formal designs of either or both procedures utilize the principles of both in their own therapy activities.

The key issue actually involves an accurate evaluation of the client's behaviors and attitudes. For some, the establishment of fluency will reduce tension and anxiety to nominal levels that ordinary transfer and maintenance procedures can deal with. For other clients, particularly in some areas of Group II and widely in Group III, failure to consider relaxation and desensitization needs may encourage failure of transfer, foster future relapse, and ultimately intensify anxiety and tension so that future therapy (if attempted) will be more difficult than before.

CHAPTER TWELVE
FLUENCY PROCEDURES: PART I

OVERVIEW

Production of speech involves the coordinated activity of the respiratory, phonatory, and articulatory systems. The reflex networks and rapid adjustments of neuromotor control depend on sensory input and programmed response patterns at cerebellar and brain-stem levels. On an interacting hierarchy, higher levels of the central nervous system influence prime movers, set synergist support groups, initiate selected motor sequences, and control the feelings associated with communication. At the highest levels, linguistic formulation occurs and establishes the sequence that motor planning must organize and generate. It has been suggested that about 100 muscles are involved in speech production, and these 100 muscles must coordinate to a high degree of accuracy and consistency at great speed. Table 12–1 suggests the complexity of this process, illustrating it at three rates of speech utterance. It is assumed in the table that each word averages 2.2 syllables in length, with an average of 2.4 phonemes per syllable. For each phoneme an arbitrary beginning, stable production, and termination phase is hypothesized so that for each muscle there are three muscle adjustments per phoneme. With these suppositions, neuromuscular adjustments are calculated and range from a low of

TABLE 12–1. Hypothetical Projection of Neuromuscular Requirements for Various Rates of Speech Utterance

MEASURE/REFERENCE	EFFECT BY RATE OF UTTERANCE		
Word rate per minute	160 wpm	120 wpm	40 wpm
Syllable rate @ 2.2/word	352 spm	264 spm	88 spm
Phoneme rate @ 2.4/syllable	845 ppm	634 ppm	211 ppm
Muscle adjustments of 100 muscles @ 3 adjustments per phoneme, per minute	253,000	190,200	63,000

63,300 per minute for a speech rate of 40 wpm, up to a possible 253,500 neuromuscular adjustments per minute at a fast speech rate of 160 wpm.

The assumptions are, of course, very tenuous and not to be taken too literally. However, they illustrate the complexity and rate factor of speech production, probably erring on the side of conservatism. The point is made that speech production requires a great deal of the controlling organism before accurate, timed, and smooth speech occurs. Many things can go wrong in the process, and fluency disruption is only one of the possibilities. Recall from discussions in earlier chapters the significance of motor planning and coordination, and the effects of rate. When a stutterer breaks the rhythm, timing, and coordination of the production process, a whole network of interlocking functions is thrown out of sequence and a neuromotor catastrophe results. One therapy approach to try to eliminate or reduce the disruption problem is to slow down the rate and/or change other production parameters in order to facilitate and simplify the motor production process.

This chapter addresses four therapy methods used in fluency facilitation: rate and prolongation, masking, rhythm, and unison speech. The methods overlap and have variable targets, but many of the effects are common. Rate and prolongation procedures affect stress, pitch, respiration, and other areas. Rhythm procedures also change rate, prolongation, respiration, and so on. Other procedures have similar ramifying effects. This complicates separating therapy procedures and saying that one is rate and another is respiration, and neatly categorizing and comparing them. The four methods discussed in this chapter, plus those added in Chapter 13, all have the significant overlaps just noted. Confusion in the literature, and classroom, results when clinicians evaluate methods, compare them, and declare one to be better than another. These overlap effects range all the way from just tainting comparative results to making them meaningless. It is possible that the increased or decreased value of one therapy technique compared to another rests, at least in part, not on the technique so much as on the clinician's ability to use it well and the client's ability or willingness to accept it. The author has had good results using relaxation therapy, but some clients resist it psychologically—yet some of them achieve very adequate relaxation as a result of successful respiratory therapy. Obversely, some clients who just cannot get the hang of breathstream management experience a satisfactory alteration in their respiratory patterns as a result of relaxation therapy. This is not to say, and it should not be argued at this point, that all therapy procedures are the same in their effects and equal in their values. But it does make questionable any tendency to debate whether one particular method is superior to all of the others. By the same token, it is difficult to support one approach within a method over all other approaches. For instance, in rhythm-timed speech which is better, syllable tapping, syllable timing by other means, metronome, carotid-pulse counting, or swinging exercise clubs? Again, for lack of better information it may depend on the particular clinician's implementation and the particular client's receptivity. The final, and most important, factors to consider are how the client modifies and shapes the method effects into fluent and normalized speech patterns and then transfers the effects into stable, maintained use. Here we can have the situation where a less effective in-clinic method is transferred more thoroughly to out-clinic use than a method that worked better during in-clinic learning and practice.

Several points have thus far been made. The first suggests that speech is a very complex neuromotor act and that as we slow down rate, the complexity demand factor lessens. The second points out that we have a number of methods that achieve a variety of effects on the neuromotor production process. It then emphasizes that each of the various methods affects not only its primary target but also the entire neuromotor process of speech production. This makes it difficult to separate the effects of procedures, and to compare them. Difficulty is compounded when we add peculiarities of approach and application by individual clinicians, and complexly compounded when we add factors of client perception, acceptance, and response. The reader should bear these considerations in mind as discussion continues across a variety of procedures and should continue to remember them over the professional years as new procedures, or combinations, are suggested for use.

We have found that simplifying motor acts, slowing them down, and altering production parameters can facilitate fluency. Whether these procedures generate normal-sounding speech is questionable, and this will be discussed at the end of the chapter. Wingate (1976) reviewed a number of the speech modification methods and claimed to find some commonality in their effects (Wingate 1984d, p. 276):

> The major common features involved changes that emphasized the prosody, or melody, of speech, those aspects of spoken language that are expressed through variations in pitch, loudness, and duration.

Wingate's conclusions require further evaluation and clarification but underscore the overlap factor discussed previously. And although the following sections necessarily consider discrete methods, the common-effects factor continues to surface along the way.

RATE/PROLONGATION

Relationships

Speech rate is typically measured in words, or syllables, per minute. Therapy of stuttering, directly or indirectly, has targeted rate for many years. As the stutterer slows down speech rate, all aspects of production are simplified. Thus, there is more time for language formulation, motor planning, coordination of diverse speech elements, and for coarticulation adjustments. Adams, Lewis, and Besozzi (1973) had stutterers read a printed passage at their usual rate, and also in a procedure presenting one word at a time so that rate was reduced to 60 wpm or less. Fifteen subjects stuttered less, two showed no change, and one stutterer increased dysfluency under the slow-rate conditions. Passage presentation on a one-word-each-utterance basis might not facilitate changes in other vocal characteristics in the same way as would slowing rate on the whole passage. However, it was concluded that speech rate and stuttering (or fluency) are positively correlated for most stutterers. Most rate control therapy involves the change of other production characteristics as well. How significant rate, and only rate, is in facilitating or creating fluency is debatable. Adams, Sears, and Ramig (1982) studied the effects of monotone speech on stuttering, when there was no significant reduction in rate. Stutterers and nonstutterers showed significant reductions in fundamental frequency, fundamental variability, vocal sound pressure level (SPL), and vocal SPL variability. In most therapy procedures, rate is not the only target. Duration factors are commonly considered, and it has been suggested that prolongation, or reducing phone rate, is more effective than simply slowing rate by increasing pause time (Perkins et al. 1979).

The variables of rate and duration affect each other, but one can predominate. The clinician cannot assume that clients will adopt a particular pattern in rate reduction. Healy and Adams (1981) evaluated children and adults, requiring them to "reduce by one-half" their utterance rate, without providing any models or instruction. The primary naive method was to increase pause duration time, although phonation duration increased generally. However, subject variability was great, ranging from a zero percent increase in consonant production time while vowel production time increased by 89 percent, while others had a zero percent increase in vowel duration and consonant production time went up by 58 percent. In other words, some stutterers slow more by pausing and others slow more by prolongation. The question of stutterer timing has been investigated, with mixed results. Gautheron and others (1972) reported that stutterers have a longer silent interval separating consonants and vowels than is normal. They suggested that there is a higher than usual vocal fold tension level that requires more effort and greater subglottal air pressure to initiate fold vibration. Janssen, Wieneke, and Vaane (1983) studied the fluent articulatory and phonatory timing patterns of stutterers and failed to support suggestions that the groups differ in speed of articulation coordination or in difference delay between articulation and vocal onsets (McFarlane & Prins 1978; Cross & Luper 1979; Zimmerman 1980b). However, the stutterers did show much more variability, that is, less consistency, on the interval between articulation and vocal onsets during identical utterances. Whether this variability is an inherent flaw in motor timing, or a result of habituated compensation from efforts to control fluency, cannot be stated. Therapy procedures that require a slower and more consistent approach to oral-laryngeal timing would probably tend to reduce this variability.

Prolongation, mixed with overt rate control (slowing down), is common to many therapy methods and procedures (Webster 1974; Runyan & Runyan 1986). Adams (1984b) describes prolonged speech as a reduction in the rate at which articulators approach, contact, and separate from their production targets. He also notes the value of an associated increase in phonation duration during this process. Adams feels that since 1979 the trend to rate control has become a firmly entrenched part of therapy. Even when duration or prolongation is emphasized, as in legato speech, rate reduction is significantly involved. In 1950 Bloodstein listed conditions under which stuttering was reduced or absent. Thirty-two years later 15 such conditions were evaluated for their effects on stuttering (Andrews et al. 1982). Except for 3 or 4, the conditions involved either slowing speaking rate, increasing phonation duration, or both.

In discussing rate/prolongation control, it is easy to identify targets:

1. Word/syllable rate is to be slowed.
2. Vowels and continuant consonants (everything but stops) are to be prolonged.

Therapy techniques frequently add two other factors:

3. Reduction in the number of syllables per phrase, although phrase duration may not drop significantly.
4. Use of continuous phonation, or legato speech, in which vocal folds are kept in continuous vibration until interrupted by a respiratory phrase break.

Additional effects will include regularization of respiratory patterns, downshifts in fundamental frequency level and variation, stereotypy in inflection and stress patterns. Thus, the easy target identification referred to previously can actually become a complex of interactions.

Delayed Auditory Feedback

One of the most published therapy approaches to rate and prolongation control has been the delayed auditory feedback (DAF) procedure. This refers to a delay in the return of the air conducted (AC) speech signal to the central auditory system. As an artifact it has existed in the echo phenomenon in certain types of acoustic environments and can plague musicians and speakers during performance. As an electronic or mechanical phenomenon, it was reported by Lee (1950a, 1950b) who coined the term *artificial stutter* and commented on its fluency disruption effects. At first DAF was produced by separating the record and playback heads of a tape recorder and engaging them simultaneously. Thus a recorded signal was played back an instant later, the delay interval being a product of the distance beween the record and playback heads and the speed of tape movement. Subsequently, units were produced that generated delay intervals by electronic means, although tape units for delay are still in use, particularly in DAF research. Recently the author tested a digital DAF unit that provided delay intervals of 1 msec to 21,000 msec in 1-msec intervals!

DAF research   More extensive summaries of DAF research are available (Wingate 1976; Leith & Chmiel 1980; Ingham 1980; Ham 1986), and only capsulized summaries are presented here. The most disruptive delay interval was found to be in the 180–200 msec range (Black 1951; Fairbanks & Guttman 1958; Zalosh & Salzman 1965: Ham & Steer 1967). There have, however, been indications that males and females respond with maximum disruption effects to different delay intervals (Spuehler 1962; Bachrach 1964; Mahaffey & Stromsta 1965). In the subject area of chronological age, effects of DAF were reported in infants as well as young children (Chase et al. 1961; Cullen et al. 1968). Chase and others (1961) reported milder effects among children aged four to six years than among those seven to nine years of age. Covering the same age ranges, MacKay (1968) reported that the younger group showed peak disruptions at 750 msec, while the older group of children displayed maximum effects at 375 msec. These and other studies, with or without critical delay times, suggest that as we drop chronologically from adult ages, the most effective (disruptive) delay time increases so that the elementary ages have a peak delay factor about double that of young adults, and preschool children have one about double that of the Group II children. It has been speculated that the age-related aspects of temporal delay disruption are linked to the acquisition and stabilization of linguistic and prosodic aspects of communication and to decreasing (with increasing age) reliance on auditory feedback to monitor speech production functions. Research generally supports a DAF loudness level of about 80–90 dB (Tiffany & Hanley 1954; Ham & Steer 1967), although clinical use tends to follow a "Loud enough?" formula. In findings that relate directly to therapy applications, it has been reported that the disruption effects of DAF tend to be related to the speaker's oral production rate (Kodman 1961; Robinson 1972); that is, the slower the speaking rate, the less the DAF disruptive effects.

Listener-speakers under DAF conditions tend to show a marked variation in their responses. Some are devastated and cannot think or talk coherently; some are affected severely but persevere; some are affected noticeably but adapt and plow ahead with some effort; some appear to be affected moderately or minimally and adapt quickly; a few seem to be momentarily surprised and then proceed (apparently) as if nothing is happening. Research has verified this variability (Beaumont & Foss 1957). It has been suggested that internal versus external cue dependence (Spilka 1954; Yates 1963a, 1963b) variables, or auditory versus tactile/kinesthetic dependence, in subjects might explain differences. However, Burke (1975) failed to secure response differences in high disfluency–slow rate persons compared to low disfluency–fast rate persons. Ham and Holbrook (Ham & Holbrook 1986; Holbrook & Ham 1988) failed to establish susceptibility based on manual/oral reactions times or on speaker self-confidence among female normal speakers. At the present time we have few or no tenable explanations for response variations to DAF, but factors to bear in mind must include the following:

1. Stuttering severity and DAF effects appear to be positively related. As stuttering is more severe, DAF is more likely to be accompanied by greater reductions in dysfluencies (at least in severity, if not frequency).
2. As chronological age decreases, the critical peak effect of DAF increases.
3. Stutterers, and nonstutterers, may show particular and individual reactions to DAF.

Effects of DAF   As noted previously, effects of DAF tend to be individual. However, there are certain commonalities. Fairbanks and Guttman (1958) reported that articulatory and fluency disruptions (substitutions, omissions, interjections, repetitions, tense pause and stoppage, and so on) were *direct effects* of DAF. Disruptions in pitch, intensity, and emotional response were designated as *indirect effects*. Chase (1958) found repetitions to be a frequent effect. Venkatagiri (1980a, 1980b, 1982) stated that PWR and disrhythmic phonation create most of the disfluencies. He also noted, in disagreement with Wingate (1976), that the PWR occurrences tended to happen on initial syllables rather than on final ones. In using DAF with nearly 1,000 normal speakers, this author has noticed no tendency for repetitions to occur on final syllables.

The wpm-rate effects of DAF are usually pronounced, but individual variations can be frequent. The slowing effect of DAF has been reported by a number of researchers (Black 1951; Spilka 1954; Brokaw, Singh & Black 1966; Ham & Steer 1967). This rate reduction tends to be accompanied by duration increments (within, rather than between, words) so that phonation time increases. Many speakers become louder under DAF, but it is quite probable that this is due to the Lombard effect, or response to the auditory masking effect from the increased dB level of the DAF signal. Intelligibility of speaker output suffers during DAF. Tiffany and Hanley (1956) reported that speakers rated as highly effective during normal auditory feedback (NAF) were, under DAF, less effective than those who were rated low in effectiveness during NAF. This undoubtedly relates to the finding that speakers with high self-confidence attitude scores, compared to low self-confidence speakers, produced more dysfluencies under DAF (Holbrook & Ham 1988).

Overall, effects of DAF on normal speakers can be catastrophic, and variable. In general there will be tendency to slow down, prolong sounds, reduce stress and other prosodic variations, lower pitch, speak more loudly, and generate articulatory and fluency errors. The reasons for the severity range of individual reactions, by and within age groups and between sexes, have not been explained.

Stutterer reactions to DAF have been a focus of research interest. Naylor (1953) found that stuttering severity and dysfluency reduction under DAF were positively related. Ham and Steer (1967) reported that mild stutterers reacted quite individually to different delay intervals, while more severely dysfluent subjects responded with fewer or less severe dysfluencies to almost any delay interval. Various studies on specific delay times, duration of exposure, signal loudness level, and comparison with other auditory conditions have been summarized in several sources, cited earlier (Wingate 1976; Leith & Chmiel 1980; Ingham 1984; Ham 1986).

Therapy with DAF   The author's first use of DAF, in 1954, was when an 800-msec delay time was used to help clients with foreign dialects develop self-correction monitoring. Later that year it was used with several stutterers. However, the author had learned the procedures from another clinician who had used it earlier. Naylor (1953) reported stuttering severity reductions under DAF. Adamczyk (1959) and Chase, Sutton, and Rapin (1961) published reports of DAF use in stuttering therapy. For a while, after the initial interest during the 1950s, there was a reduction in published research relating to DAF. Then a series of extremely significant studies were generated by Goldiamond and his colleagues, studies that led to an expansion of interest in DAF as a therapy tool with stutterers (Goldiamond 1967, 1965, 1960; Goldiamond, Atkinson & Bilger 1962). Goldiamond used DAF as an aversive contingency or reinforcer, interjected following occurrence of a stuttering dysfluency or continuously and temporarily eliminated after each dsyfluency. Webster and Lubker (1968) eliminated the response contingency aspect and had the DAF run continuously. Curlee and Perkins (1973, 1969) utilized Goldiamond's initial findings in devising a conversational-rate control therapy, which initiated the stutterer to DAF at 250-msec delay at the most tolerable loudness level. Fluency criteria (two 15-minute periods without stuttering) were applied as the stutterer moved in 50-msec decrements down to zero delay, or NAF. Results, in terms of stuttering dysfluency, seemed to be excellent. Yet Perkins (1973a) reported that follow-up studies found the majority of the stutterers suffered significant deterioration in their fluency gains following dismissal. A revised program was published (Perkins 1973b), one which increased client self-evaluation and self-consequation, breath control, prosody development, psychotherapy, and general voice and speech improvement and added a transfer and maintenance section.

Another example of DAF approaches to therapy is noted in the work of Ryan (1971, 1974, 1979) and Ryan and Van Kirk (1971, 1974). Among a variety of behavior modification formats, DAF was used in several therapy structures. Their reports of therapy results have been highly optimistic. However, a high attrition rate of clients who drop out, in-treatment conditions for data collection, and unclear specification of procedures make it difficult to assess Ryan's results, compare them to those of other programs, and replicate therapy efforts. Shames and Florance (1980) have published a popular therapy program based on the concept of stutter-free speech. Delayed auditory feedback is utilized, based on the Goldiamond steps, to institute slowed and prolonged speech. Incidentally, Shames (among others) has pointed out that DAF is not necessary in order to achieve "DAF effects" on speech (Watts 1971; Perkins 1973b; Shames 1975; Helps & Dalton 1979). The stutter-free program involves developing self-monitoring by the client, reinforced or rewarded by nonmonitoring periods that are earned by successful monitoring time. That is, the occurrence of a behavior (self-monitoring) is reinforced by periods in which the behavior does not have to occur. One can only surmise that this is a valid operant function, or that it contributes functionally to the client's progress.

A number of clinical reports on DAF use and prolonged speech application have been identified generally as the "Andrews and Ingham program" and have involved the combination of DAF speech and the use of a token economy in a controlled reinforcement schedule (Andrews 1973; Andrews & Ingham 1972; Ingham 1975a; Ingham & Andrews 1973a, 1973b). The different variations in the therapy programs are summarized and evaluated by Ingham (1984). He concluded that the token economy application was viable and that results seemed to be durable. However, most of the data were collected on an in-clinic basis, fluency definitions could be debated, and some out-clinic data (Andrews & Ingham 1972) indicated that 74 percent of 23 subjects averaged a syllable stuttering rate of nearly 8 percent at 152 spm. Nevertheless, as a fluency establishment program, the system seems to have been valuable in its applications.

Other applications of DAF therapy have occurred. Leith and Chmiel (1980) have described a "DAF-shaping" program in which analysis of rate, enunciation, easy onset, and flow of speech (REEF) is used to evaluate determinants of stuttering. This program has some similarities to those of Webster (1974, 1979) and the Hollins College Precision Fluency Shaping Program. This was not a DAF program, but it serves as a useful example of programs that secured by other means the slowed and prolonged speech pattern identified with DAF. Other clinicians have replicated, or varied, the programs identified with Perkins, Ryan, and Van Kirk; Andrews and Ingham; Shames and Florance; and Goldiamond. However, the mainstream work of this area has been to achieve the same types of effects without DAF or to use DAF only briefly. Also, a variety of supplementary techniques or procedures have been added by many clinicians.

Comments on DAF   Although there has been considerable interest in, and publication on, the use of DAF in therapy, a word of caution is in order. The caution, or concern, relates to the training institutions that prepare student clinicians. Many university programs have one, or several, DAF units that cost from $200 to $1,000 each. However, in surveying over 100 public school and private practice clinicians during a series of in-service workshops, the author found that not one of them had a DAF unit or any access to one! This is the time to reinforce a point made earlier, that DAF effects can be obtained without the use of the instrument itself. For instance, modeling and imitation can be effective methods to use and, in the section on unison speech, reference will be made to adapting that method to a rate/prolongation procedure.

Comments on Rate/Prolongation

There is no doubt that rate/prolongation is currently the most popular method of therapy, and different procedures have been used in its application. Shames (1975) compared instructed and mandated (DAF) rate control. He suggested that with both methods fluency can occur quickly, the stutterer becomes more aware of his or her speech pattern and monitoring is encouraged, motivation and attitude generally are facilitated, and rate variations can be tried for best effects. He warns that, particularly with DAF, self-perception and self-responsibility can be reduced, machine dependency can be fostered, and the expense must be considered. Brutten and Hegde (1984) reviewed various rate control therapies and commented that "though rate control by itself may not produce lasting and generalized fluency . . . , it can help reduce stuttering in a relatively short period of time" (p. 226).

The question of rate/prolongation and age is one of the reasons for its popularity. The method, depending on the procedure used, is applicable in all three age groups covered in this book, and beyond. Levels of sophistication and methods of establishment can vary with age, but the basic method is applicable at age 2, 12, or 20. Costello (1981, 1983) states that rate control, in one form or another, is probably the best method to use in enhancing fluency. She notes that DAF is the best-known method for achieving rate reduction and sound prolongation. However, she argues that DAF is usually too extreme for use with young children, who generally do not like it anyway. She feels that instruction, modeling, and practice are sufficient. Costello measures syllables, not words, per minute in rate reduction, and uses *articulatory rate,* not overall rate (Perkins 1975). Articulatory rate includes the number of syllables produced during nonstuttered speech. For instance, the overall spm rate for an utterance with three stuttered words involving a total of 12 repetitions would add 12 syllables to the overall spm rate and provide a false picture of the rate at which the child was speaking during nonstuttering moments. Costello suggests a rate of 180–200 spm for fluent speech, but notes that this is only an estimate. She also feels that slowing the spm rate below 120 is probably not necessary. It is recommended that in therapy the clinician count syllables by calculating spm-rate targets in advance and then counting client productions within short time blocks. For instance, if the spm target is 120, then the client should utter no more than ten syllables during a five-second period (10 syllables × 12 time intervals of 5 sec = 120 spm). By sampling periodically (not continuously) rate can be monitored effectively.

What is "normal" in terms of rate is difficult to establish. It has been suggested that the stutterer's average reading rate is about 123 wpm, while nonstutterers average about 167 wpm (Darley 1964; Bloodstein 1950). However, the range in each group ran to about 100 wpm. Also, reading rates differ from those of spontaneous speech, and Kelly and Steer (1949) reported that sentence rate correlates more with listener perception of speaker rate than does overall wpm rate. The type of message, emotional tone or content, and general nature of the situation also affect rate. Finally, the personality and the biological timing patterns of each individual affect speech rates. It is therefore impossible to say with even approximate accuracy exactly how fast or slow the "normal" rate for a particular stutterer should be.

This section has referred to a number of rate/prolongation programs utilizing DAF. A specific outline of therapy procedures is not presented here mainly because there are a number of them available in the literature. Those who wish to review detailed programs in which DAF is the procedure applied in rate/prolongation therapy might refer to some of those sources (Perkins 1973a, 1973b; Ingham & Andrews 1973a, 1973b; Ryan & Van Kirk 1974; Shames & Florance 1980; Ham 1986).

RHYTHM PROCEDURES

Background

As we speak, our speech has an inherent, individual cadence, although the rhythm does not follow a 1-2-3, 1-2-3 sequence. Neurophysiology and prosody combine with individual differences to produce rhythmic patterns in communication. As discussed in the Section I discussion of fluency in this book, these rhythmic patterns coincide with the timed integration of planning, formulation, and production. In stuttering, the normal speech rhythm is disrupted—some suggest as a precipitating factor in dysfluency; others feel the disruption is a result of dysfluency occurrences. At any rate, the use of artificial rhythm patterns in stuttering therapy has a long history. Ingham (1984) stated that of current therapy approaches, no other technique "has had a longer and less illustrious career" (p. 89) than has rhythmic stimulation. It has been condemned as quackery (Boome & Richardson 1939), as a distraction (Barber 1940; Bloodstein 1949; Van Riper 1973), and as a distortion of speech into unuseable patterns (Bluemel 1960).

Consider one of these criticisms—rhythm operating as a distraction, so that stutterers simply pay less attention to their speech production and its feedback. Azrin, Jones, and Flye (1968), and Fransella and Beech (1965) compared rhythmic and arhythmic stimuli accompanying speech to speech without accompaniment. In general, stuttering in the presence of "no stimulus" and "arhythmic stimulus" conditions fell into comparable ranges, while stuttering dropped sharply if the accompanying stimulus was rhythmic. The more effective rhythm rates seemed to be those below 90 beats per minute (bpm). Although not denying possibilities of distraction inherent in any alteration of or addition to feedback signals, it is clear that the sharp reductions in stuttering spasms (frequently 90+ percent) in the presence of rhythmic pacing go beyond the reduction level possible through distraction. Reasons for rhythm effects have been suggested or investigated by Dijk (1973), Watts (1973), Wingate (1969b), and others. Changes in the rate of speech do not seem to be a critical factor (within limits). It is possible, referring again to the fluency discussion in the first major section of the book, that the influence of rhythm or pause timing may remove a significant speech production variable from uncertainty and, therefore, affect syllable sequencing and phrase structuring on a predictable basis that is simultaneously different from habituated patterns. The question to be considered is how well the procedure works over time, and what the speech of the person sounds like with reference to normalcy.

Rhythm applications traditionally have been used in two forms. *Aided* methods utilize mechanical or electronic devices that produce an audible and/or visible or tactile rhythm pattern for the client to follow. *Un-*

aided methods generally provide an audible model for the client to learn and then, without further assistance, duplicate in speech. Somewhere in between are methods such as that of Van Dantzig (1940). He utilized "syllable tapping" in which the speaker rests the hand (palm down) on a surface and taps a different finger (little finger, second finger, to thumb, and over again) on each syllable spoken. Modern developments, such as the portable metronome (used in a hearing aid type device) have somewhat blurred *aided* and *unaided* distinctions, and the haptometronome (see later) and audio tape cassette models have compounded definition problems. To reduce confusion in the subsequent discussion of rhythm therapy, reference terms used are as follows:

- **Modeled Rhythm** (MR)—client is taught to imitate a model supplied by the clinician and use it without further aid.
- **Instrumental Rhythm** (IR)—client is required to coincide utterances with an electrical or mechanical device until a rhythm pattern is established, and imitates the pattern in unaided speech.
- **Prosthetic Instrumental Rhythm** (PIR)—the client maintains a rhythmic cadence in speech by wearing a portable IR device.

Modeled Rhythm

In the MR approach the clinician serves as the demonstrator and the reference for the client. If group therapy is used, then other clients may also be models. Such modeling approaches go back for centuries, but the classic report of Andrews and others (1964) will serve as an example. After evaluation, and establishment of baseline measures, clients were taught to repeat sentences modeled by the clinician. Rates were initially slowed, and there was elimination of all stress and syllable contrasts. Clients progressed to reading and then to spontaneous speech. Brandon and Harris (1967) followed a carefully graded series of steps and agreed with the previous study over the values of group therapy and treating the "whole person." Ingham (1984) summarized additional MR studies where a token economy was introduced and other variables controlled or changed. Although admitting that many stutterers improved through the use of syllable-timed speech in an MR setting, Ingham questioned whether or not their improvements transferred well and remained stable. The best results in transfer and maintenance seemed to be with children.

Instrumental Rhythm

The IR approach to timing usually involves a metronome. This device seems to relate back to de l'Isere's 1830 reports of a metronome device (Wingate 1976; Van Riper 1973; Klingbeil 1939). This was a lyre-shaped, pendulum device which could be set to produce different bpm rates. Today, many of us are familiar with the mechanical wind-up metronome that has bedeviled generations of young musicians. It has also been produced as an electronic device with the usual "tick" and/or a flashing light. An IR stimulus can also be produced with a wristwatch device that delivers a tactile pulse to the skin of the wearer (hap-tometronome). Metronomes can be used in therapy as tabletop devices and/or as portable units worn on the body. They can be a sole approach to therapy, a primary part of a mixed approach, an adjunct to a major technique, or a brief demonstration of fluency possibilities during the early stages of therapy. As fluency-inducing devices, they can be used as fall-back systems when acquired fluency patterns slip, or as the core of a patterned revision of speech timing and stress.

The hearing aid prosthesis metronome, or the PIR method of rhythm therapy, seems to have been applied first in the 1960s by Meyer and his colleagues (Meyer & Mair 1963; Meyer & Comley 1969). Data from their reports are not published, but they stated favorable results for most of their clients. In 1969 Rothman, an osteopathic psychiatrist, de-scribed use of a PIR metronome, which Brady used in earlier and revised forms, and described in a series of therapy reports (Brady 1973, 1971, 1968). He became associated with a single-procedure rhythm pacing pro-gram called Metronome Conditioned Speech Retraining (MCSR). He re-ported (1971) that 90 percent of 23 subjects improved and maintained about a 70 percent reduction in dysfluencies at the time (6 months to 3.5 years later) of follow-up studies. Other clinicians have utilized rhythm as therapy or part of therapy (Ost, Gotestam & Lennert 1976; Jones & Azrin 1969; Adams & Hotchkiss 1973; Wohl 1968; Silverman 1971a, 1971b, 1976; Silverman & Trotter 1973; Trotter & Lesch 1967; Trotter & Silver-man 1973, 1974).

Values

Evaluations of rhythm therapy have reported reservations. They have suggested that it does not function as well as DAF in reducing associ-ated behaviors, and tends to create a slower optimum speech rate (Ing-ham & Andrews 1971). Apparently not all stutterers respond well to rhythm therapy (Meyer & Comley 1969). Ingham (1984) concludes that Pacemaster PIR therapy may provide desirable results in some clients "and may certainly be a preferred mode of treatment in the case of many" (p. 113). However, he feels that reports have not supported rhythm ther-apy and notes a trend to combine other techniques with rhythm. Overall, 1960–75 seems to have been a high mark in rhythm therapy resurgence, particularly as a sole or major component in therapy. Rhythm therapy still is one of the most effective methods of inducing fluency, doing so almost immediately. Also, group and individual applications are feasible and it adapts well to either intensive or standard therapy formats. In addition, because of its portability, it can be used as an ongoing system in transfer and maintenance programs. Nevertheless, on a psychodynamics basis it is not applicable to some stutterers. Further, it tends to produce a fluency that requires extensive work before it can sound normal and may, in some, retain automatonlike speech qualities. There are also some indications that over time it may lose or reduce efficacy for some stutterers.

Opinions about rhythm therapy are varied, and sometimes strong. Some of the strong opinion is probably a residuum of recent times when many clinicians associated rhythm with quackery. Failure of programs to take the basic rhythm-induced fluency and shape it back toward normal-sounding speech may also have contributed to the criticisms of artificiality, transfer difficulty, and loss of effectiveness over time. Dalton and Hardcastle (1977) agree that syllable-timed speech is easy to learn, bypasses previously learned timing patterns, and promotes quick fluency. But they do feel that the product sounds abnormal, and only favor it as a demonstrator of fluency, as an initial establishment source for fluency, or for limited use on a when-needed basis. Brutten and Hegde (1984) state, "By and large, it seems evident that rhythm-based procedures have not been proven effective in producing normal and lasting fluency in a majority of stutterers treated" (p. 227). They reason that the imposed fluency prevents normal intonation patterns and speech seems monotonous. This is common to most rate control therapies, however, and subsequent shaping activity can lead to more normal speech. Wingate (1984d) recommends rhythm as part of his overall management program in therapy. He regards it as a "pivotal procedure" because it dramatically reduces stuttering, sounds very close to normal speech, can be fitted to various modes of speech, and can be varied easily. He recommends starting with simple, or basic, rhythms, but progresses beyond that to more varied and complex patterns rather than continuing a monotonous, even beat. "The essential objective in using rhythm is to have the patient develop a comfortable sense of command over stress pattern change" (p. 289). Wingate strongly recommends the use of poetry in therapy to reinforce the rhythm and stress pattern variations in speech, and to provide for transition into ordinary speech expression.

In spite of its long history it is evident that very little has been done overall with the development of rhythm or with specific rhythm procedures. At first this seems to be contradictory when one considers the metronome itself, portable timing units, syllable tapping, and syllable-timed speech. However, all these procedures, like DAF, produce a strongly artificial, mechanical, and unattractive speech product. The following step, to develop this fluent but abnormal speech pattern into speech that is fluent and normal sounding, has often been poorly planned and applied. Wingate's (1984d) emphasis on shaping and transfer is an exception to this. As, and if, refinement and variations of rhythm procedures occur, the method should become more popular and useful in a variety of fluency problems, not just stuttering. It may well be the next popular therapy form, once people tire of rate/prolongation.

Age Factors

Although rhythm techniques can be applied to all three age groups covered in this text, age and psychodynamics will affect the efficiency of any particular method. Children in Group I and the early ranges of Group II will probably respond best to IR procedures, that is, the use of a metronome. It is this author's opinion that they do not do as well with MR procedures because of possible attending problems, lack of syllable awareness, and other distracting factors. However, it has been argued that MR "rhythm games" and music can be used effectively in this age range, so it may be more accurate to say that this author (not the children) does not do as well with MR procedures. It also has been this author's experience that Group III adolescents often seem to resist or reject IR rhythms, but are more responsive to MR patterns, such as syllable-timed speech. Riley and Riley (1983) feel that rhythm procedures may be particularly applicable to children, especially when they fall into the oral discoordination subgroup.

 Hutchinson (1976) has provided an extensive review of rhythm therapy, as has Ingham (1984); and Wohl (1970) reports on a very detailed program of rhythm therapy. The author himself (Ham 1986) has published a step-procedure sequence for IR therapy. This procedure (pp. 311–16) starts with the selection of clients for rhythm therapy and describes each step of therapy up through dismissal and maintenance. It is written at an adult level of use but can easily be translated into acceptable, comprehensible forms for even preschool children. Its performance levels fit into a behavior modification structure or into a more loosely structured and interactive therapy form. With Group I children, following Wohl's pattern, rhythm activities can include marching and other physical movements performed in a cadence, if there is a need to generally improve timing and coordination of neuromotor movements of the body.

AUDITORY MASKING

Description and Effects

As with so many other methods, auditory masking is not new. Van Riper (1973) referred to the use of "therapeutic deafening" early in this century. Shane (1955) and Cherry and Sayers (1956) had reported reductions in stuttering as a result of masking noise during the speech of stutterers. Subsequent research explored various aspects of masking noise and stuttering. It was reported that masking was most effective in the low-frequency range (MacCulloch, Eaton & Long 1970); and that the masking dB level and the amount of stuttering decrement were positively correlated (Maraist & Hutton 1957). Extensive summaries of masking-noise research, and evaluations of masking, are available (Ham 1986; Ingham 1984; Wingate 1976; Van Riper 1973).

Auditory masking in stuttering has typically involved the use of binaural earphones receiving the output of a low-frequency broad-band noise generator. The noise usually has an intensity level within the 70–100 dB SPL range. As an aversive stimulus it can occur following stuttering spasms, and it has been used as a continuous signal to facilitate fluency. A variation of the latter application has been the voice-activated noise generator (see later), which is silent during speech pauses or other nonspeaking intervals. The typical noise effect is the so-called Lombard effect—or an increase in speaker vocal loudness and frequency of the vocal fundamental (Atkinson 1958)—an increase in phonation duration, and a decreased speech intelligibility (Garber & Martin 1974). Effects reported on rate of speech have been equivocal.

Explanations of Effects

Explanations for masking-noise effects on stuttering have varied. Distraction effects have been suggested and must be considered, though distraction cannot explain completely the dysfluency reductions that occur. Some clinicians have speculated that the vocal signal changes (Lombard effect) cited in the previous paragraph produce an altered motor planning and production sequence which can explain stuttering reduction through alteration of habituated speech patterns. Others have suggested that masking simply reduces auditory feedback and, perhaps, requires the speaker to concentrate on proprioceptive signals. In an example of the search for explanations, Garber and Martin (1977) compared the effects of noise when stutterers spoke with normal loudness during masking and when speaking loudly during masking. They found little change in stuttering when speaking loudly or normally under nonmasking but recorded stuttering decrements when either normal or loud voicing was masked. They concluded that the decrease in auditory feedback was the critical factor affecting stuttering. This conflicts with hypotheses expressed by Wingate (1976) that stuttering decrements might be linked to altered vocal parameters. It is possible that the decreased auditory feedback impairs cerebellar and brain-stem automatisms and requires a higher level of attention in the central nervous system because of the interference. It is also possible that distraction, altered vocal variables, and reductions or revisions in habituated monitoring patterns combine; further, they may combine with differing degrees of importance and effects across different speakers.

Comparisons and Variations

The effectiveness of masking as a fluency aid has been considered and evaluated. Since stuttering is associated, by some, with significant anxiety levels, there was a question of whether or not changes in anxiety occur as changes in stuttering happen. Adams and Moore (1972) measured anxiety levels and vocal variables during normal and noise-masked feedback. Anxiety was measured through the palmar sweat index, one time, during the end of the first paragraph of a 176-word passage. As expected, stuttering decreased and vocal intensity of speech increased during masking. The palmar sweat indexes for masking and nonmasking were nearly identical, and it was concluded that masking did not affect anxiety. It also would have been appropriate for the authors to conclude that reading a prose passage under laboratory (not social) conditions was not particularly stressful for the subjects. Other studies have compared masking with simple amplification of the stutterer's own voice, instead of using noise. Martin and others (1984) reevaluated the use of amplified auditory feedback, comparing it with normal feedback and to various dB levels of masking noise. They reported on previous research suggesting reduction in stuttering during amplified sidetone, and this author (Ham & Steer 1967) had observed similar responses in 1955, while evaluating the effects of various sidetone alterations on stuttering: Amplified sidetone reduced stuttering, but it was not as effective as external masking noise in fluency induction. Evaluating more familiar methods, Brayton and Conture (1978) reported that vocal loudness in stutterers increased significantly during noise masking and that stuttering dropped from 0.69 during no masking to 0.29 under masking. However, these results were compared to rhythmic pacing at 60 bpm. In the rhythm condition, vocal loudness barely changed, while stuttering frequency dropped to 0.02. Also, the vocal fundamental went up 16 percent under masking but dropped only about 5 percent during rhythmic stimulation. Interestingly, vocal duration increased by about 10 percent under masking, but it increased almost 50 percent under rhythmic cadence. One can speculate that this duration increase was due to expansion of the duration of unstressed syllables and of pauses. On the other side, rhythm reflected an almost total loss of duration times attributable to moments of stuttering. Martin and Haroldson (1979) compared masking noise to TO, rhythm, and operant conditions (interjection of a loud "wrong" following each stuttering). Metronome and TO were almost equal in reducing the frequency of stuttering the most, while masking was least effective. In measures of stuttering duration, TO was decidedly more effective (reducing duration by 74 percent), metronome was second (46 percent), and noise was least effective (12 percent). Since voice initiation and nonvoice-voice transitions have become a point of interest in stuttering, Hayden, Adams, and Jordahl (1982) compared masking and rhythmic stimulation on the speech initiation times

(SIT) of stutterers and nonstutterers. The results: In normal and in experimental conditions stutterers' SIT scores were slower than were those of nonstutterers. Rhythm-stimulated SITs were faster during pacing than during either the normal feedback or masked conditions, and masking SITs were slower than those during either normal or paced conditions.

Effectiveness

As evident from the previous section, masking frequently does not function as well in reducing stuttering as do some other techniques. In diagnosis and assessment activity with stutterers, the author always has the client talk or read for several minutes each during DAF, unison speech, metronome timing, and masking noise. This is done to demonstrate fluency and also to evaluate client responsiveness. Using this method, the author in the past ten years found that masking noise was highly effective in a few instances, totally ineffective in a few instances, and most of the time was the least effective of the four procedures. MacCulloch, Eaton, and Long (1970) evaluated matched stutterers and nonstutterers, ranging from about 3.5 to 16 years of age, with an average age of about 12 years. Masking at 300 Hz was used for 12 to 24 therapy sessions, and posttreatment testing was conducted. Stuttering decreased from an average of 41.6 percent pretreatment to 15.5 after 12 sessions, but it dropped only to 15.0 following 12 additional sessions. The authors were impressed favorably by their results and felt that the procedure avoided the undesirable rate reduction of DAF or the cadence effect of rhythm therapy. However, a 63 percent reduction in dysfluencies after 12 sessions cannot be regarded as a great achievment in fluency, and a further 3 percent reduction in dysfluency after 12 additional sessions is even less impressive. The DAF, and rhythm, effects on speech variables can be shaped rather easily into normal rate and rhythm patterns, and a 16 percent stuttering rate that still is at 5 percent after 24 therapy sessions does not compare well to other techniques. Brutten and Hegde (1984) reviewed the use of masking in stuttering therapy, including earlier applications (Van Riper 1965), and more recent uses of the Edinburgh Masker (Dewar, Dewar & Barnes 1976). Their conclusion was that masking noise fails "as an impressive procedure for modifying stuttering" (p. 229). They also felt that masking effects tended to disappear once the noise was turned off, that portable units carried an "earpiece stigma" many stutterers were unwilling to accept, and that it also was possible that prolonged use of masking (portable units) could result in decreasing effectiveness over time.

Therapy Applications

Masking can be used as an in-clinic therapy in order to establish fluency and then be shaped toward normalized speech. In such instances, it is usually mixed with other fluency procedures. A possible sequence might be the following:

1. Client practice to learn the mechanics of turning noise on and off, to acquire easy-onset skills to coincide with speech and masking attempts, and to speak with normal vocal loudness during masking (shifting attention to proprioceptive rather than auditory monitoring).
2. Development of fluency on an ELU basis starting with single words. Each word is repeated twice, with and without masking. An adequacy criterion is set and must be met before moving to two-syllable words, short phrases, sentences, and so on.
3. Monologue speech is started with a set period of masking (for example, one minute), followed by five minutes of unmasked speech. Any stuttering is punished with one minute of masked speech, which does not count toward the fluency total criterion. Three five-minute periods of fluency are required before moving to conversation. The clinician works to continue shaping the client's speech in masked and unmasked speech efforts.
4. Conversational speech in five-minute (client talking time) segments, as in step 3. However, the total fluency time requirement is 30 minutes. By that time the client should be able to monitor speech and shape it to maintain fluency.
5. Transfer, using a fear hierarchy, is initiated progressively to increase ability to use fluent speech outside. Masking is used to assist in-clinic practice; it is not used on an out-clinic basis.

Auditory masking can also be used in portable forms, in which the stutterer uses a manually triggered or voice activated masker that feeds noise to hearing-aid receivers. Earmolds are required, preferably of the skeletal type (to facilitate listening to other people and to environmental sounds). A sample program using the portable aids is described by the author in another source (Ham 1986). Portable masking units were reported on without enthusiasm by Van Riper (1965), although initial credit is assigned to Derazne (1966). Other clinicians have experimented with portable maskers, but most attention has been paid recently to the Edinburgh Masker (Dewar et al. 1979). This device has an external laryngeal contact microphone which will activate the masker during speaker phonation. It can also be triggered manually for first-speech efforts and has a 0.5 second lag before turn-off in order to bridge silent gaps during voiceless productions and respiratory phrase breaks. Reports by Dewar and associates are highly favorable, but the adequacy of their data has been challenged (Code & Muller 1980) and rejected (Ingham 1984). However, the author has never found a client willing to use it long enough to accept the wires, straps, neckband, and other paraphenalia (or the noise) and dropped using it in his graduate class (as an assignment) because of similar complaints. But the author has met two stutterers who use it consistently, are fluent and normal sounding, and say they are very pleased to "use it forever."

Age Factor

As with DAF, masking is not recommended for Group I children, nor for many in Group II. If it is to be used, Group III should be its main area. It can be used in diagnosis and assessment and in fluency demonstrations. During other therapy procedures, masking can be used to facilitate tactile or kinesthetic monitoring; it can also be used as a penalty for errors in whatever fluency modes are being practiced and as penalty for stuttering errors that occur. Further, Gruber (1971) reported the maskers to be helpful in symptom modification therapy during the pullout stage (see Chapter 14).

Masking Summary

As with many procedures, we do not really understand why masking operates to reduce stuttering. As a major or central method, it seems inferior to most of the other methods that have been or will be discussed. Nonetheless it does have some values as an ancillary aid in diagnosis and assessment, as well as in certain therapy procedures. Of course, and always, there will be the particular stutterer who will respond more favorably to masking than to any other procedure.

UNISON SPEECH

Overview

Unison, or choral, speech involves two or more speakers delivering the same utterances synchronously. It has existed for many centuries in dramatic and religious productions and today is practiced widely today in certain prayers, pledges, and rituals. In many parts of the world unison speech is still used in classrooms as students answer or practice in a chorus. Ingham (1984) noted that unison speech has a long history in stuttering therapy, and that by the twentieth century it was known to most prominent clinicians. In early elocution-oriented stuttering therapy, unison speech was found to be quite effective. Research, however, has been limited. Johnson and Rosen (1937) reported excellent fluency effects. Barber (1939) used 14 different choral reading combinations and found that all reduced stuttering, although two persons reading the same material together seemed most effective.

The explanations for effectiveness of unison speech in reducing stuttering have varied. Bloodstein (1949) suggested that speech pattern alteration, or reduced communication responsibility, were possible explanations, and many other clinicians have expressed similar views. Cherry and Sayers (1956) suggested that unison speech (and shadowing) required the stutterer to listen to the other sound source rather than to her or his own auditory feedback. Wingate (1976, 1969b) stimulated renewed interest in unison speech and shadowing, proposing that the effects were rate reduction, phonation emphasis with sound-stress reduction, and conformity of articulatory movements to the source pattern. Ingham (1984) provides an excellent review of studies that have tested Wingate's modified vocalization hypothesis (Ingham & Carroll 1977; Adams & Ramig 1980; Andrews et al. 1982). He concluded that

> quite obviously, the chorus-reading effect does not depend on either reduced reading rate, increased vowel durations, phonation continuity, or vocal level. (pp. 183–84)

In spite of this, it should be noted that stutterers vary in their responses to unison speech (and shadowing), and small-sample studies (the four studies reviewed by Ingham totaled only 25 stutterers ranging from early elementary to mature adult age) have left weak spots in our understanding. It is quite possible that different stutterers respond well (reduced stuttering) to unison speech for different reasons or for a different mix of the same reasons. Children seem to respond particularly well to unison speech, although clients may be less accepting in and above adolescent age levels.

Applications

Unison speech is easy to apply and can be used with any age level, although reading ability by the client is very convenient. The clinician can use earphones on the client or sit very close and "overwhelm" the client's own auditory feedback with the clinician's speech pattern. Commercial megaphones, cupped hands, rolled up paper tubes or cones, and stethescopes have also been used. Van Riper (1973, 1971a, 1971b, 1959) has described the use of unison speech, and Falck (1969) has recommended basic steps in using it to establish fluency. Gregory and Hill (1984) cite unison speech, or choral speaking, in their therapy program for school-age stutterers, while Culp (1984) utilizes unison speech with preschool children. In her sequence, choral speaking is used as a first step of performance modes, followed by immediate modeling responses, immediate modeling with disruptions, and on up to the seventh (fluent) step of spontaneous speech during disruptions. As an indication of the method's flexibility, Gregory (1968) described a comprehensive therapy program combining unison speech and symptom modification, with shaping and attitude revision added. In the *first step*, the child and clinician read together, moving from words to phrases to sentences, and then to paragraphs. This is recorded and played back. Every session, regardless of purpose, starts with the first step, and then it jumps to whatever is the current step or level. The *second step* is a repeat of the first, but the microphone is placed near the child so that his or her voice is predominant on playback. In this day of built-in, omnidirectional microphones, it is becoming more difficult for the clinician to control placement of the microphone. However, the clinician can sit very near the child, back from the table, incline her or his head near the child's ear, and, if necessary, mask his or her mouth with one hand or a sheet of paper. A brief summary of the other steps is as follows:

3. Microphone near clinician, who fakes several stutterings as they read together. Playback is evaluated, and mirror analysis made of the spasms.
4. During unison readings, clinician fades or drops out intermittently, until several child stutterings have occurred. Playback evaluation and mirror analysis again.
5. Unison readings, where the child fakes stutterings as the clinician did earlier. Playback and analysis.
6. Unison readings, from single words on up, to teach one of the controlled disfluency modes of utterance (see Chapter 14). This step is rigorous, exploring various phonemes, phoneme combinations, syllables, stress factors, and so on.
7. Refine the new control model; reinforce other areas of speech.

Where it is appropriate in the various steps, question-answer and conversation modes can be added. Gregory emphasizes that every therapy session starts with step 1, but that particular other steps can be abbreviated or omitted as progress makes them less relevant. He also states that relaxation therapy or other procedures can be integrated into the overall therapy structure.

Where the Gregory approach has emphasized some of the classical elements of symptom modification therapy (pseudostuttering, negative practice, spasm analysis, modified disfluency, and so on), the author has used unison speech to design a prolongation–rate control procedure (Ham 1988). This was done primarily to aid public school clinicians who do not have DAF units but who do have access to various types of tape recorders. The procedure begins at wpm rates approximating those imposed by a 250–300-msec DAF delay and progresses to faster rates. Pretaped unison speech models (clinician) are used so the clinician is free to evaluate, interrupt and correct, guide, reinforce, and collect count data for baseline comparisons. The program runs from initial establishment phases up through transfer, dismissal, and maintenance. In another source (Ham 1986), the author has outlined a more general unison speech program that is applicable to various modes of fluency reinforcement and also runs through the transfer stage (pp. 320–23).

Shadowing

Many readers have no doubt played the game of talking simultaneously with another person but lagging behind his or her utterances by one or more syllables. Freund (1966) has reported that this game was used as a therapy method in the nineteenth century. Apparently, the label *shadowing* was created by Marland (1957). However, credit for its modern organization and use belongs to Cherry and his associates (Cherry 1953; Cherry, Sayers & Marland 1955; Cherry & Sayers 1956; Cherry 1957). One might almost wish it had been related to DAF and called DUS (delayed unison speech). There have been limited reports on the use of shadowing in therapy. Walton and Mather (1963) described the case of a client for whom shadowing was used. After 48 sessions normal speech could be obtained during in-clinic sessions, but transfer efforts were unsuccessful. An additional 47 sessions were devoted to relaxation and desensitization procedures; they produced satisfactory results. Also, use of shadowing with children in Czechoslovakia has been reported (Kondas 1967, 1968). Most were in the 8–16 year age group, but several preschool children also were evaluated. Kondas reported that the method was easy to use and resulted in good fluency results, but transfer was a serious problem. Other researchers, Peins and her associates (1970), have used shadowing as part of a tape-recorded home therapy program, which was applied initially to adolescents.

Attitudes toward shadowing have been, at best, restrained. Van Riper (1973) suggested it had value in reinforcing fluency, especially with very young stutterers, and Fiedler and Standop (1983) expressed a similar opinion. Ingham and Andrews (1973a, 1973b) suggested that to achieve effectiveness it needs to be combined with other techniques. When Ingham (1984) reviewed choral speech and shadowing, he concluded that interest in its use had declined (this author feels it will cycle back up again). He also noted, as have others, that a particular value may lie in its use with young children.

A possible shadowing sequence is suggested as follows:

1. Evaluate the child's speech to determine rate, melody, stress, technique, characteristics, dysfluency characteristics, and decide what speech mode or modes will be used to model.
2. Instruct the child that she or he is to "shadow me" by one to five syllables as the clinician talks or reads aloud. Practice with commonly used phrases. Instruct the child also to imitate the manner in which the clinician speaks.
3. Read or talk at a very slow rate (50–70 wpm), so client will have an easy time shadowing. Stop frequently and coach, criticize, and reinforce. Consistently use the speech mode selected.
4. When the child is performing well (specific criteria can be set), maintain the overall rate but introduce variations such as:

    • And soooooo, I wennnt downnnn the sssstreeet, buuut Sssaaammmm did not seeee the treee braaannnch fffall.

Variations in loudness, inflection, and so on, can be used also. Stop and evaluate performance as needed.

The child is being taught a high level of auditory monitoring, slow rate, prolongation, plus any other fluency modes desired, as well as flexible use of prosodic and other vocal factors.

5. Increase rate by 20–30 wpm, and repeat steps 3 and 4. Insert breaks during which no shadowing is done, but both clinician and child speak in the current mode and at the current rate.
6. Continue increasing the wpm rate until a desired rate is achieved.

Therapy must include other considerations as they are needed. For instance, parent counseling and environmental manipulation are usually important, and parents can be trained for home practice in shadowing. Also, shadowing is a useful vehicle if the client has subclinical or more significant levels of oral discoordination.

Section Summary

Unison speech and shadowing are not, and have not been, predominant methods of therapy. Either method, in various forms, promotes a high level of fluency and does so quickly. Although it is most amenable to use in shaping a client's speech patterns, it has not been as popular as some other methods already discussed. Because it is so easy to do, and requires so little in the nature of special equipment or materials, it has possible values that we may have overlooked in our enthusiasm for other methods.

CHAPTER SUMMARY

This chapter has looked at methods that focus on the rate, duration, and prosodic elements of speech—methods that probably cover a large number of the core therapies used today. However, there have been significant problems resulting from these methods, or others, being used as a total or near-total therapy without adequate regard for preparatory steps before and transfer and maintenance steps after. In some cases the result has even been a failure to adequately shape the client's speech toward normalcy once fluency has been achieved. Wingate (1984), in discussing DAF, rate, metronome rhythm, masking, singing, unison speech, and other procedures used to develop fluency, commented that "all of these conditions result in speech that is unlike ordinary spontaneous speech" (p. 275). His objection is not to their use per se; rather, his objection is to their use as programs of therapy without regard for their place in a framework of linguistic prosody or their modification (as fluent speech) into a normalized pattern of production. However, many clinicians have realized that a procedure is not a program of therapy, and they have integrated the methods discussed previously into total therapy programs. An example of this is Adams (1980) writing favorably about breathstream management therapy interwoven with a GILCU linguistic structure. He notes that the management of speech respiratory patterns occurs most favorably if the motor speech act has been simplified. Slowing of rate is regarded by Adams as the optimal approach to motor simplification, particularly if prolongation is utilized as the primary slowing agent. The Adams example is an illustration of how one method may have its own values for fluency yet also be used to support or facilitate other methods. As another example of combinations, Weiner (1978, 1984a), in her vocal control therapy (VCT) program, describes a complex therapy that focuses on good vocal usage to support fluent, normal speech. Embedded in the VCT program, particularly in early stages, are elements of rate reduction, prolongation, easy onset, rhythmic patterning, and so on.

In the following chapter, other examples of combined methods within an overall program are discussed, and the reader is reminded that oversimplification and reliance on a very limited technique can result in very limited effects. Therapy parsimony is a two-edged sword—it may reduce "shotgun" procedures and save time, but it may also leave gaps or weak spots in terms of the normalcy of the speech, in efficacy of transfer, and in stability of maintenance.

CHAPTER THIRTEEN
FLUENCY PROCEDURES: PART II

OVERVIEW

This chapter was developed simply to avoid a Chapter 12 that ran on far too long for convenient reading and teaching. An effort has been made here to organize sections around the respiratory and phonatory systems and their coordination with the articulatory system. For instance, rate decrements and/or prolongation require a timing and coordination of the respiratory system patterns. It is therefore obvious that changes in respiratory patterns, in onset forces, or in other production areas will have associated effects on speech rate, timing, rhythm, stress, and other factors. As much as possible, therapy methods are not to be repeated, as it is assumed that the reader has already covered Chapter 12.

Respiration

Most speech and language pathology students, usually as undergraduates, study the anatomy and physiology of speech, with major coverage of respiration. Students are instructed concerning the interactive linkage among the respiratory system and the valving or modifying components of the vocal tract. As shown later in this book, dysarthric oral structures can force changes in respiratory patterns, and deviant or inadequate respiratory support relates to phonatory and articulatory problems. Thus it is no surprise that respiration and stuttering occur as related problems. Researchers have reported greater variability in the breathing of stutterers (Murray 1932), that stutterers exhibited abnormal behaviors or inadequacies in respiration (Weller 1941; Starbuck & Steer 1954), and there may be irregularities in the nonspeech breathing of stutterers (Schilling 1960). In a review of respiratory studies Sheehan (1970) reported that stutterers tend to be more variable in breathing, have less coordination between thoracic and abdominal respiratory movements, breathe less deeply when having speech difficulty, and display other nontypical or abnormal patterns. He also concluded that there was no set or stereotyped respiratory pattern for stutterers; instead, they showed considerable variability.

Respiration for life and respiration for speech involve the same space and structures but differ in their characteristics. The smooth, even cycles of vegetative breathing are more irregular for speech, longer in expiration, and usually shorter during inspiration. Where elastic recoil of the thorax and lungs account for most of expiration in quiet breathing, involvement of expiratory muscles is required for speech. This is because motor planning sets speech initiation timing and air pressure requirements, and the steady leakage of air during sound production requires constant adjustment of thoracic and abdominal musculature to obtain sustained, balanced phonation. We typically have a speaking posture, or respiratory set, which is linked to phonatory and articulatory sets. Disturbance of these sets disrupts the respiratory pattern, and pattern disturbances can alter the various sets. Typically, airflow rates during speech are in the range of 150–200 cm/sec (cubic centimeters per second), while the average speech inhalation is 500–800 cm (Daniloff, Schucker & Feth 1980, p. 148). Under ordinary circumstances this rate of airflow is more than adequate for "a smooth stream of explosions, frictions, buzzes, silences, and combinations thereof" (p. 145). The rapid adjustments to produce all of the effects just mentioned tend to occur at the midvolume range of thoracic expansion because that is the range in which the least amount of physical effort can produce the most effect within the shortest period of time. If we are driven out of the midvolume range, to speak with too little expiratory reserve or with high thoracic air pressure, strain is placed upon the respiratory system and disruptions can occur all along the timing and coordinating effects of the vocal tract. Indeed, any amount of stuttering can interrupt the basic inspiration-expiration cycle and significantly alter the timing, pressure, and airflow rate during speech.

However, there are varying points of view as to whether respiratory anomalies are a causative factor of stuttering, whether any breathing disturbances are only symptomatic and related only to the moments of stuttering, or whether the nonstuttering and nonspeech respiratory patterns of stutterers are basically flawed. Points of view about the value of respiratory therapy procedures with stutterers also vary. Some approaches attempt to revise the entire breathing sequence, starting with vegetative respiration, while, at the other extreme, other procedures target only the airflow past the several points of constriction in the vocal tract during the act of speaking. These therapy variations are reflected also in the differing attitudes that exist concerning the overall value of working with respiration. We begin with that consideration as in the next section we examine these varying points of view.

Values of Therapy

Consideration of respiration variables and effects has been involved in most therapy of stuttering, directly or indirectly and as either a primary or a secondary procedure. Therapies that deal with desensitization, anxiety reduction, attitude change, relaxation, and so on, have an effect of slowing, altering, and regularizing respiratory patterns as a concomitant of other changes that occur. Direct therapy with stuttering spasms requires alterations in the inspiration-expiration cycle and the controlled release of air. Fluency procedures that slow rate, alter phrase timing, distribute syllable stress, or otherwise change production variables all have mandatory effects on the intake and release characteristics of the breathstream. It is therefore moot to consider whether or not breathstream management is involved in the therapy of stuttering. It always has been, and it always will be. The point of argument is whether or not direct therapy of respiration is necessary and, if so, to what degree and in what form. In this argument generations of clinicians have attended to the respiratory state. Gutzmann (the younger) was a powerful influence in Germany during the early twentieth century. In his book on communication disorders (23 editions), he suggested self-induced relaxation, easy onset of phonation, and control of the breathstream (Fiedler & Standop 1983). This rather sensible and restrained approach can be found reappearing in some of the "new" therapy approaches that have surfaced in the past decade. However, during the first half of the century, a number of therapy methods expressed what I call the "better breather" approach to stuttering. Many exercises were developed that might have been applied to persons training to be opera singers or underwater swimmers. Stutterers strained to develop enlarged vital capacities and turned faint shades of purple as they practiced prolonged expiration until they either reached the residual air barrier or fainted. Breathing exercises developed a bad odor and so-called reputable clinicians swung away from the formal programs, even though their own programs typically affected respiration in ways discussed at the beginning of this paragraph.

Classical symptom therapy was not generally supportive of classical breathstream therapy, and the author, early in the 1950s, received no training at all in any direct therapies for airflow. Van Riper (1973) was not an advocate of breath control therapy, and he recalled his own end-less hours of futile exercises that did little more than cause him dizziness from hyperventilation. However, the cancellation-pullout-preparatory set sequence of symptom therapy, the "Iowa bounce" technique, and other symptom procedures require adequate respiratory support and controlled release of the breathstream. As the supposedly new therapies began to appear in the 1960s through the 1980s, a number of them targeted respiration as a major goal in revision efforts, and many reactions to this respiratory renaissance have not been favorable. Sheehan (1979) was quite explicit in his evaluation and stated:

> We hear of stutterers cured in half an hour through "discovery" of an airflow technique . . . that turns out to be an elaboration or variation on discredited breathing exercises. (p. 184)

Evaluation of the modern breathstream programs has not been particularly favorable, as will be seen in the application section following.

> Most researchers now agree that stutterers do not generally need lessons in correct breathing. In fact, breathing exercises have been rarely used during the past several years. (Brutten & Hegde 1984, p.229)

Ingham (1984), in reviewing airflow therapy as a variant among the prolonged speech methods, found little data to support efficacy claims.

In spite of the negative comments breathstream management has increased, not decreased, in the present decade. Research by Adams, Runyan, and Mallard (1975) suggests airflow rate and consistency; further, the rate and duration of articulatory production relate to the ability to maintain or manipulate breathing. More and more, therapy programs have included respiratory and breathstream management elements, either directly or indirectly. Miller (1982) reviewed therapy programs by Perkins (1973a, 1973b), Webster (1974), Schwartz (1974), Ryan (1974), and Shames and Florance (1980). These programs were called, respectively, breathstream management, precision fluency shaping, airflow, Monterey fluency program, and stutter-free speech. All of the programs have unique characteristics, mix in different therapy sequences, and present commonalities in different ways. Miller stated that all the programs utilized some form of rate control to establish fluency or to facilitate the learning of other procedures. A second common factor was breathstream readjustment, usually in an easy-onset pattern of phonation initiation. She concludes that many stutterers will profit from an airflow therapy but that the speech improvements may reflect manipulation in several dimension, not simply from respiratory changes. Miller also warned against exaggerated claims for respiratory therapy and noted that speech results may be fluent but far from normal. The therapy trend has moved away from respiration-only therapy, and generally it has moved away from separating respiration and the speech act. Some therapies use a breathstream orientation to facilitate changes in rate, relaxation, phrasing, and so on, while other approaches slow rate and simplify other motor speech aspects in order to revise and normalize the speech breathstream. Several of these approaches are reviewed next.

RESPIRATORY/BREATHSTREAM APPLICATIONS

General Approaches

There can be no question that the moment of stuttering introduces abnormalities into the inspiration-expiration cycle and the flow of the breathstream during speech. Research does not support such firm statements about stutterers' fluent speech or vegetative breathing. However, normative distribution possibilities argue that a certain number of stutterers will fall into one or more of the following subgroups:

1. Disturbed or inadequate vegetative breathing patterns, for reasons related or unrelated to stuttering.
2. Disturbed or inadequate breathing patterns during fluent or nonstuttered speech.
3. Specific stuttering symptoms that involve significantly abnormal patterns in respiration and breathstream management as an identifiable aspect of stuttering spasms.

There will be stutterers who display no significant alterations in their use of air and others for whom breathstream deviations are a secondary concomitant that appropriate fluency or symptom modification procedures will normalize without special attention. But there are those stutterers for whom more specific approaches appear to be valuable.

Generally using the popular garden hose analogy, Conture (1982) described an airflow therapy used with child stutters as their stuttering reaches noticeable levels. Water source, pressure, release, and so on, were compared to breathing, and simple line drawings were used to illustrate points. The pressure points of hose nozzle (lips), hose (tongue), and faucet (larynx) were emphasized in the analogy. The therapy uses relaxation to facilitate ease at tension points, while continuant sounds, such as /s/, are used to demonstrate open and continuous release of air, the effects of gradual vocal tract constriction, and stoppage. Another approach is used by Fiedler and Standop (1983), who present an overall training program with two levels, speech and social. Among other procedures, the speech level includes progressive relaxation and practice on easy breathing. Other fluency aids can be added as needed. The social level works to transfer developing fluency and is a mixture of desensitization, role playing, and other procedures. This first phase is accompanied and followed by cognitive therapy to develop, modify, and maintain therapy gains. Wells (1987) recommends routine evaluation of respiratory patterns. If there is a problem with shallow breathing, she initiates a program to develop respiratory adequacy. Simplified explanations of respiratory basics are followed by the following steps:

1. Proceed in oral breathing with minimal movement of the chest and shoulder area.
2. Repeat each breathing cycle, using a voiceless consonant.
3. Repeat each cycle, using an open vowel or voiced continuant consonant.
4. Vary postural positions while voicing.
5. Progress to words, sentences, monologue, conversation.

Wells notes that the clinician may need to determine if there is an appropriate release of air prior to the onset of phonation. Adams (1980) has targeted initiation and maintenance problems in airflow or phonation as one of five criteria for differentiating dysfluent and disfluent children. His therapy formulates a selective breathstream management, targeting the particular problem (for example, initiating voice) or problems. Also, rate reduction is employed to slow down and simplify motor planning so that revisions can be taught.

The preceding examples involved various degrees of concern with respiration and speech, generally mixed in with an overall program of therapy which did not particularly emphasize respiration ahead of other concerns. Next we will look at some procedures where respiration is more specifically emphasized.

Specific Approaches

Some therapy programs emphasize a broader approach to respiration and breathstream management while still integrating it into a larger program. The organization reported by Gronhovd (1977) is an example of the ways in which standard breathing exercises can be applied. In the breathing, rate, airflow, tension (BRAT) management method, the client is to lie supine through all steps of the first phase of therapy. Deep muscle relaxation is achieved, followed by production of voiceless sighs, and then by voiced sighs. The client is then to count up to four numbers while breathing in a moderately deep and easy respiration cycle. Rate is slow, and relaxation is to be maintained so as to allow for an easy glottal attack and a breathy voice. When counting performance is satisfactory, the client moves progressively to words, phrases, monologue, and dialogue. With the client shifted to a semisupine posture, the entire phase is repeated again, and then repeated once more with the client moved to a sitting posture. Rate is now increased to a more normal speed, and any needed changes in prosodic elements or vocal characteristics are secured. A similar but more complex sequence is described by Overstake (1979) and has been summarized previously by the author (Ham 1986). Overstake also begins with deep relaxation and then moves into respiratory adjustment. He states that the majority of stutterers have disturbed vegetative breathing patterns that are the result (not the cause) of stuttering. Overstake teaches "block breathing" in which, timed from the client's cardiac pulse, the client is to inhale-hold, exhale-hold air until an even, steady cycle is obtained and stabilized, both in and out of clinic. Following block breathing, Overstake works to coordinate thoracic and abdominal movements in respiration and, when this is achieved, turn the exhalation into a loud whisper. Production is to be relaxed and prolonged while there is good vocal quality and relaxed exhalation. Vowel production is introduced, shifting from a "sigh" to normal production. Then it moves into a counting sequence, starting with 1 and progressing to 8. Easy onset, by releasing a small amount of air prior to an utterance, is used to blend respiration and phonation. Therapy progresses to phrase production, still on one breath, seeking to expand the utterance length through relaxed and effective use of air. More complex speech is introduced as the client continues to develop the ability to maintain adequate respiratory support and use it in the most efficient and relaxed way. Overstake emphasizes that this breathstream management is not a dysfluency control method: It is a respiratory control method that, when learned, allows the stutterer to profit from fluency therapy approaches dealing with rate, time, and stress.

During the 1970s Schwartz (1974) expressed the contention that stuttering is caused by inappropriately timed contractions of the posterior cricoarytenoid muscle, the prime (or only) vocal fold abductor. This contraction was stated to be a distorted residuum of the primitive infantile *airway dilation reflex* (ADR) that protects the very young from blocking and choking in the airway. This contention led Schwartz, in *Stuttering Solved* (1976), to the development of the *passive airflow* program. A general summary of the Schwartz therapy indicates that 40 hours of therapy in five eight-hour days completes the primary program. Over the next 12 months the client is to practice one hour each day, divided into 15-minute sessions. One minute out of each 15-minute session (28 minutes per week) is to be recorded, and the audiotape mailed to the clinic for evaluation and feedback. A telephone access number is provided, and motivational procedures and materials are presented to the client. Elsewhere the author summarized the airflow aspects of the therapy (Ham 1986):

The client seems to be asked to emit a prolonged, relaxed, audible sigh. This is produced immediately following inhalation so there is no intervening "set" or transition period between inhalation and exhalation. Then the client, midway in the passive sigh, "releases" a one-syllable word without any interruption, change in tension, or other alterations in the passive ongoing flow of air. Articulators are not preset and should move into position during the airflow. The number of one-syllable words is increased progressively on each breath, and then turned into sentences. Syllables should be slowed (prolonged). Acquisition, then, is practice, error correction, and private sessions. (p. 266)

The passive sigh technique certainly is not new or unique, having been used for at least 200 years (Jonas 1977). However, the therapy sequence and its presentation mode were different, and there have been efforts made to replicate, or modify, the airflow program for evaluation purposes. Falkowski, Guilford, and Sandler (1982) took the five-day, 40-hour Schwartz program and applied it over a four-week period to two stutterers. Although reading fluency stayed relatively stable after dismissal, spontaneous speech fluency relapsed to pretreatment baseline measures. Andrews and Tanner (1982a, 1982b) also evaluated Schwartz's passive airflow technique; they reviewed a modified form involving eight-hour sessions for three consecutive days, and then on the eighth day and thirtieth day. Initial results were variable, and all six stutterers experienced regression in the subsequent year. The researchers did not feel the approach was as effective, in the short-term or long-term, as other therapy techniques such as prolonged speech or precision fluency shaping. Gregory (1979) criticized Schwartz's airflow publication (1976) for "omission of references and bibliography" (p. 13), and for premature generalization from his hypothesis about the cause of stuttering. Fiedler and Standop (1983) also found Schwartz's claims to be unacceptable, but because of an absence of control data. Cheasman (1983) evaluated Schwartz's airflow therapy, after critizing his unsubstantiated ADR theory and the lack of data to give credibility to his therapy claims. He found fault with the procedure of slowing production only on the first syllables of words, with a failure to provide for a rescue response if stuttering does occur, and doubts whether the procedure can overcome strong word and phoneme fears by the stutterer. However, Cheasman allowed that the Schwartz program might be best for stutterers who do not have strong fears related to sounds and do have particular problems initiating speech. He suggests that the technique originator's charisma might be a major factor in any therapy success and that although many stutterers might be helped "by aspects of the technique, for most it simply is not enough" (p. 85). However, Ingham (1984), after criticizing Schwartz's data inadequacies, concluded that quite probably the technique might be effective in the modification of stuttering, but there were no data to support any claim to generalized, maintained speech that sounded normal and was free of stuttering.

Azrin and associates published reports concerning a regulated breathing therapy of stuttering (Azrin & Nunn 1974; Azrin, Nunn & Frantz 1979). In this program various incompatible behaviors are combined to block stuttering. The authors claimed that one two-hour therapy program resulted in stuttering decrements that reached 99 percent in post-therapy follow-up studies. During the 120 minutes of therapy, the following steps are accomplished:

> recall, visualize, and discuss stuttering history; identify and analyze stuttering and associated behaviors; construct a fear hierarchy for words, people, and situations; develop awareness of stuttering; establish basic relaxation in sitting and standing postures; learn speech control; secure desensitization through incompatible relaxation while recalling unpleasant situations; learn a new general pattern of breathing; plan maintenance.

One is tempted to suggest that a stutterer who can achieve all of the foregoing in 120 minutes might comprise an entirely unsuspected subgroup among mainstream stutterers. The stutterer is taught to let stuttering spasms act as signals to stop, relax, and slowly inhale, formulate the intended word, and begin speaking as soon as inhalation is complete. Respiratory retraining involved uttering one word per respiratory cycle, consciously relaxing after each utterance. When this can be done consistently, two words per breathing cycle are uttered, and so on.

Reports on the Azrin program have been varied and not consistently supportive. Ingham (1984) criticized the basic reports by Azrin and his associates, stating that "absolutely no objectively collected speech behavior data were obtained" (p. 361) and that there was a failure to consider how normal, as opposed to fluent, the client speech sounded. Replication studies by Ladouceur and others (1982) have been disappointing, and Fiedler and Standop (1983) suggest that the lack of credible data fails to support the authors' optimism. Posttreatment speech in one client has been observed by the author (three months after therapy), and the results were interesting. No overspasms were observed, although prespasm tremors would occur, be caught, and consciously smoothed out. The rate was extremely slow (estimated at about 50 wpm), prosodic stress was lacking, and production quite breathy.

It is probable that respiration and breathstream, as an integral part of speech production, can be an integral part of stuttering. Their significance in stuttering and therapy will vary as long as the characteristics of different stuttering syndromes vary. Therefore, their effectiveness and importance as a therapy method must also be variable. Where therapy appears to run into trouble is in programs that single out respiration, pull it from its integral relationship with running speech, and force it to carry most or all of the remedial burden. The same comment can be made about rate control, chunking, pullouts, or relaxation. If, in addition to the overemphasis, a therapy programs fails to deal with other elements (attitude, environment, tension, fears, transfer, monitoring) of therapy, then less favorable outcomes and relapses can be anticipated with some frequency. This does not, however, negate values of respiratory revision and breathstream management when they are applied where there is need, and when their use is integrated properly into an overall therapy program.

Group I

Typically, preschool children do not show a generalized disturbance in their basic respiratory patterns, so no suggestions are offered here for major revisions of them. However, it has been this author's experience that the young may show more breathstream anomalies during dysfluencies than will many more mature stutterers. This seems to reflect that the young child, when truly "stuck," is less efficient, more random, and more wasteful in his or her struggles to break dysfluencies. Older children tend to become more efficient and focused in their struggles. As a result, one older child may have very little in the way of breathing anomalies during speech, while another has specific and exaggerated breathstream problems. Younger children, on the other hand, seem to present a wider range of speech breathing problems and to be less consistent.

Group I stutterers can be taught the importance of respiration in speech, and they can be practiced in activities to increase breathstream awareness and control. The garden hose analogy, mentioned several times already, can be used where water and air are equated and relaxation encouraged at the various constriction points. Other activities might include the following:

1. Having child blow through soft plastic tubes so that the free end directs air onto the child's own hand, cheek, and so on. Clinician varies slowly and quickly pinching the tube shut as the child blows, so that she or he can feel the back pressure and reduction or stoppage of the airstream.
2. Release air through an open mouth and then play with stopping it at the lips, at the linguapalatal and laryngeal locations.
3. Practice talking with different respiratory patterns: with interrupting inhalations, with a large exhalation before phonation, with very breathy speech, and with "residual air."
4. Blowing exercises and games; breathing while supine, sitting, standing; timed prolongations of air release, or prolonged vowels, of continuants; games with s/z ratio, and so on.

The activities in the preceding list are not intended to change respiratory patterns, to redirect the breathstream, or to increase vital capacity. They are used primarily to make the child aware of respiration, of different pressures and timing efforts, and of constriction points in the vocal tract, and to develop some initial capacity to monitor breathing.

Relaxation activities of all types are an avenue to changing respiration patterns in young children. The decrease in tension reduces or eliminates dysfluencies temporarily, and this typically brings respiratory patterns into line. If speech utterances are elicited during relaxation, the utterances will be slowed, prolonged, lowered in pitch, reduced in stress, and produced with less energy. These changes involve a respiratory pattern that uses less air for speech, uses air more economically, and promotes a more rhythmic timing cycle in speech breathing. Subsequent to relaxation activities, there can be variable carryover periods where effects continue, depending on the particular child and the nature of the following activity. The relaxation efforts can be formal, use of quiet music and suggestion, simple relaxation games, and so on. Relaxation can also be practiced through pseudopersonalities (lazy man, rag doll, scarecrow) adopted at particular times in therapy. Dramatic play stories (Rip Van Winkle, Snow White) can be used also. If feasible, the child's attention can be drawn to breathing for speech during relaxation, with efforts made to extend it.

In addition, clinicians also can use easy-onset speech patterns (see later) as a direct mode of securing smooth expiration if initiation is a problem. If a young child displays broken breathstream patterns, improper timing, or other specific difficulties, these will need direct attention. Fluency therapy of the ELU type can be used. In such control of utterance length, the clinician can restructure the child's breathing pattern as needed. The clinician can also control for difficult words, voiceless and voiced transitions, and initial phonemes that will facilitate easy-onset use.

Group II

The children in Group III can start at the same types of activities described for Group I, but with explanations and requirements upgraded to their maturity level. In Group II the clinician is more likely to find dysfluencies that are marked by prolongations, tense pauses and stoppages, struggle, and associated behaviors that alter air use. In such instances breathstream anomalies may proliferate. Explanations and analogies can be more direct and explicit, the clinician can demonstrate desirable and undesirable breathing behaviors, and the child can practice specific changes. Activities that carry respiration changes as part of their performance or as effects of their activities can still be used profitably, but direct effects can often be used as well. Finally, the clinician should observe for anomalies during fluent speech. If these are found, then some of the restructuring activities outlined in the discussion section on general methods and techniques can be utilized.

Group III

Children in Group III, and some in Group II, can be dealt with cognitively in terms of respiration function and therapy. Analogies can be used, if presented in an age-appropriate fashion, but factual information should be used to structure a rationale that is clear to the client. Clients can be assigned to observe and categorize breathing in other persons. As part of self-analysis (see Chapter 14), the stutterer can be taken through evaluation of his or her own breathing patterns for speech. Many of the procedures described earlier can be used, totally or in part, as long as they are part of an overall therapy program.

Client Selection

Selection of clients for breathstream management should involve application of several basic criteria and not just the clinician's preference to use the method. Adams (1983) has stressed that failure in therapy can come from the clinician making erroneous assumptions about client needs. He has used airflow therapy as one of several examples where a perfectly valid therapy technique can be applied to the wrong client. There is no set of established criteria for selection, but the following suggestions are offered to indicate when breathstream management is worth considering specifically:

1. Basic disturbances in speech respiration, evidenced by frequent and shallow inhalations, noticeable releases of air prior to initiation of phonation, or inhalatory interruptions during a phrase.
2. Visible/audible signs of laryngeal tension during stuttering. Vasodilation, flushing in the neck area, and hypertension of the neck strap muscles may be visible. Hard glottal attacks, glottal fry, and tense vocal tone may be audible.
3. Specific individual respiratory patterns that interfere with easy, fluent speech.

In many instances stutterers may exhibit mild or intermittent occurrences of some of the behaviors cited in the preceding list, or they may exhibit problems in oral tension, phrasing, and so on. When this occurs, the clinician may wish to use certain portions of conventional breathstream procedures or use a method only long enough to resolve the particular problem.

EASY-ONSET PROCEDURES

One of the most consistent problems the stutterer faces is that of initiating an utterance. Difficulties in timing and coordination are complicated by any anticipation or apprehension they may feel about initiating speech. Falck, Lawler, and Yonovitz (1985) studied prespasm vocal activity of stutterers and reported that prior to stuttering symptoms the phonation characteristics of stutterers tended to show identifiable acoustic differences from nonstutterers. Whether this is part of a faulty motor pattern or a previously unidentified segment early in a stuttering spasm cannot be stated. Fifty or more years ago, some clinicians would have identified it as a distorted vocal preparatory set (Freund 1966; Van Riper 1937).

Easy onset has a history before this century, and it is an important aspect of most symptom modification therapies, where the moment of stuttering is the target. It has been used as one form of cancellation, as a possible method of relaxing in pullouts and converting a hard onset into an easy termination, and as a pure easy onset in preparatory sets. Symptomatic therapy generally condemned continuous use of easy onset (or any other fluency controls) on the grounds that it would ultimately become an habituated speech pattern, fall from conscious control, and probably become incorporated into a return of the dysfluency pattern as Jost's law applied (that is to say, over time, older responses tend to displace more recently learned responses). In fluency enhancement, stuttering is targeted indirectly in that easy onset is used more or less continuously, used on initial words and syllables, used at syllabic stress points, used after clause boundaries, used on feared or typically troubled words, and so on. Often it is taught in conjunction with airflow techniques that have been used with stutterers in the past (Azrin & Nunn 1974; Van Riper 1973; Gifford 1940), and has been more recently applied to stuttering in children (Adams 1984a, 1980; Adams & Runyan 1981; Adams, Runyan & Mallard, 1975). Costello (1983) feels that easy onset may be particularly applicable where a child's speech is marked by glottal stops, prolongations, tense pauses, and so on. However, she feels that inserting the pattern into the child's production may be difficult and that eliminating it or phasing it out may present problems. She also notes the opinion that easy onset usually causes a drop in talking rate, although she is not sure which, or both, is most responsible for the dysfluency reduction that results.

Easy-onset procedures can be taught at any age level if applied with the appropriate degree of simplicity or complexity. As noted, these procedures are an essential part of a number of respiratory therapy methods. They require, first of all, that the speaker have an adequate degree of relaxation, whether all-body or localized around the speech mechanism. A reduced rate of speech will facilitate easy-onset production, since it sup-

reduction and reduces the strain on motor-timing and coor-
        .ivities. This reduction allows the speaker to integrate more ef-
        the articulatory and phonatory systems of production. The
si..   .ace of timing and coordination between articulatory and phonatory muscle groups was underscored in the research by Commodore and
Cooper (1978), in which the stutterers read aloud with whispered speech
and read with mouthing (no air stream). Stuttering in ordinary vocal
reading was significantly greater than during the other two conditions,
and stuttering during whispered speech was significantly greater than
during mouthed production.

When the stutterer can relax, slow rate, and have adequate respiratory support (mandatory prerequisites), easy onset involves

1. Easy inhalation combined with conscious relaxation.
2. Then prompt release of air (do not "set" and release), which is accompanied
   by gentle closure of the vocal folds if the first sound is voiced. If the first
   sound is voiceless, vocal fold closure is delayed. However, the voiceless
   sound can have some sonancy added near the end of its production in order
   to slide easily into the sound following.
3. Movement of the articulators from a neutral, relaxed position to shape the
   vocal tract for the initiating or following consonant sound.
4. Continuing movement of the articulators, rather than coming to rest at stop
   or pressure targets.

The foregoing are a combination of several variations of easy onset (Ham
1986), and the clinician can vary them at need. Easy onset, or variations of
it, has been used by many clinicians (Irwin 1972; Webster 1974; St. Louis
1979; Perkins 1983). The limitations in its use occur under several possible conditions, or combinations thereof:

1. Preliminary relaxation, respiratory support, and so on, are not adequate.
2. The client inadequately understands his or her own speech production
   habits.
3. Physical skill and practice is not established adequately, particularly on
   complex phonological combinations.
4. Transfer is not carried out in a planned, graded sequence.
5. Self-monitoring and evaluation are not trained adequately.
6. Maintenance is not guaranteed through fear hierarchy use and client
   confidence in technique efficacy.
7. Adequate desensitization to stuttering has not occurred.

In fluency reinforcement therapy, the client can become bored with effort
and time required. In symptom modification procedures, the danger is in
overuse (use when stuttering is not actually anticipated), and resultant ha-

bituation of the easy-onset behaviors. The latter situation is likely to de-volve into stuttering spasms that are a distorted version of easy onset.

BREATH CHEWING

If you observe people as they talk, you will see quite a range of jaw, lip, and tongue movement. At one end of the range, people barely seem to move their articulators. Conversely, some speakers almost seem to relish their words physically—talking with lip smacking, licking movements of the tongue, and expanded mouth openings. One can only speculate as to why these variations occur. This author has observed a similar range in stuttering spasms, from tight and tremorous contacts to grossly open and exaggerated movements of the articulators. Again, one can only speculate as to why. My speculations have led me to observe people covertly as they eat and talk, and my empirical data suggest to me that "tight jaws" and "loose jaws" tend to eat and speak in similar fashion. That is, the restricted-movement talker seems to take smaller bites and to chew with restraint, while the wide-movement talker eats with bigger bites, wider movements, and more open-mouth chewing (they also seem to be more frequent in talking while food is still in their mouths!). Where this all lead is not clear to me, but it might preamble the topic of breath chewing as a form of therapy.

The activity called breath chewing is credited to Emil Froeschels (1952a), although its history undoubtedly is longer. Chewing and swallowing of food must be coordinated with the respiratory system so that epiglottis deformation is timed with vocal fold adductors, such as the lateral cricoarytenoid muscle, to allow liquid or a food bolus to pass into the esophagus without entering the trachea. However, interspersed with chewing and swallowing will often be inspiration-expiration actions of the respiratory system whereby glottal adductors must relax and the posterior cricoarytenoid muscle contract for air passage. As the reader knows, everyone occasionally commits an error so that food or liquid is inhaled into the trachea with uncomfortable and/or embarrassing results. Most of the time, though, people perform with amazing laryngeal dexterity, without thought, this complex interaction of the linked systems.

Since speech, in all aspects, is overlaid on primary biological functions, Froeschels suggested that deliberate practice to coordinate and time breathstream release, vocal fold vibration, and articulator movements could be achieved through "chewing" the breathstream. It has been suggested that such an activity would facilitate relaxation (Hollingsworth 1939) and that also, because of its difference from usual speech movements, it might induce fluency (Van Riper 1973). Certainly breath chewing alters rhythm, rate, timing, stress, and other characteristics. Because the breathstream is propelled through articulator movement, respiration tends to be retimed and regularized.

In therapy of stuttering (also when used with certain phonatory disorders) breath chewing has had limited exposure over the past 40–50 years (Froeschels 1952a; Froeschels & Jellinek 1941; Kastein 1974; Ham 1986; Van Riper 1973). Nevertheless, it has persisted, probably for two reasons: A few clinicians use it with what might be excellent results, and more clinicians don't use it but suspect that there is more in it than we presently understand. It is also simple to teach; the following sequence, for example, could be used with Group I and younger Group II children:

1. Demonstrate and play with expiration to make child aware of the breath stream.
2. Using animal allusions practice "savage chewing" without deliberate sound (many children will tend to growl or make other noises). Make sure that lips, jaw, and tongue move in exaggerated chewing motions. Chewy (soft raisins) or crunchy food (unsugared cereals) can be used to improve movement.
3. Combine expiration and chewing. Excess body movements and gestures may help. Instruct the child to feel the strong movements and touches; keep the movements savage; maintain a good level of respiration. It is usually wise to discontinue chewing food bits because some overenthusiastic children will spray the clinician with them.
4. Add voicing to the breathstream. Steer away from growling and have the child chew vowels. This is done best by having child shadow clinician's model. Add continuant consonants; then vary them so that nonsense syllables are produced.
5. Convert to words, easing up on the vigor of chewing but retaining exaggerated, continuous movement and stable respiration. Examples are *hello, one man, who me, see some,* and *vinegar.*
6. Expand to phrases, use questions and answers, pay attention to prosody, and reduce the chewing extent. However, if dysfluencies occur, immediately drop back to more exaggerated levels.
7. Progress to conversation in which air release and articular movements are coordinated, articulators stay in motion, phonation is extended, and respiration matches phrasing.

Young children usually enjoy breath chewing very much—if the clinician does. It may help overall neuromotor timing and coordination problems and could improve tactile and kinesthetic awareness.

Older Group II, and Group III, children may feel ridiculous using breath chewing. When the author demonstrates breath chewing in class, student reactions range from frozen efforts not to giggle to hysterical collapse. Some adolescent clients will feel threatened. Nonetheless the method can be used with any age, depending on the enthusiasm and charisma of the clinician.

VENTRILOQUISM

In 1951, in his first therapy course, the author was required to purchase a "bone prop." This device was a small piece of plastic, slotted on each end, and drilled for a string that ran through it. The slotted ends were fitted between the cutting edges of upper and lower incisor teeth. Intended for use with clients who have flaccid articulator muscles or subnormal oral cavity openings, the bone prop has also been used to force stutterers to change and reduce the degree of their articulator contacts. In a variant form, without a mechanical aid, *light consonant contact* has been used for many years. Unlike easy onset, the breathstream is not involved; rather, the strength and duration of contact between articulators is targeted. The stutterer is to use light contact to change abnormal preparatory sets and reduce or eliminate prespasm tremors of articulator muscles.

An interesting approach to light consonant contact was devised by Froeschels (1950, 1952a) and called ventriloquism speech. The label is very misleading, since ventriloquists attempt to have no movement of visible articulators, whereas light contact is unconcerned about visibility while stressing exaggeratedly reduced contacts. The procedure has been taught in many ways, but one possible sequence is the following:

1. Practice talking with mouth completely open, using words that minimize articulator contact. Articulator contacts are avoided so that articulation is made up of modified vowel strings. In this pattern, "Who is he?" becomes "ooo iiii eee?" Effort is concentrated on smooth movement, prolongation of vowels, and developing the sensation of moving vowel to vowel without interruption of consonants. Inflection, stress, and other production variables should be retained or exaggerated.
2. Reduce the degree of oral opening so that consonants are just barely touched or stroked. Emphasis is still on movement from vowel to vowel.
3. Further reduce the oral opening until consonants are formed accurately, but with significantly less pressure than usual. Contrasts between strong pressure and light contact can be made to aid in tactile differentiation.

As an isolated technique, ventriloquism or light contact is relatively valueless, as are most methods. It tends to result in total or near-total fluency quickly, but transfer is rare. However, it can be used as a supplement to easy onset and passive airflow and in various forms of symptom modification. It helps children with oral discoordination problems, aids in respiratory revisions, and places significant stress on prosody factors. Also, applications are possible in localized relaxation therapy and with clients for whom tactile and kinesthetic awareness needs enhancement. The age and acceptance factors discussed for breath chewing apply equally to this area.

SINGING

When a person sings, speech output changes markedly. Melody, inflection, stress, and rate usually vary. Vowel duration and consonant duration (to a lesser degree) may change markedly. In particular, the rhythm of speech utterance is changed significantly. With all this, respiratory patterns change significantly. All these changes can be demonstrated using ordinary speech pattern to recite a few lyric lines from almost any song, and then singing them as written in the music. Wingate (1976) and Miller (1982) have suggested that duration changes, related to vowel production, are the major influences on speech. Wingate has also felt that rhythm was not particularly significant, whereas Van Riper (1973) and Starkweather (1982a) have disagreed with this contention.

The salutary effects of singing in reducing or eliminating stuttering have been known for a long time (Bloodstein 1949). However, it apparently is not true that "people never stutter when they sing" (Healey, Mallard & Adams 1976; Colcord & Adams 1979). Van Riper (1973) provided an extensive summary of singing therapy, particularly as used in Europe. Although not a strong advocate of the method, he summarized a number of favorable reports. On the other hand, Galloway (1974) strongly criticized singing therapy and stated that past history and lack of relevant research fail to justify its use. It is probable that the clinician would need some level of vocal music ability and also that the client should have at least some naive capacities in that area. Singing can be particularly useful with Group I and Group II children, especially in group therapy. Where Wingate (1984d) stressed the use of poetry in therapy to secure control of timing, rhythm, and stress variations, singing can be used for similar reasons. Singing can be applied to encourage relaxation, improve frequency range, increase oral resonance, improve rhythm and timing patterns, alter stress patterns, and so on. In developing a therapy method, one could move to intoning, or chanting, as the next stage.

Chanting and intoning in fact involve production in a rhythmic pattern, often a stereotyped one, where stress is usually reduced and distributed equally. Vowel prolongation is usually involved, and the method can merge with legato speech, which is discussed elsewhere.

CHAPTER SUMMARY

Many stutterers display breathstream anomalies during moments of stuttering, and some appear to have irregularities of the general respiratory process. Over the years therapy of stuttering has involved respiration in a variety of ways. There is little support today for respiration-only therapy, however, even when linked to relaxation and transfer efforts. When breathstream control is related to timing and strength of phonatory and articulatory movements, there is a more efficient therapy result in many instances. Whether one area is more influential than another is unclear, and the clinician probably should be prepared to rearrange emphases to provide for the particular combinations of individual clients.

The chapter has also discussed several other therapy methods, all of variable relationship to respiration. Breath chewing and easy onset, which carry close ties to breathstream management, have received particular attention here. Easy onset is widely used in a variety of control systems, and it, along with rate control, probably account for nearly all of the fluency therapy done today. There is danger in using these methods as if they were total programs, however. Also, their popularity has probably reduced interest and research in other methods such as breath chewing, ventriloquism, and singing or singing-element therapies. The author would encourage readers to experiment with the range of methods described in this and other chapters, rather than adhering rigidly to the method or methods currently most popular.

CHAPTER FOURTEEN
SYMPTOM MODIFICATION PROCEDURES

OVERVIEW

Background

Symptom modification therapy (SMT) is limited to one chapter in this text because of the book's age orientation to stuttering. The author was educated and trained when most of the current therapy approaches labeled fluency reinforcement were regarded as useless or, worse, as quackery. At that time therapy of stuttering was usually aimed at parents, in the Iowa diagnosogenic model. If children received direct therapy, it often tended to be play therapy with vaguely stated objectives of increasing speech interaction, self-confidence, emotional release, and so on. When speech was targeted, then variations of standard adult symptom modification procedures tended to be used (Luper & Mulder 1964). This was true from Group I up through Group III clients. However, times change, and so should therapy. These concepts and practices were upset or rearranged as the values of early intervention were proved and the possible efficacies of fluency reinforcement therapies were demonstrated.

What, exactly, is SMT? If one speaks of goals, definitions are fairly uniform, although frequently misunderstood. Overly zealous opponents of SMT have attempted to hang a derisive "stutter more fluently" label on the approach, while frequently defining the "fluency" as so many SW/M or a certain %SW figure—in other words, the approach suggests to the stutterer, "Be more fluent as you stutter." Symptom therapy does in fact target the dysfluent, not the fluent, moments of speech. It is, moreover, concerned with feelings, attitudes, interaction, counseling, and the other psychosocial aspects of communication. Acceptance of and tolerance for dysfluency are focused on in therapy. Finally, although most SMT clinicians agree that fluency is possible (however defined), therapy is structured on the assumption that the client may always need to exercise variable degrees of self-monitoring and speech control.

The preceding statements are philosophy, variations of which occur among SMT clinicians. Even wider differences occur when methodology is considered. In fact, there is no such thing as one SMT approach that can be evaluated and compared with one fluency reinforcement therapy (FRT) approach. The author practiced as a symptom clinician for two decades before FRT developed any significant impact on the profession. During those early years my procedures were varied in many ways—which ones were used, the sequences of use, the way steps were presented, and the various ancillary methods comprising the remainder of the therapy program. However, with all the variations, the basic goals remained the following:

1. Development of client analysis and evaluation skills relative to communication.
2. Development of insight and understanding concerning feelings and attitudes, relative to communication.
3. Reduction or elimination of avoidance behaviors exhibited in psychosocial interactions, particularly with reference to communication.
4. Acquisition of speech production patterns that provide for control of dysfluency in a form that is acceptable to the client.
5. Transfer and stabilization of nonavoidance behaviors and speech control skills in such a way that the client has complete responsibility, as well as the capacities to carry it.

Chapter Coverage

This chapter is somewhat longer than other parts of the book because there are so many areas to cover. The more limited use of SMT with children requires much more space for FRT and related therapy procedures, even though it has been emphasized a number of times that the two therapy philosophies actually overlap to extremes in a number of areas. Several topic areas have been discussed elsewhere in the book and thus require only brief coverage in these sections. Nevertheless, the one-chapter limitation restricts the depth of coverage, and so the reader is referred to other sources if more information is desired (Ham 1986; Van Riper 1973, 1971a; Luper & Mulder 1964). Symptom therapy relative to

age is considered first followed by a section dealing with skills or procedures that cut across most of the different methods of dysfluency control.
These dysfluency methods, or disfluency controls, separate into those
used to control stuttering and those in which faking, or pseudostuttering,
is learned. With these background factors explained, an outline of a sample program is presented as one possible way to organize SMT. The section following flows from the sample outline and describes specific procedures, with references made to age factor and management techniques.
Finally, the remainder of the chapter deals with related procedures and
transfer and maintenance approaches.

AGE FACTORS

During the heyday of SMT very little direct therapy of stuttering was conducted with children younger than nine or ten years of age. This philosophy, or pragmatism, was compatible with learning theory semantogenic
models where stuttering origin and early development was blamed on the
environment. It was felt that direct therapy could exacerbate child anxieties and possibly increase dysfluency. Also a consideration was that
direct-therapy early intervention often failed or, if satisfactory, was followed by relapse. Symptom modification therapy tended to be most
efficacious (and still is) when the stuttering spasms are more severe in
terms of duration, struggle, and complicating factors. With exceptions,
many child stutterers have shorter, simpler stuttering spasms, and their
predictability or consistency may be less. Symptom modification therapy
also functions best when the client has sufficient maturity to develop and
use behavioral insights into self and other people, can apply objective
principles to evaluation, and can develop self-therapy planning, execution, and evaluation strategies when needed. Again, with exceptions, these
factors tend to be correlated negatively with decreasing age.

   Clinicians vary in their willingness, or ability, to use SMT with children. Conture (1982), in considering therapy for the older child (about
9–12 years) who is overtly aware of stuttering, has suggested that direct
efforts aimed at symptom control be considered. These methods could be
of the precision fluency shaping (Webster 1979) type, or the cancellation-
pullout-preparatory set sequence. Dalton and Hardcastle (1977) considered symptom modification and stated, "It demands the utmost patience
and concentration and is more appropriately applied to severe blocks,
prolongations, and repetitions" (p. 104). They suggest that milder stutterings pass too quickly and that SMT efforts take too much time for real effectiveness to occur. As noted earlier, milder spasm patterns are often
characteristic of young children. On the other hand, Turnbaugh (1983),
while stressing the need to change therapy philosophies and methods, ex-

pressed the feeling that stuttering modification was more reality-oriented than is FRT. She perceived an incongruity between training for fluency and simultaneously trying to increase tolerance and acceptance of fluency disruptors. Some clinicians will not consider SMT at all, others age-divide it, and yet others apply it routinely. The author has joined the centrist group and applies SMT with age discrimination. It is difficult to justify symptom therapy as an overall approach for most Group I children if the stuttering pattern is fairly simple and the attitudes manageable and if any needed environmental manipulation can be achieved. When the situation is favorable, the time efficiency, the speech results, and the stability of results tend to favor fluency reinforcement therapy.

Children in Group II present a more difficult choice, but school settings (where most Group II clients are seen) often impose therapy duration and frequency constraints that militate against the often slower pace of symptom therapy. Also, the factor of insight maturity cited for Group I still operates, even though it may be less of a problem. However, some Group II children will be good candidates for SMT procedures. Even for those who are not, or where situation mandates would make it unfeasible, aspects of symptom therapy can be integrated easily into other types of therapy programs. Situational constraints aside, Group III children can be excellent candidates for symptom therapy. The interactive psychosocial aspects of therapy frequently fit Group III needs quite well, and their stuttering patterns are more likely to respond to symptom procedures. Where down-the-line symptom therapy is not planned, techniques from SMT can meld easily with other approaches at various stages of therapy.

Overall, symptom therapy is age related, but not age bound. It places great stress on the interactive and client manipulation skills of the clinician, and this capacity allows for considerable variation in how particular procedures are structured. In the hands of an experienced clinician, SMT has values with children, either as a whole program or, in parts, within a fluency reinforcement program, relaxation program, or counseling approach.

DISFLUENCY METHODS

Rationale

A core aspect of FRT and SMT has been the utilization of disfluent speech. In some fluency therapies the client is taught prolongation, syllable-timed patterns, easy onset, or other disfluencies, which then are shaped toward normal utterance patterns. In some symptom therapies the client is taught prolongation, bounce, light consonant contact, and other disfluencies, which then are shaped toward controlled utterance of stuttered words. All of the currently used disfluency procedures have been used by past generations of clinicians, for various purposes. In SMT, disfluencies can be used for any of the following:

1. Practice analyzing and evaluating different forms of disfluency.
2. Experimentation in modifying stuttering spasms in a variety of forms.
3. Learning to use voluntary disfluencies in different control techniques.
5. Analysis and evaluation of environmental reactions to disfluent speech.

Other rationales exist for using disfluencies in therapy, especially among FRT clinicians. However, the preceding list covers most of the symptom modification rationale. The next step, once rationale is established, is to examine disfluency uses more specifically in terms of characteristics and use. The applications in the preceding list involve two major categories of disfluency. One category, generally serving as speech goals or acceptable disfluency forms, is called control disfluencies. The other category involves the recreating or simulation of stuttering spasms and will, for the moment, be called pseudostuttering.

Control Disfluencies

As described earlier, *control disfluencies* are typically characterized by

rhythm, timing, duration, and/or pressure changes in the manner in which sounds, syllables, or words are produced. Usually occurring on the initial or stressed syllable of an utterance, they generally have the effect of slowing rate of production, altering prosodic and vocal parameters, and changing the timing and contact patterns of vocal tract constriction and modification actions.

Because of motor planning simplification, changed neuromotor patterns, and increased feedback-monitoring cues, the stutterer is better able to control these voluntary disfluencies and not have them slip into the habituated motor patterns of stuttering spasms. A general rule of thumb in teaching control disfluencies has been initially, to use control disfluencies that are unlike the typical stuttering spasm patterns. Therefore, *prolongation* might be used with a stutterer presenting a strongly clonic (repetitive) spasm pattern, and *bounce disfluencies* could be used where a tonic (prolongation or stoppage) spasm pattern usually predominates. Later on, control disfluencies quite similar to the usual spasm form can be practiced. In all instances production begins at exaggerated or extended levels, and then is shaped into briefer or less obvious forms. Some clinicians have even recommended a final shaping where the disfluency becomes a "mental image," with no audible or visible characteristics. However, this has not been common. Most of the control disfluencies assume or require a relaxed production mode so that stuttering spasms are not triggered easily, and speech avoidance or other associated behaviors should be eliminated or reduced. Many control disfluencies have been described, but nearly all of them fall into one or more of the categories described in following subsections.

Bounce disfluency The bounce, or "Iowa bounce" (Van Riper 1958a), actually has a long history. In simple form, the speaker is to repeat the target syllable (usually, but not necessssarily, the first) in an easy, slow, rhythmic pattern. This rhythmic repetition, or bouncing, is to continue without any pause or alteration until the word is completed. The correct vowel is to be used on the bounces, not the schwa sound. Easy-onset or light consonant contact procedures can be combined with bounce production, if desired. Initially, the stutterer may use 6, 8, 12, and so on, bounces before moving into the word. During prolonged bouncing the stutterer works on targets such as relaxation, airstream release, eye contact, maintaining control, and so on. As skill develops, the number of bounces is reduced progressively until they either disappear or are at a minimum (some clinicians have carried the process to silent or "mental" bounces).

Symptom therapy may also use bounces, or any other control disfluency, to increase client tolerance for disfluency. For instance, a stutterer who has learned the technique might be assigned to collect 25 occurrences in out-clinic speech situations where words are to be bounced on at least six times before completion. If any of the practice bounce patterns slip into real stuttering, then the client is to use a cancellation. As a penalty for having "slipped," two more bounce-words are to be added to the original target of 25 words. The foregoing was an example of one possible assignment, and many others are used. Bounce also can be used as a method of pullout (see later) by slowing a real spasm (or a faked one), relaxing it, and turning it into a bounce. This works particularly well with clonic spasms.

Production errors in bounce use tend to cluster around a few patterns: tense bouncing, using too few bounces, jerking the final bounce, accelerating the final few bounces before uttering the word, and irregularities in the bounce rhythm. As a rhythm-based procedure, the bounce can be extremely effective if properly used. However, it is an obvious disfluency, and many mild and moderate stutterers will find it too noticeable unless they develop the invisible bounce referred to earlier. Indeed, Berlin and Berlin (1964), comparing bounce procedures to prolongation and pullouts, reported that lay persons rated bounce lowest in terms of listener acceptance.

Easy-onset disfluency The control disfluency known as easy onset is one of the most popular methods used in FRT today and has been used in SMT for many years. It has been particularly adaptable to use in preparatory sets, after the stutterer has learned to control and manipulate dysfluency patterns. Easy onset has been discussed previously, and so will only be summarized briefly here.

Many programs use easy onset in one form or another (Webster 1979; Weiner 1978; Perkins 1983; Shine 1980a, 1980b) as part of fluency shaping. In symptom therapy, it has three primary application areas:

1. **Cancellation.** After a stutter, analyze and evaluate the dysfluency behaviors that occurred. Then relax the vocal tract, inhale, and release the airstream while moving the articulators easily so as to achieve the desired air-voice coincidence.
2. **Pullouts.** During a stutter, analyze the dysfluency tension points and relax them as you slow down production rate. From the relaxed state slip slowly and easily into the rest of the word. Very likely the last portion of the stuttering spasm will be "easy" pseudostuttering that tapers off into easy completion.
3. **Preparatory Set.** This is closest to fluency reinforcement use but directed only at words on which stuttering is anticipated. Relaxation, inhalation-exhalation, and articulatory movements are applied as described elsewhere in this text.

Failures in easy onset can occur in basic relaxation, respiration, and articulation through inadequate relaxation or return of tension, inadequate air support or release, hurried movement, excessive speed or pressure on articulations, or performance of habituated articulatory postures that tend to trigger stuttering spasms.

Light-contact disfluency   Light contact, or light consonant contact, has been discussed previously, along with ventriloquism speech. It is not the same as easy onset, since it concentrates on reducing the force or pressure with which contact speech sounds are produced. However, it is often integrated into easy-onset programs. In SMT the stutterer has analyzed his or her spasm patterns so thoroughly that articulation postures, form and pressure, are known well. Attention is then paid to lightening the contact to the point where tactile receptor feedback and alpha motoneuron signals no longer conform to habituated patterns. This change presumably eliminates, or at least reduces, the neural patterns or codes that might trigger stuttering spasms. In its extreme form, during early practice, light-contact speech is difficult for the auditor to understand. Proficient use results in a slight slowing of rate before and during production of the target word, a more precise mode of utterance, and, of course, the lighter contacts. As with all fluency or symptom methods, light contact is subject to overuse and habituation. The author has observed stutterers who fell into this avoidance trap and relapsed with a light-contact stuttering pattern.

Prolongation disfluency This control disfluency has also been discussed previously. It is very often combined with continuous phonation, so that vowels and continuant consonants are elongated and blended. This combination tends to lead to a droning, chanting, or intoning type of production. It is, of course, interrupted by phrase breaks and tends to have reduced value at those points. However, prolongation can be paired with easy onset or light consonant contact to facilitate initiation or moving from voiceless to voiced contacts. In both symptom and fluency therapies, stutterers can be taught (or learn spontaneously) to use prolongation (or any other method) only on the words or syllables, or linguistic points, where stuttering is most likely to occur. Van Riper (1973) was skeptical about the value of prolonged speech, but research comparisons have generally been supportive of this form of disfluency (Ham 1986).

Strong-movement disfluency The strong-movement method of control is not well known and actually combines elements of several other methods. Production of sounds is prolonged and tends to be continuous. Indeed, the key element is production as a *continuous movement.* Yet articulatory contacts are not made lightly or easily, for they are produced as if the tongue and lips and other surfaces were being "scraped" together in a continuous movement. One analogy that has been drawn is to imagine that the articulators have been coated with peanut butter, and you must talk while scraping off the peanut butter (no hands) at the same time! Sounds slide in slow, strong movement so that even stops such as /p/, /b/, /d/, /k/, /g/ are moved through without a stopping point ever occurring. There are similarities between strong movement and certain stages of Froeschels's breath-chewing therapy. The presumed effect of strong movement, aside from prolongation and continuation, is thought to be the elimination of prearticulatory sets or in-production postures that, historically, tend to trigger stuttering spasms. The method has been used particularly with, or after, work on preparatory sets when increments in tactile and kinesthetic awareness will aid in monitoring and control of articulatory motor patterns.

TYPICAL SYMPTOM MODIFICATION

There are many variants of SMT, since it has predominated in our profession for several decades. (Some forms, as with Sheehan's avoidance-reduction therapy, have been discussed elsewhere in the book.) So-called classical symptom modification therapy was an Iowa product and probably is exemplified best in the writings of Charles Van Riper (1971a, 1973, 1978; Van Riper & Emerick 1984). Van Riper tends to be labeled as representing a particular method of stuttering therapy, but this is erroneous. He routinely varied his therapy programs every year, and every fifth year amalgamated the most successful components from the preceding four years. A diary of two decades of such experimentation has been published (Van Riper 1958a), and one could wish that more clinicians would test and try as did Van Riper rather than holding on to monothematic therapies. A representative illustration of Van Riperian SMT can be found in his MIDVAS program (1978), referred to in Chapter 11. The elements of the MIDVAS acronym (motivation, identification, desensitization, variation, approximation, stabilization) are summarized briefly in the following subsections.

Motivation

Motivation is the initial stage, in which client-clinician rapport is established and the client is made to feel that the clinician is interested in her or his problem and cares. The clinician's competence and confidence is displayed, and the stutterer is encouraged to express feelings and to stutter without emotional stress. The clinician uses pseudostuttering to help illustrate discussions and to expand the client's acceptance of dysfluency. Goals are identified by the stutterer, and an agreement is reached as to what the therapy goals are to be. Finally, the clinician lays out very clearly what the steps, and procedures, of therapy will be so that the client understands what will happen and what each of them, client and clinician, must do to move through therapy steps and reach the agreed-upon goals.

Identification

The identification stage involves an aggressive program in self-analysis. Basic aspects of the stuttering spasms, and their variability, are studied. Also, feelings of guilt, fear, anger, frustration, and anxiety are explored. Extensive use of out-clinic assignments is made, and the client starts self-therapy responsibility by learning to identify therapy target areas and design assignments to explore them. The overall scope, and characteristics, of the individual client is explored—with emphasis on the stutterer finding out about himself or herself, rather than being instructed by the clinician.

Desensitization

In desensitization, basically the stutterer is taken through his or her own fear hierarchy, *as a stutterer*. This step has close similarities to Sheehan's avoidance-reduction therapy. Clinicians, acting as stutterers, are expected to model real situations and then help the client experience them. Skill and empathy are required of the clinician, and this phase is difficult for both client and clinician. The desired result is the client's increased tolerance for stuttering, increased knowledge about his or her own behavior and about the reactions of the environment, and reductions in avoidance behaviors within speech proper and in psychosocial interactions.

Variation

Variation can be a relatively brief step and involves using the information gathered in the two previous steps. The client is to take his or her own stuttering behaviors and deliberately vary them. If "uh" is used as a postponement, then something else must be used; if eyes are shut during a spasm, then they are to be blinked or kept open; if repetitions usually evolve into a prolongation, the process is to be reversed. Situation and personal behaviors are also to be varied. The target is to enable the stutterer to control the stuttering, rather than the other way around. When this has been achieved, the client is ready to learn new responses that will reduce the stuttering.

Approximation

The client is to move, in approximating stages, to alter stuttering into more acceptable forms. The clinician may model techniques, such as unison speech, and pull the stutterer along in the change process. Cancellation, pullouts, and preparatory sets are learned (these will be discussed further in other sections of this chapter). Meanwhile, client counseling is used to deal with fears and other feelings during this stage.

Stabilization

In the previous step the client learned to modify stuttering into a disfluency form that he or she can accept (even if only temporarily). This form may be readily identifiable by auditors as stuttering, or it may be fluent sounding in terms of reference to current FRT modes. The difference (type or degree) is not important at this stage as long as it is accepted and tolerated by the client. Stabilization is planned to shift all therapy responsibility, in stages, to the client and to equip her or him with the resources to maintain gains. Fluency practice, such as through shadowing, is used to improve general speech. Faking, or pseudostuttering, is employed by the client to maintain tolerance, increase evaluation skills, and provide for practice in pullouts or other control systems. Monitoring and evaluation plans are worked out. Finally, the stutterer undergoes "resistance therapy" in which efforts are made to induce stuttering. Unison reading with the clinician pseudostuttering, DAF reading or talking, particularly difficult situations or topics, and so on, are used. In all of these the stutterer is to use the learned skills to maintain speech control. Also, to the degree possible, the client is to try to "resist stuttering." This does not imply avoidance; rather, it could be stated, "Since you have learned to tolerate stuttering, have learned to control it, have learned to turn it into acceptable forms, and can deal with any situation now, *don't stutter.*"

Starkweather (1973) concluded that "Van Riper therapy" is based on the assumption that stuttering is an avoidance response. Harking back to the idea that stuttering is what the person does in order to avoid stuttering, therapy is seen as a psychological approach to minimizing or eliminating the avoidance behaviors. Although Starkweather's basic contention is true, he would be wise to contrast Van Riper and Sheehan. The latter individual is almost totally committed to reduction of avoidance; whereas Van Riper, on the other hand, combines avoidance reduction and control of the physical behaviors that have become an habituated aspect of the avoidance. Not only must avoidance be reduced, but the stutterer must learn to control the struggle behaviors and reshape them so that avoidance drives are reduced. Other SMT approaches could be summarized, but that is not necessary, for sequences, and emphases within sequences, can vary from program to program. The variations cited in the five-year cycles discussed at the beginning of this section involved some drastic additions and omissions to what some have labeled as being classic symptom therapy. Just as avoidance-reduction can be achieved in many different ways, symptom modification and control is accessible in a wide range of approaches and with different techniques. And so although in the following section some "classic" techniques are discussed, it should be emphasized that they are presented as examples of ways in which SMT can be implemented, not as a final description of how it must be done.

SYMPTOM MODIFICATION METHODS

After the preceding statements, it may sound somewhat presumptuous to declare that certain procedures are symptom modification procedures. In fact, every method described in the following subsections can be found among various FRT programs today. Recall that in the consideration of fluency therapy the author discussed the use of portable noise maskers and cited Gruber's (1971) reported use of a portable masker in SMT. Similarly, relaxation, principles of reward and punishment, breathstream management, and other areas can be found in both therapy approaches.

In the following subsections six method areas have been focused on because of their frequency of use, because of their unique characteristics as methods per se, and/or because they relate particularly to overall goals of symptom therapy: acceptance of self, tolerance for fluency disruption, and voluntary control of dysfluencies. The areas surveyed are the following:

Stutterer self-analysis   Cancellation
Desensitization   Pullout
Pseudostuttering   Preparatory Set

Stutterer Self-Analysis

Self-analysis, or self-evaluation, has been discussed extensively in Chapter 10, with procedures and applications suggested. The process will not be repeated here, but it may be helpful to look at the method in context. It coincides with Van Riper's MIDVAS step of identification and is paramount in bringing the stutterer into contact with her or his speech and speech behaviors. In SMT it is mandatory that a thorough self-evaluation be performed. If it is lacking, or incomplete, the stutterer can never take responsibility for self-control of speech. He, or she, is reduced to following by rote whatever procedures the clinician devises and teaches. This does not always have to have bad results, philosophy aside, as long as the system works effectively and does not break down over time. If the breakdown occurs, then the stutterer may have no resource except to try harder to use what has just failed, and that usually leads to greater failure because the reasons are not known, the subtle aspects leading to breakdown are in limbo, and the stutterer has no past history of self-correction and evaluation. SMT expresses the view that you cannot fix something unless you know what is wrong with it. This knowledge makes it possible for classic techniques to be individualized to the peculiar stuttering and social characteristics of each client, rather than using rote acquisition of a rote procedure.

Self-analysis also provides for motivation, in which the client simultaneously feels that she or he is doing something, personally, about stuttering, and also is reducing any feelings that stuttering is an entity that controls the behavior of the client. Self-analysis projects forward into desensitization by requiring the client to become objective, accurate, and analytical about behaviors that previously were unknown, avoided, suppressed, or masked by facades. Finally, self-analysis is a mandatory step preceding direct-symptom control work with cancellations, pullouts, and preparatory sets. These and other procedures require thorough knowledge by the client if they are to be used in proper form with anticipated effects.

Chapter 10 divided self-analysis in terms of its use among the three age groups, and so those divisions will not be repeated here. In general, the clinician decides how much time and emphasis to spend on self-analysis, based on the following factors:

1. Age of the client.
2. Severity and complexity of the stuttering pattern.

3. Existing level of awareness and self-analysis ability.
4. Psychosocial adjustment of the client in terms of covert patterns and social avoidances.
5. Degree to which subsequent methods will rely upon the information gathered, skills developed, and attitude changes initiated during the self-analysis process.

The self-analysis process is not conclusive in duration. There is no exact time period in which it should be the sole or major focus of therapy; it is also true that self-analysis continues and resurfaces in every step of therapy. The clinician should set initial goals in terms of the following: awareness of stuttering, location and description of stuttering spasms (including struggles), associated speech behaviors, attitudes and feelings, auditors and environment. These initial goals should be apportioned into subgoals so that criterion levels can be set, data counts made, and progress measured. When therapy focus shifts to other methods, self-analysis should continue on a recurrent basis so that client sophistication keeps pace with the growing demand, and potentials, of therapy. Obviously, the basic structure of self-analysis, and many of its components, are quite compatible with fluency therapies of various types.

Desensitization

Desensitization was considered earlier also, in Chapter 11, and so its discussion will be limited here. In SMT the assumption is made that the stutterer has become overly sensitized to dysfluency experiences and tries to avoid them. Avoidances may be speech-specific, such as postponements and substitutions, or they may be behavioral in that behavior patterns and psychosocial interactions are altered by the stuttering. As noted earlier, some clinicians maintain that the establishment of fluent speech will eliminate the cause of avoidances and, therefore, the avoidances or other undesirable behaviors. With many Group I children, and some in Group II, this can happen. However, some preschool and Group II children are more stress-sensitive than usual and can benefit from some desensitization therapy. Group III children probably have been stuttering for anywhere from 7 or 8 to 10 or 15 years. During these years very nearly all of them have experienced personal embarrassment, guilt, shame, and anger and have had auditors react with surprise, fear, amusement, imitation, ridicule, and rejection. Some survive this experience remarkably well, but others have developed strong feelings, covert patterns, reduced or distorted psychosocial interactions, and will not be changed significantly by the magic gift of fluency.

Desensitization can be limited to experience in resisting or tolerating fluency disruptions (Luper & Mulder 1964). In typical SMT it involves deliberately creating or seeking out experiences that create communication stress. The activities involved in self-analysis are basic desensitization steps, since few stutterers like to think about, listen to or watch, and discuss their stuttering and behaviors. Where to start varies with the client. Some require desensitization even to discussing their stuttering with an accepting, understanding clinician. One client, during assessment, quit on the second adaptation reading because he could not tolerate so much stuttering! Other clients, at the outset, cope with nearly all situations except those that would make most speakers feel uncomfortable or nervous. A fear hierarchy is constructed, and the stutterer is guided through it, not to change speech, but to face the situations. Usually types of counting behaviors or observations are required in order to measure progress and engender feelings of accomplishment. Desensitization can be linked with self-analysis and other methods, emphasis depending on the client and the therapy stage. A hypothetical set of activities for several therapy sessions might be the following:

1. In-clinic discussions of experiences client has had in talking with father, or other persons.
2. Refinement and analysis of the fear hierarchy.
3. Role rehearsal of answering questions in class, talking with an opposite-sex peer on the telephone, and ordering a meal in a fast food restaurant.
4. Out-clinic assignments to
   a. Smile and wave at five to ten classmates the client does not know well.
   b. Deliberately exchange conversations with three people in class.
   c. Have a long conversation with a good friend and look at her or him each time stuttering occurs.
   d. Call mother from school to make some request. Count stutterings and try to remember what each one was like.

As you can see, the "worst" fears (talking with father) are just being analyzed, role rehearsal is in the stage of probing how to deal with situations in the near future, and actual assignments are scattered among a number of less-feared activities. In addition to facing fears, the various methods and techniques described in Chapter 11 can be used as needed.

Desensitization, like self-analysis, is not a step with set termination. For a period of time it is the main focus of therapy, but activities continue throughout all subsequent steps of therapy. The clinician will find some clients for whom desensitization is a major problem, while others grimace and do what is necessary. In his clinical experience this author has found mild stutterers more likely to be resistant to desensitization because adroit mixtures of avoidance, covert behaviors, and mild spasms enable them to get by 90 percent of the time. Where time pressures and client motivation combine to create problems, FRT may become an elective or fall-back therapy. It seems that most stutterers at more severe levels, since they cannot hide their stuttering, are more accepting of desensitization needs.

The clinician must decide when sufficient desensitization has occurred for therapy focus to shift to another area of emphasis. The basic criterion is that out-clinic practice and transfer cannot occur if the stutterer is not sufficiently desensitized *at some level.* If clients are not prepared adequately, they cannot plan, perform, and evaluate to generalize the desired behaviors. If clients are not successful in desensitization, therapy will not succeed.

Interim Note

In Van Riper's MIDVAS program, variation follows desensitization. The stutterer practices varying the form of stuttering and learning to produce and control various types of voluntary disfluencies. The author has no quarrel with this step but has tended to collapse it into the cancellation, pullout, and preparatory set series rather than having it as a separate step.

Voluntary Stuttering

Pseudostuttering, faking, voluntary stuttering, negative practice, all reflect different meanings. Note that the timing of use depends partly on definition and partly on use in therapy. Some clinicians start with the activity in the first therapy session, some wait until transfer stages, some place it in or after desensitization, and some slowly develop it in every stage of therapy. Its age applicability roughly parallels desensitization: rarely in Group I, occasionally in Group II, often in Group III. With these contexts, let us consider definitions.

The author has defined voluntary production of dysfluencies before (Ham 1986), and there are a number of applications:

> **Voluntary stuttering**—being willing to stutter openly; some add the removal of avoidances and covert behaviors. The stuttering is real, not imitation.
> **Pseudostuttering**—imitating genuine stuttering, under voluntary control; may faithfully duplicate real spasms or deliberately include or exclude certain elements.
> **Faking**—same as pseudostuttering.
> **Negative practice**—pseudostuttering that faithfully replicates the speaker's real stuttering spasms.

The preceding are the author's personal definitions, and others exist. Bryngelson (1935) is credited with applying voluntary stuttering to therapy and used it in the fullest sense of the definition given here. Others (Emerick 1963; SFA 12) have defined voluntary stuttering in different ways. Negative practice, identified with Knight Dunlap (1942) involves faithful replication by the stutterer of his or her own stuttering spasms. In Dunlap's work the effect could result from a complete fake replica, a fake

that turned real, or a real spasm that was converted into a fake, as long as the original spasm was duplicated. Dunlap applied learning principles in that deliberate practice of an error facilitated changing or reducing that error.

In this text, discussions are limited to pseudostuttering by the client and clinician. Voluntary stuttering is covered in self-analysis and in desensitization areas, and elements of negative practice appear in some of the control methods discussed. Pseudostuttering has many applications, depending on clinician preferences:

1. In self-analysis, to study behaviors more precisely. Both the client and the clinician duplicate spasms or parts of spasms, slow down stuttering rates, reduce spasm tensions, and eliminate various avoidance behaviors to facilitate evaluation of various spasm components.
2. In desensitization, to stutter in easy situations where pressures are less, to increase stress, and to test tolerance for stuttering.
3. To serve as a vehicle, in-clinic and out-clinic, for practice of various control disfluencies.
4. To serve as a vehicle, in-clinic and out-clinic, for practice of various control methods.
5. In maintenance, to test for stability of improvement, quality of control methods, adequacy of monitoring, and viability of tolerance.

In speaking of pseudostuttering Falck (1969) has described it as "perhaps the most successful (and often the most difficult) technique in analyzing stuttering behavior" (p. 68). Other therapy applications have occurred. Gregory and Hill (1984), in discussing therapy for confirmed (older) stuttering children, accept the use of pseudostuttering if it is needed to aid in analysis and control of errors. It also can be used to practice control methods. They do not suggest a generalized use of pseudostuttering in every case. Also, Gregory (1968) described using negative practice and voluntary stuttering (as defined earlier) in stages of unison speech therapy. In general, faking and voluntary stuttering seem to be regarded as synonymous, and reference is made to bounce or slide (easy-onset and prolongation) disfluency techniques, with at least half of the fakes occurring on nonfeared words.

Exactly how pseudostuttering is used in therapy will depend on many variables, so it is difficult to describe a recommended sequence. However, following are some suggestions based on applications the author has used at various times:

SELF-ANALYSIS

- Reproduce the more obvious associated behaviors for identification, description, and evaluation.
- Practice some simple, easy fakes in reading and talking in order to under-

stand basic spasm patterns, practice postspasm analysis, and sharpen monitoring skills.
- Reproduce own stuttering patterns in their complete forms and in various modified styles that eliminate or change covert patterns and associated behaviors. This pinpoints evaluation areas, is early desensitization, prepares for later control systems, and builds self-confidence. If the spasms (at any time) turn real, there is no failure and the client is to use them as evaluation material.

DESENSITIZATION

- In-clinic stuttering usually has dropped, sometimes to near-zero levels. Faking offsets this and requires overt disfluency by the client.
- Role-play activities to simulate how the client can stutter and still cope with situations. Clinician-accompanied and -modeled activities to help the client start on what will become self-supervised assignments in the future.
- Stuttering targets, such as directing client to "keep entering situations until _____ (50, 75, 100, and so on) fakes are collected" or to produce a certain number of each of several types of spasms," and so on.
- Negative practice of various behaviors, such as to exaggerate and overuse a postponement device or, in reverse, duplicate real spasms with some typical component lacking, reduced, or altered.

CONTROL METHODS (Cancellation, Pullout, Preparatory Set)

- Use on an in-clinic basis to practice the various methods of spasm control. This can lead to further variations in real stuttering spasms, variations that will facilitate the effectiveness of controls.
- Out-clinic practice, in easy situations, where stuttering is usually rare.
- Use in early learning stages, usually in-clinic, by having a real spasm, immediately duplicating it with a fake, and then practicing a control on the fake.
- Use as a penalty. If the client fails to use a designated control method, or fails to use it properly, the same word or next word must be pseudostuttered and the control method used. Penalty also could be in the form, "Each time you _____ or fail to _____, there is a penalty of 5 fakes to be produced and you must _____ on each fake."

TRANSFER AND MAINTENANCE

- Psuedostuttering plans can be laid, behavioral contracts drawn up. For instance, "Each week you will produce at least _____ pseudostutterings for practice evaluation. If you fail to do this, then you cannot _____. If you are successful, the next week you can reduce the number of required fakes by 10 percent."
- Review assignments if the stutterer feels that control has started to slip, avoidance behaviors have reemerged, or feelings of anxiety have returned.

Clinician Pseudostuttering

There are few absolutes in this world, but it is true that pseudostuttering should not be used in therapy unless the clinician is competent in the skill. The author would go further and advise the reader that the clin-

ician should be willing to perform any pseudostuttering assignments he or she designs for the client and should actually do some of them. The client needs the emotional reinforcement (and pressure) of seeing the clinician do what the client is asked to do. Also, teaching a cognitive-mechanical skill is facilitated by live modeling. It should be understood that pseudo-stuttering is a real skill that requires hard work, practice, and intellect. The author always assigns students in fluency disorders class a project to use various associated behaviors (slowed rate, postponement, retrial, substitution, and so on) in everyday, otherwise normal, speech. Every report submitted contained variations of "It took so much planning . . ." "This really disrupted me while I talked . . ." "It was hard work!!!" It helps to understand, client and clinician, how much time and effort goes into even the simpler aspects of stuttering. A step-by-step procedure for learning to pseudostutter (Ham 1986) has been published, and variations in the format are introduced each year. At present the author uses the following sequence:

1. A series of five or six assignments covering evaluation of disfluencies in normal speakers, use of the associated behaviors (as described earlier), practice in retiming speech rate, analysis of real stuttering on audiotape, analysis of real stuttering on videotape.
2. Word, sentence, paragraph, conversation (with a partner) practice to learn simply repetition, prolongation, and stoppage patterns. Partners continue from this point on.
3. Repeat the previous step, but practice producing the three types of spasms at mild, moderate, and severe levels.
4. Varying severity levels, add prescribed associated behaviors.
5. Make designated number of telephone calls, selecting from an option list of stuttering patterns to fake.
6. Videotape speech while pseudostuttering. Samples will be played back in class for student practice in analysis and feedback to speakers.
7. Outside assignments, with partner, in stores, and so on.

Students find learning to pseudostutter challenging but not enjoyable. The author observed that even though he has taught many of the students in prior classes, instructor-student rapport noticeably reduced for several weeks. This is because the author as instructor is associated with the stress of the assignment. Klinger (1987) tested one aspect of the author's rationale by collecting data on 55 student clinicians assigned to learn pseudostuttering. The students' self-evaluations of their own inner and outer "beauty" was evaluated before and after pseudostuttering assignments. Pseudostuttering experiences were followed by significant downshifts in "beauty" self-concepts, with undergraduates showing a greater change than did graduate clinicians. If this fractional, brief experience can produce such strong reactions, one wonders at those who claim that FRT eliminates any need to be concerned about the attitudes, feelings, and communication adjustment of stutterers. Having the clinician learn to be a convincing, not a token, pseudostutterer is of great value, even if only to help the clinicians understand their client's behaviors and to appreciate the mechanical complexities of a well-integrated stuttering spasm and its associated behaviors.

Cancellation

The use of cancellation in therapy has been varied, partially due to how different clinicians define it. For purposes of further discussion, cancellation is described as follows:

> A *completed* stuttering spasm is followed by a *pause*, during which immediately preceding undesirable behaviors are *analyzed* and decisions made relative to eliminating or controlling these behaviors. From a *relaxed* state, the word is *repeated* so that the decisions are implemented.

The stutterer is not to interrupt or prematurely terminate a dysfluency, but carry it to completion. Any desire to continue talking or to escape is countered by a pause that lasts long enough for the stutterer to realize what was done during the spasm. It is then necessary to decide what behaviors should be eliminated completely, what can be retained in altered form, and what should be added in order to improve performance. Ensuring that relaxation and adequate breath support exist, the stutterer then repeats the word while applying the various decisions that were made; for example,

- **Spasm:** "Ruh-ruh-ruh-Richard." This spasm was repetitions with a schwa vowel, high tension, loss of eye contact, jaw tremor, rising loudness, and a nervous arm gesture.
- **Pause:** The analysis takes place, the planning occurs, inhalation and overt relaxation occur.
- **Cancellation:** "Rrrrrichard." An easy onset with prolongation and a quiet voice. Facial and arm muscles are relaxed, eye contact established with auditor, and the schwa vowel replaced by correct vowel.

Other cancellation modes could be used. The tense, jerky, schwa vowel repetition could have been turned into an easy, rhythmic, correctly articulated bounce. For various reasons, part (but not all) of the original spasm could have been canceled, a totally different pseudostuttering spasm could have been used, and so on. A more comprehensive view and discussion of cancellation (and pullouts and preparatory sets) has been published previously by the author (Ham 1986).

The rationale for use of cancellation is probably derived, although there is justification of it as an isolated technique. It is credited to Van Riper (1958a) in terms of its present place in the therapy sequence. Although often taught as the first major control method, its ultimate value (others will be cited) was as the last line of defense for failures of preparatory sets and/or pullouts to be used successfully. That is, the stutterer who failed to anticipate and control a stuttering spasm (preparatory set), or who failed to gain mastery of a stuttered word and convert the spasm into a controlled finish (pullout), had the opportunity to reestablish control and demonstrate it in an iterative production of the word. Aside from the practicality of cancellation in a symptom therapy triad, it also has validity based on Wischner's (1950, 1952) theory that stuttering is self-reinforcing. In this frame of reference, cancellation prevents the reward of relaxation and completion that follows stuttering. Research indicating that TO periods following dysfluency were greater among stutterers than among non-stutterers would tend to support this idea (Yonovitz, Shepherd & Garrett, 1977). Pause time aside, one can also speculate that being required to iterate a word and be disfluent again is punishment, which would place cancellation within the operant framework of behavioral modification.

Luper and Mulder (1964) regarded cancellation as "one of the most fundamental all-purpose tools in stuttering therapy" (p. 131), and it certainly can be found in several FRT therapies today. However, Luper and Mulder comment that cancellation per se is abnormal and cannot function as a total therapy. Their instructions for performance, learning steps, and evaluation points faithfully reflect traditional SMT methods. Ryan (1971, 1978) has utilized a form of cancellation as part of a programmed sequence of what he called traditional therapy. Shames and Egolf (1976) also used a type of cancellation, which will be described later in this chapter. Falck (1969) describes a variant use of cancellation in which, as accurately as possible, the stutterer recreates the initial aspects of the stuttering spasm, and then stops. At this point, pullout procedures are mixed into cancellation, and the word is to be finished with the equivalent of easy onset or relaxed production. As this can be accomplished, the stutterer turns to the re-creation of spasms and selects one spasm characteristic to alter. For example, eye contact might be improved. As one characteristic is returned to normalcy and controlled, another spasm facet is identified for change, and so on. Wingate (1984d) has recommended the use of cancellation as therapy progresses and fluency is expected. Instead, if stuttering occurs, "have the stutterer re-do the word, especially the site of the stutter, utilizing the principles he should know by this time" (p. 292).

If there is a traditional method of learning and using cancellation, the author has described it elsewhere (Ham 1986). The description covers six to eight pages for the technique itself, without variations and qualifications. In abbreviated form, the sequence is the following:

1. Mastery of self-analysis, ability to stop completely after a stutter, basic competence in various control disfluencies, basic competence in pseudostuttering.

2. Starting with word lists, and progressing to conversation, develop in-clinic skills in cancellation. Use a mixture of real spasms and fakes. Require variations in cancellation forms, moving toward a disfluency form that will be preferred for use in pullouts and preparatory sets.

3. Before step 2 is completed, begin transfer to outside situations. Clinician must model some of these and help with evaluation. Errors and failures must be dealt with. Considerable motivation and counseling may be required, and desensitization values can be extensive.

4. As other control methods are acquired, maintain some use of cancellation (if only as a penalty) so that it will not fall into disuse and be lost.

Flaws in learning cancellations, or using them, can occur, and the clinician needs to be alert in order to identify the problem or problems accurately. These problems might be any of the following:

1. Inadequate grounding in the preliminary skills cited earlier in 1 step. Failure by the clinician to pace progress adequately.

2. Attempts to cancel too quickly so that the word iteration is tense, hurried, and jerks back into a renewed spasm.

3. Inadequate cancellation in that all undesirable behaviors are not limited or eliminated.

4. Lack of motivation, rejection of the "double dysfluency" aspect of cancellation.

Cancellation is not an easy procedure to learn and use. A student answering a test question commented that cancellation "must be the castor oil of symptom therapy." It doubles the fluency disruption and stresses the speaker. After starting with a 100 percent use of cancellation, the author evolved to a yes-no decision state on its use and then altered to a yes-no-variable option pattern. Mild stutterers often do poorly with cancellation, and their brief spasms can be almost impossible to catch (to stop afterward) in the normal neuromotor speech timing rate. Age also is a related factor, with younger children usually showing less ability to perform, or profit from, cancellation. Some adolescents react too strongly to the perceived social penalties of cancellation. At times I have waited to bring cancellation in until after pullout skills have been acquired, at which time clients usually can perceive its values more clearly. How well a client should perform cancellations is variable with age of client, severity of spasms, situations, and uses of cancellation. Gregory (1968) has stated that it is difficult to use, and he is satisfied with a 50–70 percent cancellation rate on an in-clinic basis. If I use the model of a moderately severe to severe stutterer in Group III to adult age range, cancellation expectations might reflect those shown in Table 14–1. The lowered out-clinic percentages for mild and moderate spasms reflect reality, as well as the value of the cancellations. However, this does not imply that the stutterer is to be unaware of the uncanceled spasms.

TABLE 14–1.

SITUATION	SEVERITY OF SPASM AND PROFICIENCY EXPECTATION		
	MILD	MODERATE	SEVERE
In-Clinic			
All modes and, or situations	60%	85%	98%
Out-Clinic			
Favorable situations	20%	60%	90%
Moderate stress	40%	70%	95%
High stress	20%	50%	85%

Pullouts

The pullout technique can be, and often has been, used as an independent procedure in therapy, although here it is presented as the second step of the triad sequence. The label for the technique is credited to Van Riper (1958a), who stated that his therapy clients invented the term (1973), and he did not particularly like the label (1978). There have been efforts to change the name to "in-block correction" (SFA 12), but recent publications about therapy continue to use the original term.

Pullouts have been used in therapy far longer than the present label has existed. The basic procedure is for the stutterer to gain control of an involuntary stuttering spasm and to complete the stuttered word while in full control of the utterance. Completion may occur in one of three forms: normal or fluent production, controlled disfluent production, controlled continuation of the original spasm (in voluntary form). The controlled disfluency will be one of the forms, or a combination of them, currently popular in FRT programs. Where cancellations are a problem in motivation for many stutterers, pullouts are usually very attractive to them because they

1. Reduce the duration and severity of stuttering spasms.
2. Can be developed to occur sooner until over time pullout moves near to the initiation of the spasm.
3. Increase client self-confidence and feelings of efficacy in that they actually can control stuttering spasms.

There are some age limitations in pullouts, motivation notwithstanding. The age factor relates to the spasm characteristics and to client skills, so that effective application of pullouts generally requires the following:

1. Stuttering spasms of sufficient duration.
2. Awareness and spasm analysis skills by the client.

3. Ability to relax tensions, at least in the speech mechanism areas.
4. Skill in being able to produce various control disfluencies in a relaxed form.

Many Group I children will fall short on one or more of these factors, particularly if straight-line FRT procedures can produce effective results. However, a few preschoolers will present spasm patterns in which pullouts can function well. Application possibilities increase rapidly as we move through Group II and up into the adolescent group.

Luper and Mulder (1964) recommended using pullouts with children after they have demonstrated a thorough competence in cancellation. As with cancellation, their criteria and development stages follow familiar SMT lines and will not be repeated here. They devote considerable space to pullouts and provide a number of procedural and evaluation suggestions. Conture (1982) expresses the opinion that stuttering is a problem of sound production entry and release, with the latter being more significant (and operating during presumed fluent, as well as dysfluent, speech). He suggests that Van Riperian (1973) pullouts may be feasible, although there can be problems with undue prolongation and having the child understand transitional speech movements. Conture may use therapy analogies, where tense and strong grapheme formations are compared to easy, flowing initiation and completion of written letters. This author has used the same analogy and finds the old technique of simultaneous talking and writing can be useful. By starting with all continuant words, such as *sum, father,* and *fan,* and having the simultaneous verbal and graphic productions slightly slowed and exaggerated, the concepts usually become clear (if the child can write). Then stop-sound words can be added, and the functions of light contact, easy onset, and continuous movement applied. Other applications of pullouts in therapy will be discussed in the summary at the end of this chapter.

As with cancellation, the author has published a more comprehensive discussion of pullouts elsewhere (Ham 1986), but the basic procedures are not difficult to explain. It would be possible to say the following to a client:

> Now, from now on every time you stutter, I want you to try and slow the spasm down, relax your speech mechanism, and finish the word with a . . .

Some stutterers could take the minimal direction and with practice and modeling develop an adequate pullout capacity. However, broken into steps, a more comprehensive description of pullouts is useful:

1. The occurrence of a stuttering spasm is to signal an approach response in which the speaker analyzes what she or he is doing and how the auditor is responding.

2. Decisions are made in terms of what must be eliminated and changed in order to bring the spasm under control and cancel its negative characteristics.

3. During the first two steps, the stutterer is to start slowing down the rate of spasm utterance and reducing tension by relaxing the speech mechanism. When this is achieved, the stuttering will turn into faking as a slowed and relaxed version of the real spasm.

4. As the spasm becomes a fake, struggle activity disappears and elements such as lost eye contact, head jerks, and so on, are to be corrected or terminated.

5. The slowed, relaxed fake is to blend smoothly, without pause, into a completion of the word. Completion may be the faked real spasm or, preferably, through use of a control disfluency.

Completion with typical articulation patterns is not recommended; this author has seen too many clients jerk back into a stuttering spasm as monitoring reduced and/or habituated neuromotor trigger points along the vocal tract were stimulated.

Preparation for pullouts extends all the way back to motivation and awareness training where the stutterer practices "catching" stuttering spasms. Pullouts are of no use after a spasm has occurred. On an in-clinic basis, moving from single words up to conversation, criterion levels can be set on the basis of spasm severity as follows: severe = 90 percent, moderate = 60 percent, mild = 20 percent. One must be flexible. The low criterion for mild spasms is practical, since they do not last long enough for pullouts to occur, or if pullouts occur, they may be disfluent longer than the original spasm. A possible sequence could be followed in various speech modes as follows:

1. Use fakes to practice stopping during a spasm and then verbally analyzing type, location, tension points, and associated behaviors. Then shift to doing the same with real spasms.

2. Starting again with fakes, move from stop-go to stop-freeze where the stutterer stops but holds the articulators, for example, "frozen" in the posture of that moment. Hold for a few seconds and then slowly relax back into the spasm pattern, but with a slow and easy production. Shift to real spasms.

3. Again with initial fakes, practice slowing down the spasm and relaxing it until the fake sounds and looks fake. Then practice with real spasms.

4. Starting with fakes, follow step 3 but turn completion of the word into a control disfluency. Experiment with various forms and combinations. Check to see if the phoneme shift point from dysfluency to disfluency affects the control form used; for example, a vowel might pull out better with an easy-onset style, a stop plosive do better with a bounce, and so on.

5. Work to pullout sooner. At first, even in step 4, many pullouts will require more time than the original spasm would take. However, skill development progressively reduces the time until the first spasm tension can signal a pullout.

If cancellations have been taught to the client, it is useful to require that every missed pullout be followed immediately by a cancellation in which the original spasm is duplicated and a pullout performed. This can be softened by setting an initial criterion of "severe spasms only," without efforts to use the pullouts on mild spasms or all moderate spasms. As skill, and enthusiasm, develops the client can move into briefer spasms, the criterion levels depending on spasms and clients. That is, the author has had clients whose mild spasms were five to ten sec in duration, as well as other clients whose severe spasm was four seconds with a mild spasm that could not be timed by conventional devices.

Pullouts, like any technique, are subject to errors. This is particularly true because the client is literally in the middle of the things feared most, a stuttering spasm. Tension, anxiety, covert behaviors and avoidance devices, all these are maximal right around and in the spasm. Also, spasm patterns become as habituated as any other speech production pattern, and it can be difficult to break into them. Generally errors fall into one or more of the following categories:

1. Pullout is missed completely or occurs on the nonstuttered completion of the word.
2. Pullout occurs too quickly, without adequate analysis, planning, slowing, and relaxation. Rebounds into a renewed or continued stuttering spasm.
3. At the transition point from controlled spasm to control disfluency, the stutterer "jerks" and rebounds into a spasm.

A number of other errors can occur, plus individual variations. All can be addressed and dealt with, usually by backtracking to required basic skill areas.

Transfer of pullouts is critical because it is so important to many stutterers, offering a real opportunity to diminish and control stuttering for the first time. Clients should be warned against premature efforts to utilize pullouts. If they do anyway (and some will), success will greatly increase their self-confidence and foster independence from the clinician. Failure can be turned to therapy benefit and motivate better practice efforts; rarely does failure undermine faith in the technique. Faith in self will need more attention and careful consideration in transfer. Once the stutterer has reached basic skill levels, the clinician should combine role play, accompanied out-clinic assignments, and careful progress up the client's fear hierarchy. Pseudostuttering in all types of activities can be of assistance, and the clinician should provide frequent models on an in-clinic and out-clinic basis. Psychological support of the stutterer is important, and the client should have a problem-solving rather than a do-or-die approach as he or she works through the transfer process. Problems routinely will occur but should be amenable to resolution as long as the client's motivation (usually high) and self-confidence (often uncertain) are kept under control. Clients often experience a noticeable reduction in stuttering as transfer develops.

During transfer activity, in-clinic time can be spent on refining pull-out skills, resolving special needs such as specifically feared phonemes, words, and situations, and dealing with out-clinic problems or questions that arise during transfer. This also is the time when a particular problem, if it is going to occur at all, will start to surface. That problem is client fear of the results of fluency. As a generalization, it never occurs in Group I, rarely in Group II, and can occur in Group III. Fear of fluency is the realization that the loss or control of stuttering removes a valuable crutch or alibi for failure and nonperformance and thus eliminates the rationalization that allows one to avoid being fully responsible and socially interactive. The author feels this may be a possible element in at least some of the individuals who could fall under Cooper's (1987) description of the CPS syndrome (chronic perseverative stuttering syndrome). Clinicians need to be alert for the occasional fear-of-fluency pattern and be ready to deal with it or to prepare the groundwork for future counseling referral if and when the problem becomes major.

The preceding descriptions and steps have been targeted primarily at the Group III level of insight and capability. It is possible to simplify pullout procedures for use with younger children and to use pullout for various other purposes. However, it is a key aspect of symptom therapy and establishes the foundation for the next step, preparatory sets. Although it is possible to terminate and transfer a program at the pullout stage, and stutterers occasionally do this independently, pullouts are not usually structured as a final goal. When used properly and with skill, a stutterer's overall dysfluency can drop by as much as 90 percent, and auditors may prefer pullouts to fluency systems such as bounce and prolongation (Berlin & Berlin 1964). The fluency of well-done pullouts will more than equal the most effective FRT results that have achieved 0.5 SW/M or its equivalent.

Preparatory Sets

Speakers constantly use, or have, preparatory sets in posture, respiration, phonation, and articulation. Watch any speaker preparing to interrupt or jump into a discussion, and you will see speech structures postured for implementation. Preparatory sets are probably a reflection of cerebellar and basal ganglia activity occurring prior to initiation impulses from areas 4 and 6 of the cortex. As we mature from early childhood our commonly shared preparatory sets acquire characteristics that are individually unique and strongly habituated. This is part of the reason that in articulation therapy, it is easier to correct omissions than substitutions, and usually easier to replace substitutions than amend distortions. It is also part of the rationale supporting early intervention. These comments apply equally to stuttering and the development of abnormal preparatory sets. One can argue whether such sets are a cause or an effect (this author leans to the latter), but many stutterers can be observed to have preproduction distortions of articulatory sets, articulator muscle tremors before movement occurs, prephonation maladjustments of laryngeal muscle tension, and inappropriate respiratory preparation.

Fluency therapy actually is more or less continuous alteration of preparatory sets. By changing tension, rate, timing, rhythm, and so on, habituated set patterns are altered or destroyed and conscious voluntary speech production results. If limbic interference (anxiety fears) is dealt with, the speaker can shape fluent production into normal-sounding speech patterns and no longer stutter. If Jost's law does not intervene, or limbic factors reappear, relapse will not occur, and maintenance is a success. The same can occur in symptom therapy. However, the SMT target is, not all speech, but that portion of speech on which stuttering is anticipated.

By the time clients reach the preparatory set stage of therapy they have usually eliminated "all" associated behaviors, eliminated most of their avoidance behaviors, and reduced the overall frequency and severity of stuttering. They can cancel effectively and pull out almost immediately from nearly all severe, and most of the moderate, stuttering spasms. Self-confidence is usually high, and the stutterers talk much more than they did during pretreatment life. Preparatory sets are intended to extend and expand gains and to establish a final dysfluency that is acceptable to the client.

The procedure of preparatory sets involves the factor of spasm consistency and predictability, as well as early signals. Recall that previous chapters have covered consistency and predictability considerations (spasms tend to occur within the first three words of an utterance, and so on). Given these considerations, the self-analysis and other therapy activities of individual clients tend to increase predictability averages and accuracy. At the same time clients learn the "early warning signs" characteristic of their individual dysfluency patterns. Changes in rate, premonitory muscle tremors, autonomic changes, and so on, presage many stuttering spasms. These two general areas (predictability and signals) help stutterers minimize their need to use preparatory set control in shotgun or wholesale fashion. To this can be added behavioral predictability, where the specific stutterer has come to know what people, situation types, topics, emotional feelings, and so on, are most likely to precipitate stuttering.

Preparatory sets are associated with Van Riper (1937), although Freund (1966) claims to have formulated the concept in 1932. Actually, the basic procedure has probably a lineage measured in centuries. In symptom therapy they apparently were an early development, and pullouts then developed as a method to deal with spasms that were missed or where "prep sets" failed, just as cancellation can be used to compensate for missed or failed pullouts. Luper and Mulder (1964) wrote briefly of using prep sets with children, suggesting prolongation of initial vowels or consonants. Weiner's (1978) vowel-focus therapy is a variation of preparatory sets, and Ryan and Ryan (1983) and Shames (1978) have utilized aspects or versions of preparatory sets in therapy (see "Chapter Summary"). Falck (1969), unlike many clinicians, regards prep sets as a temporary technique to be learned in conjunction with relaxation therapy. The client is taught to produce a sound (vowel or consonant) that is not part of the target word and use this as a carrier to move into the word itself. Falck suggests that the technique be kept available "in case," but that it should not be used routinely on many words.

Implementation of prep sets is more individualized than previous techniques discussed, but basic steps might be the following:

1. Anticipate the occurrence of a spasm, based upon cues or factors discussed previously.
2. Slow speech utterance rate on the two or three words preceding the word on which stuttering is expected.
3. While slowing down, make sure that respiration is sufficient and rhythmic, and that vocal tract muscles are relaxed and not forming into habituated postures.
4. If feasible begin the altered preparatory set within the word immediately preceding the target word.
5. Use a preferred control disfluency, such as easy onset or bounce. The type used may vary with the phonological contexts of different words.
6. Move through the word with a slow, easy, controlled disfluency, extending it to the following word in decreasing degree until production returns to normal patterns.

The learning process is relatively simple on an in-clinic basis because of all the previous work on pullouts and cancellations. Pseudostuttering is not needed, but early practice in reading with target words underlined will help develop skills. Target words should have many different phonetic contexts, centering around "most likely" words on the basis discussed previously in this section. Out-clinic assignments should be frequent and extensive, as, for example, in the following:

1. In five speech situations, use a prep set each time you start a new utterance. Pull out on any real spasms.
2. Make ten telephone calls. In each call use at least three prep sets, each one with a different control disfluency. Cancel any real spasms.
3. Take a paragraph and underline 50 likely words in it. Read the passage aloud, using prep sets on the underlined words so that 10 are bounce, 10 are easy onset, light contact, prolongation, and strong movement.

Take the client on out-clinic assignments and emphasize finding out three things: which disfluency forms work best on what words, how prep sets need improvement, and what spasms are missed and why.

OTHER THERAPY APPROACHES

While cancellation, pullouts, and preparatory sets procedures are the core of SMT, they are still production techniques that depend upon self-analysis and desensitization to be practicable for use, transfer, and maintenance. There are, of course, other procedures that are important to symptom therapy, all of which have been included in various discussions in this and other chapters. These procedures are highlighted next.

Assignments

Many years ago the author, as a student, was told, "Never send a client home without some assignment to perform." With some flexibility, I have followed this dictum with all communication disorders. Assignments provide for practice, skill refinement, and habituation of new behaviors that have been learned. They favor improvement in the client's monitoring and evaluation skills. Self-evaluation and adaptation skills are enhanced, and the concept of consistent and expanding transfer becomes accepted. Finally, the client's feelings of responsibility and self-efficacy are increased with every assignment as the clinician strives to transform the client into being her or his own clinician.

Assignments should start with the very first session, be part of every session plan, and be designed as thoughtfully as the therapy session itself. The principle also applies to parent-counseling programs. Group I children can be given assignments—"Father will read you a bedtime story and then ask you some questions. You must answer him in your easy speaking voice"—just as older clients are given them. Whatever the main focus of therapy at a particular stage of therapy progress, relevant assignments can be made. As the therapy focus shifts, continued development of the preceding step can be managed primarily through assignments. Literally anything can be subject for assignments: autobiography, observation, tolerance, practice on skills, and so on.

In the squeeze of time pressure or the confines of package programs, or for other reasons, assignments can be misused. At best they may become busy work and be boring for the client. At worst they can cause client alienation, create failures, hinder transfer, and prevent or erode the development of client self-confidence. An assignment should be relevant, cover areas or abilities in which the clinician feels the client has displayed competence in on an in-clinic basis, and be planned so that the probability of success greatly outweighs that of failure. For Group II and

Group III children, the author prefers assignments that give the stutterer a choice in the level of difficulty. Thus, for example, the following might be used with them:

- Collect 20 pullouts by next therapy session (elect one):
  a. Conversations with family or friends.
  b. Telephone calls to friends.
  c. Telephone calls to businesses.
  d. Conversations with strangers.
- Establish good eye contact each time you stutter (elect one):
  a. With a girl or boy in English class.
  b. After class, asking teacher about something.
  c. In class, volunteering to answer a question.

The assignment must be of such type that the client can be aware of and evaluate results, and a report (written or verbal) should always be requested. Principles of reinforcement and penalty for success and failure are to be established and observed. Periodically, structure solo assignments that can be replicated during a clinic session so that client reliability can be checked (teacher, parent, and so on; reports also can be solicited).

Occasionally, assignments are punishing, and this can happen through the clinician's inattentiveness or failure to accurately empathize with the client. This author has found it valuable to have the client regularly design an assignment for the clinician to perform, pseudostuttering if necessary. The only caution issued to the client is, "Think carefully and be fair because, after I finish, I may turn right around and ask you to do the same." As therapy progresses, clients can be encouraged to take over assignment planning, under supervision, progressing to semiindependence in transfer work, and to total independence as maintenance develops.

Monitoring

Monitoring has been cited frequently in previous sections, and there will be further discussion in the final chapter on transfer and maintenance. Yet monitoring needs to be considered briefly here in terms of symptom therapy, since monitoring is stressed in every phase of therapy and is one of the major keys to the self-therapy goal. In appropriately adjusted demand levels, it can be applied to any client regardless of age. As the maturity level goes up, the definition of *monitoring* expands. In its most complete sense, monitoring will include the following:

1. Physical tension and respiratory patterns.
2. Overall speech rate and production characteristics.
3. Presence of, or warning signs of, dysfluency.

4. Use and efficacy of control procedures.
5. Influence variables of particular situations and ongoing reactions of auditors.
6. Personal feelings of the client, and strength of autonomic and skeletal accompaniments of those feelings.

Speech Improvement

Many fluency reinforcement programs include a step of improving overall speech production. Although this subject will be discussed in the next chapter, it must be mentioned here as part of symptom therapy. As clients progress to preparatory sets, they usually need general improvement as communicators. Specific inadequacies of voice, resonance, articulation, and expression may have coexisted with stuttering and/or hung around as residual traces of associated behaviors and avoidance behaviors. This is particularly true with Group III stutterers, while those in Groups I and II are more likely to have coexisting speech and language problems (Blood & Seider 1981).

Counseling

This text has devoted space to attitude, feelings, and counseling activities to be applied in any therapy mode. Symptom modification places special stress on the interactive relationship between client and clinician, in addition to the psychological abilities of the client. Counseling needs increase as the client grapples with facing stuttering, tolerating it, and accepting responsibility for its management. Self-analysis and desensitization are, in and of themselves, counseling-oriented stages of therapy. Subsequent steps from cancellation to final maintenance involve the psychic growth of an individual from dependence to communication maturity, and counseling is required. To simply teach symptom control, or to only provide fluency methods, without psychological support is to contravene essential tenets of learning psychology and to ignore the needs of human beings who have placed trust in us.

TRANSFER AND MAINTENANCE

Transfer has been stressed throughout this chapter on SMT as something to be nurtured and specifically planned for. Spontaneous generalization is never assumed! Maintenance is also planned for if therapy is properly developed. In SMT philosophy the stutterer is dismissed as what she or he was at the onset of therapy—a stutterer. Overt dysfluency that remains may be better, or worse, than the residual stuttering from FRT programs. Further, the speech fluency may be better, and sound more normal, than the "fluency" of fluency reinforcement therapy. The important factor in both models of therapy will be long-term stability and continued improvement. For this reason, further discussion of maintenance occurs in the final chapter.

CHAPTER SUMMARY

This chapter has attempted, in a relatively short space, to capture the essentials of symptom modification therapy. Certainly not all aspects of symptom therapy have been covered here, but an attempt has been made to set up a format structure in which to display therapy methods. One must keep in mind, however, that other clinicians would likely structure or arrange SMT in different ways. Shames (1978), for example, presented a rapid version of cancellation, pullout, and preparatory sets. Cancellation is covered in the first two steps. First, the client must learn to stop after every stuttered word and then repeat the word. When this is done adequately, the word is to be repeated with prolongation of the initial sound. In the third step the stutterer is to stop during, not after, the spasm and say the word again, prolonging the initial sound. The fourth step involves prolonging the initial step at the time of spasm onset and then working to reduce the duration of the prolongation. As an example of operant procedures applied to SMT, Shame's approach is disappointing. This version also can be found in earlier publication by the SFA (1970), and the presentation is similarly disappointing. Shames subsequently modified the four-step core program into a ten-step program (Shames & Egolf 1976). A baseline is established, and the client works to a point where a stuttered word is repeated, with the first syllable bounced on three times before utterance. The next step duplicates the previous one, except that the client must keep saying the word over again (and bouncing three times) until it is said fluently (or disfluently). From this level, the client moves to securing bounce fluency on the first reutterance, remaining in this step for two cycles. The client then is to shift the three-bounce pattern to initiation of the stuttered word itself. When fluent completion is mastered, the step is repeated with a two-bounce initiation, then with one bounce, and finally merges into fluent speech without bouncing. In the last stage, dysfluencies are punished, while all previous stages provide reinforcement only for successful utterances.

The foregoing description is not the only way in which SMT has been applied. The Ryans (1983, 1974) have described a "PT," or programmed traditional, therapy sequence. This program provided three identification, or analysis, steps, two cancellation steps, a step dealing with pullouts, one prolongation step, and one fluent speech step. These 8 steps were to be repeated across the speech modes of reading, monologue, and conversation, for a total of 111 steps. In one source (1978) Ryan describes one (not two) cancellation steps and moves from there directly to prolongation (preparatory sets?), since prolongation is also included as part of cancellation. Other variations are described in a second-case illustration. As described in various sources, it appears that the therapy procedures were "programmed," but their "traditional" nature leaves the author in some confusion. Basic concepts or structures were present, but the applications, variations, and step-by-step aspects of transfer were not present or were not clear. This does not necessarily question the efficacy of Ryan's program and certainly does not object to putting particular therapy methods into operant structures. However, there is that recurrent question of what "traditional therapy" really is. The author has taken the cancellation, pullout, and preparatory set sequence that was described earlier in this chapter and wound up with about 50, not 8, steps. Which approach is right, or best, or most traditional, is arguable, and will be forever.

Symptom and fluency therapy have totally different targets, stuttered moments and fluent moments. Outcomes of therapy may be described either as 5 percent dysfluent or as 95 percent fluent. Both systems use most of the same fluency and dysfluency control methods, which existed before SMT and FRT had formal recognition. I do not suggest that the differences between the two systems are apparent rather than real. I have noted that fluency approaches seem to be most appropriate for Group I children and through the early ages of Group II. With children over about nine or ten years of age, it may well be that the clinician needs to elect a therapy philosophy that fits the client best. Within the elected philosophy there is a range of procedures that can be structured to build the most effective therapy program. If it is inappropriate to apply FRT to every child who stutters, then it is equally inappropriate to argue that SMT is the only route to communication effectiveness. Cooper (1987) argues that at least 40 percent of adolescent and adult stutterers are chronic perseverative stutterers (CPS syndrome) and, therefore, incurable. Such a contention has surface validity but requires further delineation and, most of all, explanation. Until that time, it seems best to state that SMT will be the best form of therapy for certain children who stutter, that FRT will apply best to others, and that a willingness to combine and borrow from both will provide the most effective results for those stutterers who do not fit one therapy pattern or the other.

CHAPTER FIFTEEN
OTHER THERAPY CONSIDERATIONS

OVERVIEW

In any text there are topics that are difficult to fit into a particular chapter in terms of its theme though the author wants to include them. This chapter collects four such topics—areas that are important but have not seemed to fit other chapters. The first topic is response-contingent stimulation (RCS), or *punishment*. Punishment has been misunderstood, misapplied at times, and certainly debated intensely. This topic is followed by a discussion of the values and problems of using *group therapy* with stutterers, which needs to be addressed because the prospect of working with a group of stutterers may be quite daunting to many clinicians. The third topic area considers briefly the therapy areas of *hypnosis* and *drug treatment*, the latter having particular applications to the neurophysiological subgroups of stutterers. This concern leads to the fourth topic, *cluttering*, and some comments from the author about our classification or labeling systems in stuttering.

PUNISHMENT

Punishment receives separate attention because of its popularity, the confusion surrounding it, and the polarization over its use among certain clinicians. Punishment has been associated with operant or behavior modification therapy, and some have condemned it as an unwarranted cruelty and/or as a mislabeled procedure. At this point it is important to note that punishment per se is not an operant technique. It can be used operantly, but its association with structured behavioral modification techniques has been due to its scheduling and to its advertisement in therapy literature. The term *punishment,* as Costello (1983, p. 76) remarked, is unfortunate because of its connotations of anger, pain, and other negative feelings. Actually, punishment is a response-contingent event that tends to interrupt or depresses response (Shames & Egolf 1976, p. 24). By this reasoning, any event, utterance, facial expression, and so on, that is used contingent to a response and interrupts, alters, or reduces that response is punishment. Sheehan (1968) inveighed against the use of punishment, stating:

> Therapists who use punishment are probably incompetent to use anything else, or they have a neurotic need to assume the role of the punisher. (p. 132)

It appears that Sheehan applied the Costello-lamented definition of punishment (pain and suffering), and it must be admitted that some clinicians have used such punishment forms. In the general therapy scene, however, RCS has been applied in the broader sense of the definition supplied here. In the debates that have occurred over the use of punishment, preoccupation with implied pain and suffering of clients has not facilitated the exchange of views and the interpretation of data.

Basically, punishment occurs when a response is followed immediately by an aversive stimulus that is intended to reduce or eliminate the future occurrence of that response under similar conditions (Mowrer 1977). It has been proposed by Holz & Azrin (1966) that a "punishing stimulus" should have certain features, namely, precise physiological specificiation, uniform constancy of application, control of opportunity for the recipient to escape the stimulus by an elective change in behavior, minimal physical responses that might mask or confuse the behavioral responses, and a variable aversive stimulus that can range from complete response reduction to one of no effect. Williams and Martin (1974) questioned some of the foregoing stipulations, using electroshock as the aversive stimulus. They concluded that punishment may not need to be both contingent and temporally contiguous in order to be effective, and that rewarding and neutral stimuli also may reduce stuttering. They very likely were pointing to what Shames and Egolf highlighted, the confusion between *suppression* and *punishment*. Further, one may question whether the punishment element is as important as the punishment effect. That is, an electroshock hurts and, in addition to any other effect, does punish the person; whereas, a loud "stop" may create the punishment effect of stopping the ongoing speech effort of the communicator. In stuttering, aversive stimuli have clustered around intense auditory stimulus (noise), aversion-relief (electrical shock), TO or time-out (enforced silence, isolation, and so on), verbal aversive stimuli (for example, "wrong"), and response cost (usually, subtraction of secondary reinforcers).

Noise and electrical shock have had some attraction in therapy in that their strengths and durations can be controlled with some precision. They often do not result in complete reduction of the response, may require expensive equipment and technical skill to utilize, raise questions of liability concerning possible injury to the client, and could result in the client suggesting the clinician try sitting there and being deafened or subclinically electrocuted as the client leaves! Verbal punishment has been found to reduce stuttering, but Cooper, Cady, and Robbins (1970) found that positive, negative, and neutral words (*right, wrong, tree*), all, resulted in stuttering reduction. This creates the question of whether or not any verbal interjection is a "punishing" interruption, that is, a distraction or a break in the motor speech planning process. Time-out has been used frequently (Costello 1983; Martin, Kuhl & Haroldson 1972; Curlee & Perkins 1969; Haroldson, Martin & Starr 1968), and so it will be discussed separately.

Flanagan, Goldiamond, and Azrin (1958) are remembered for their use of punishment in therapy of stuttering, and other punishment studies have been published (Biggs & Sheehan 1969; Martin & Siegel 1966b; Siegel & Martin 1967). Other clinicians have combined reward and punishment (Moore & Ritterman 1973; Egolf, Shames & Blind 1971). Fiedler and Standop (1983) find punishment, as a therapy program or method, to be of limited value because restoration or recovery of the punished response (stuttering) occurs with regularity. However, that does not eliminate its use as an auxiliary procedure accompanying other methods. Nittrouer and Cheney (1984) reviewed punishment use in operant procedures, including most of those cited previously, as well as research by other clinicians (Daly & Cooper 1967; Reed & Lingwall 1980; Siegel, Lenska & Broen 1969). They concluded that punishment was effective in decreasing stuttering, thus disagreeing with Daly and Kimbarow (1978). The latter used the words *right, wrong,* and *tree* as contingent responses to stuttering and found that all three reduced stuttering. Nittrouer and Cheney argued that *interruption,* not the semantic content of words, was the punisher, that is, whatever results in the reduction of a response is, *ipso facto,* a punishment. Other clinicians have tended to turn to the interruption factor and favor its use. Ingham (1984) presents the most lengthy and complete review of RCS principles in stuttering, devoting about 60 pages in a major discussion of the general topic, and then going over specific areas again in other sections of his book. (The reader interested in the topic is referred to this source.) Ingham does not hesitate to criticize methodological shortcomings of punishment studies and provides a balanced evaluation of those who have been critical of RCS applications. He comments that good therapy and bad therapy practices can occur in any philosophy, and that compassion for and sensitivity to client needs are not the unique characteristic of any one approach and missing from all other approaches.

TIME-OUT

Background

Shames (1975) stated that the effectiveness of contingent aversive stimuli (punishment) depends on the promptness of its presentation, its duration and intensity, the degree to which it stands out or draws attention, the frequency and variability of its occurrence, the availability of alternative responses with which to avoid punishment, and the client's previous response history to punishment. Siegel and Martin (1965b, 1966, 1967, 1968) would add consistency to the value factor. Stimuli do not have to be explicitly aversive, and Siegel (1970) has concluded that any event that brings dysfluencies up to attention will decrease their frequency of occurrence. The use of time-out procedures, or TO, has fitted quite well into the criteria cited and usually avoids the onus of tormenting the stutterer.

Time out has existed for centuries but received attention only recently as a variable with aversive values in a therapy reinforcement schedule (Leitenberg 1965). Haroldson, Martin, and Starr (1968) seem to have generated the first published TO study in stuttering, but many other studies have followed (Martin & Haroldson 1969a; Adams & Popelka 1971; Egolf, Shames & Seltzer 1971; Rustin 1978). The use of TO, in various forms, is simple. When a speaker stutters, he or she is required to stop speaking for a measured period of time before resuming speech. The signal to stop can be quiet and neutral, a loud "stop," a buzzer or other sound, flashing lights, and so on. Anything is possible, and the clinician may or may not use vocal and/or facial expressions to strengthen the signal. Where situations allow, the clinician can physically turn away (Costello 1980), the client can be required to turn away (Rustin 1978), or other behaviors can be performed. Curlee and Perkins (1969) had the therapy room lights turned off during the TO period. Length of TO can be set at any particular duration, but it typically has ranged from 5 to 30 seconds.

Review of Studies

The initial study referred to in the previous section (Haroldson, Martin & Starr 1968) involved four stutterers who received a balanced, rotated therapy design that encompassed non-TO and TO procedures. The TO procedure was a red light signaling the client to stop until it turned off (after ten seconds). Results suggested the efficacy of TO use. In a subsequent comparison over a period of eight sessions, Martin and Haroldson (1969a) matched TO against "information attitude" therapy. Among the ten counseling clients eight sessions failed to alter significantly either attitudes or stuttering. Unfortunately, the TO group (who also did not change attitudes) lost the extinction or reduction values on stuttering after the eight sessions, for their stuttering returned. Martin, Kuhl, and Haroldson (1972) extended TO application (at that time) to Group I children, reporting on two clients. A talking puppet was used to conduct therapy. When each client stuttered, the puppet stopped verbalization and dropped out of sight for ten seconds. The authors reported an outcome of zero stuttering on an in-clinic basis and a fairly consistent fluency during follow-up evaluations.

Yonovitz, Shepherd, & Garrett (1977) reported that stutterers tend to relax during the initial time period of a 30-second TO, becoming more anxious toward the end of the TO period. This recalls previous discussion about how the effects of SMT cancellation procedures deny the self-reinforcement of stuttering spasms (Wischner 1952). This question of a critical time factor in TO was approached by James (1976) when he divided 45 stutterers among a control group and four TO periods of 1, 5, 10, and 30 seconds. As expected, TO measures in terms of %SW were significantly less than those in the control group. Intra-TO differences were not significant, but each increase in TO duration was accompanied by a greater reduction in the %SW average. Rustin (1978) has used TO in group therapy, whereby a stuttering spasm exacts the penalty of one minute of silence by the speaker while he or she turns away from the group. Rustin does not recommend TO for children who generally have high anxiety over speaking because, she feels, the pressure of TO is likely to cause further deterioration in speech.

Other studies include those by Martin and Haroldson (1979), who compared TO and four other procedures (masking, DAF, metronome, "wrong" punishment) in terms of effects on stuttering percentages and spasm durations. The TO condition was slightly more effective (76 percent) than was use of the metronome (75 percent) in reducing spasm frequency, but it was more effective (at 74 percent and 46 percent) in reducing spasm duration. Costello (1980, 1975) has described a very structured TO procedure in which the client talks until a stable baseline is established. After that point, TO is introduced and consists of "stop" followed by ten seconds of silence with the clinician's head turned away from the client. The final 10 minutes of the session is a reward period in which stutterings are not penalized. Each session starts with 15 minutes of baseline monologue, followed by TO therapy, and ends with the reversal period. Costello reported that at first the reversal period was accompanied by a return-to-baseline resurgence of stuttering. But by the sixth session fluency began to stabilize, and the client was instructed to increase self-monitoring and fluency efforts. As improvement continued, duration of the reversal phase increased as TO therapy decreased. In an evaluation of client control of TO, James (1983) reported that adolescent and adult stutterers displayed significant improvements under a TO program, even when the TO was self-initiated and when clients set the TO duration themselves. However, the clients typically selected brief duration times, and were significantly less reliable in applying the procedure.

Other Applications

The previous discussion indicates some of the ways in which TO has been used. Many other applications are possible, and it can be combined with other reinforcement schedules. The stimulus form and TO duration can be adjusted for the age of the client, and it can be suspended or revised during therapy progress. Equipment can be used, but is not necessary, and training of the clinician is minimal. Not all clients will respond favorably to TO; some find it too punitive, some find it amusing, and a few will be angered by it. The author has found the fewest TO problems among Group I children (although one child dove under the table as each TO occurred), and the main problem has been overreaction and anxiety in the child. Group II children generally respond well, with "the giggles" being the most common problem (especially in group therapy). The most frequent problems observed by the author were with Group III adolescents, with more expressions of anger, feelings of being ridiculed or treated as a child, and elevations in anxiety. Yet the author has also observed TO, or used it, as an effective procedure with all age groups. Nittrouer and Cheney (1984), in their review of time-out methodologies and other operant methods, suggest that because of the possibilities of spontaneous generalization, these methods should be the first choice in planning therapy with children.

CLUTTERING

Background

If stuttering could be said to have a poor or neglected relative, cluttering would be nominated. Despite European interest and a surprisingly large number and range of publications, many U.S. clinicians are uninformed about cluttering. Daly (1986) has stated that, in this country people

> have not, by and large, accepted cluttering as a clinical entity, nor have they incorporated information about cluttering into their decision-making process. (p. 156)

He reports that many major sources on communication disorders in general, and on stuttering in particular, give only cursory attention to cluttering, while some ignore it completely. Daly has stated that cluttering prevalence estimates may equal that of stuttering, or it be more involved with stuttering than many realize. However, he reported that his records of fluency assessments over a period of about ten years disclosed fewer than 5 percent pure clutterers, with about 55 percent pure stutterers and 40 percent who displayed mixed stutter-clutter symptoms. This distribution would approximate that reported by Dalton and Hardcastle (1977).

Description

Definition of cluttering is more nebulous and varied than is our own present state with stuttering or fluency (see Chapter 1). It presents itself as a fluency disorder, with tachylalia (excessive rate) as an outstanding and consistent symptom. Repetitions, usually of larger units, are often seen, and there may be prolongations and struggle. However, more so than in what we tend to label as stuttering, in cluttering various clinicians have reported articulatory problems and language inadequacies. As will be seen subsequently, many other behaviors have also been suggested. Complications are added further when stuttering behavioral components are added. Although a number of literature sources on cluttering list reduced or absent awareness as part of the clutterer syndrome, environmental and learning factors appear to operate also, so that we can have stutter-clutterer and clutter-stutterer syndromes, depending on the predominance of symptoms.

Diedrich (1984) has nominated five factors that may help establish the existence of cluttering. These factors include the age of occurrence (early), problems in language formulation, the presence of other speech production problems, lack of awareness by the speaker, and an hereditary

or familial pattern of occurrence. Unfortunately, every one of these factors can occur among stutterers, singly, in combinations, or totally. St.
Louis and Hinzman (1986) reviewed six literature sources covering
1964–86 and listed 65 symptoms supposedly characterizing cluttering. Of
the characteristics, 46 appear in Weiss's (1964) writing; and of those, 15
occur only in that source. Overall, only 4 of the 65 characteristics appear
in four or more of the six sources. If we drop to a 50 percent (3 or more)
criterion, we find the following characteristics:

Tachylalia (rapid rate)	Language delay
Precedes stuttering	Grammatical errors
Prosodic monotony	Lack of awareness
Articulation errors	Reading and writing disorders
Poor handwriting	Family history
Short auditory attention	Hyperactivity

St. Louis and Hinzman were struck by what they felt was a similarity between the scattered array of cluttering symptoms and those associated
with specific learning disabilities. Perkins (1980a) implied a similar back-
ground-disorder complex in postulating a "central language imbalance"
with other associated problems. St. Louis and Hinzman asked 156 speech
and language clinicians to rate symptoms they felt were essential for a
cluttering diagnosis, and also to rate symptoms they felt were optional
(possibly present). The median-plus (50 percent or more) responses included tachylalia, run-on sentences, disorganized thinking, irregular
speech rate, lack of awareness, and repetitions of phrases, words, and
sounds and syllables. Median-plus responses on optional features included misarticulations, neurological problems, family history, language
delay, motor coordination problems, and academic difficulties.

   Just as we have been presented with growing evidence of genetic
and familial influences in stuttering, we see that cluttering has consistently
received similar observations. Writers have noted a genetic and familial
pattern in cluttering (Weiss 1964; Luchsinger & Arnold 1965; Daly 1986),
and Op'thof and Uys (1974) have suggested that cluttering follows a dom-
inant-gene inheritance pattern. Roman (1963), orienting around a con-
genital dyspraxic concept, suggested that cluttering tends to include
graphic handwriting skills as well, a characteristic also noted in several
other sources. Wolk (1986), reporting on a single-case study of an adult
clutterer, stated that EEG evaluation identified a lesion in the left fron-
totemporal area of the cortex; in addition the client's mother and brother
also presented clutter symptoms. Results of a dichotic listening task suggested a problem in auditory processing, possibly in the area of place perception. These various studies reinforce the concept of a central neurological disorder with variable symptoms. If one would establish a fluency

disorders continuum, it might be quite feasible to see stuttering and cluttering on the same continuum. Some (Weiss 1964, for example) have suggested a central-language-imbalance core (as a submerged iceberg analogy) with variable peaks of language dysfunction, reading and writing problems, behavioral anomalies in attending and responding, cluttering, and so on. Some possible revisions of, or additions to, this model would provide for stuttering, for mixtures of stuttering and cluttering, and still allow for the full impact of environmental psychosocial interaction effects.

Comparisons with Stuttering

Separation of cluttering and stuttering can present problems at times. From formulations developed in 1934, Freund (1966) summarized differences he felt separated stutterers and clutterers: Clutterers are supposed to have little or no awareness of their dysfluency, as opposed to awareness by stutterers. However, when the clutterer pays attention to his or her speech, it is supposed to improve, while the stutterer's dysfluency worsens. Similarly, strangers aggravate stuttering dysfluency, whereas they improve the fluency of clutterers. The stutterers are supposed to have more trouble when asked to repeat or to speak in short sentences, whereas clutterers improve under such conditions. The consistency of these various effects can be questioned, but data are lacking to settle the questions. Langova and Moravek (1964) compared stutterers, clutterers, and stutterer-clutterers on several factors. In electroencephalographic studies, clutterers displayed abnormal records in 50 percent of the cases, the mixed group in 39 percent, and the stutterers in 15–16 percent. They also reported that in using delayed auditory feedback, 92 percent of the stutterers improved, only 23 percent of the mixed group improved, and 85 percent of the clutterers worsened in terms of errors, repetitions, and monotone speech patterns. Reports of DAF effects on clutterering have varied, and, indeed, the author has seen it affect them in different ways and to be of variable value in therapy with them (see later). Rieber, Breskin, and Jaffe (1972) compared stutterers and clutterers in on-off speech time patterns and reported that stutterers tend to have longer average pause times and lower average phonation time scores. This would be in agreement with the overall rapid speech rate reported for clutterers.

St. Louis, Hinzman, and Hull (1985) attempted to establish criteria delineating clutterers, stutterers, and normal (control) speakers. Evaluating spontaneous speech samples, they reported that clutterers were generally lower on language measures than were the other two groups, especially with reference to complexity and completeness of utterances. As expected, the controls were more fluent, and the other two groups were marked by phrase and word repetitions. However, compared to stutterers, the clutterers were much lower in occurrence of sound and syllable repetitions, sound prolongations, and the presence of struggle. Weiss (1967) has summarized, in table form, about 20 comparative differences between stutterers and clutterers. The summary is a mixture of empirical and designed research results, and a few items are debatable; for example, stutterers' school performance is described as "good to superior" while clutterers are "underachievers." At the present time there is no clear delineation on all aspects of difference between the two groups, and often clinicians rely upon cumulative impressions to develop a diagnosis of cluttering. This means that some "stutterers" who have performance and behavior patterns that differ somewhat from those a clinician usually expects may be clutterers or stutter-clutterers. Similar occurrences might explain why some "stutterers" fail to respond to particular therapy techniques in a familiar pattern. For instance, Daly (1986) recounted several instances of clutterer clients who not only were quite poor at self-monitoring but resisted monitoring and blamed unfriendly or perfectionistic auditors for labeling them speech disordered.

Assessment

Diagnosis and assessment of cluttering has not been organized into a particular structure, much less into formal approaches such as the Riley SSI (Stuttering Severity Instrument). This is reflective of the attention given to cluttering in training institutions and the overall lack of an agreed-upon description or summation of the characteristics that signify or suggest the presence of cluttering. The material from Chapter 4 can be combined with the following information to provide suggestions for identification and evaluation. From the clutterers seen over the years, and sources such as Weiss (1967, 1964), Luchsinger and Arnold (1965), and Daly (1986), the author offers the following suggestions as aids in identifying and assessing cluttering in fluency evaluations.

History and interview   Pay particular attention to family histories of stuttering, speech and/or language problems, rapid rate, sloppy speech, or any other reported communication disorders. Information about neuromotor problems, in general, among family members and in the family history may be useful. With regard to the client, close attention to early developmental history is wise, along with greater attention to items such as hyperactivity, distractibility and attention span problems, sleep disturbance patterns, enuresis, behavioral problems, learning disabilities, and so on. In particular, the development of the fluency problem should be turned over and over to elicit recall of origin and pattern of development. Probe the awareness and memories of the clients and any other informants, to compare similarities and differences among items reported. If age-appropriate, interview about reading, writing, and school experiences. Some of the foregoing will be picked up by most standard interview procedures. However, after observing or eliciting some clutter be-haviors in a client, this author has had to return to parents or other informants in order to re-cover certain areas more thoroughly.

Physiological factors In respiration (vegetative and speech) watch for disrhythmic patterns of irregular, poorly timed breathing cycles. While examining the speech production mechanism, observe to see if there are inconsistent, groping movements often found among dyspraxics, or if there are dysarthric characteristics. With the child's eyes closed, check for tactile sensitivity to touch on areas of the lips and tongue, and check for kinesthetic awareness as the client is directed to move articulators into dif-ferent postures and positions. Diadochokinesis should be evaluated with reference to the stimuli and time-rate factors presented earlier in this text. Evaluate rhythmokinesis, ability to imitate rhythm patterns, and ca-pacities in repeating various timing and stress patterns. Throughout the evaluation, observe overall motor coordination in gait, posture, and skilled movements. Check laterality (eye, hand, foot), observe for festinat-ing gait or movements, and watch for signs of tremor, perseveration, and motor overflow.

Behavioral Hyperactivity, perseveration, distractibility, and other as-pects have already been mentioned. Behavioral patterns of unawareness, resistance to awareness requests, and denial or minimization of any prob-lems may occur.

Speech and language Employ a thorough language assessment, be-ginning with attending, perceptual, and auditory processing skills. Be sure that expressive and receptive function areas are evaluated, and that spontaneous speech is recorded and analyzed for aspects of utterance length, complexity, completeness, and grammatic-syntactic adequacy. A thorough, painstaking articulation assessment will be needed. As errors occur, review them carefully to determine why they were errors, check for place and feature factors, and always retest several times for consistency. Determine length factor effects by sequences such as

fund   fundament   fundamental   fundamentally
sum   summer   summary   summarizing

Check stimulability and error correction, watch for dyspraxic and dysarthric patterns, and compare carefully spontaneous speech to con-trolled test utterances.

Fluency Presumably the usual measures and evaluations of stutter-ing (see Chapters 3 and 4) will be applied and need not be repeated here.

In analyzing dysfluencies, watch for phrase and word repetitions predominating over syllable and sound ones, and for departures from the usual loci for disruptions to occur. At times repeated readings for adaptation-consistency measures will actually show a negative adaptation, with dysfluencies increasing on successive readings. If equipment is available, check to see if amplified NAF decreases dysfluencies and whether DAF appears to increase or decrease stuttering. Client ability to follow metronome or other syllable-timed cadences should be evaluated, along with their effects on fluency. Without instrumental aid, instruct and practice the client in self-monitoring, observing effects on speech and the client's ability to do the self-monitoring.

Therapy of Cluttering

Therapy of cluttering, as might be expected, is not presented well in our literature. In their survey of speech and language clinicians, St. Louis and Hinzman (1986) reported that about 60 percent of those working in school systems felt inadequately prepared, usually by their university training programs, to work with clutterers. On the other hand, of the speech and language professionals in teaching and research positions, nearly 80 percent felt adequately prepared to deal with cluttering. This disparity is too great to tolerate, particularly in view of possible cluttering prevalence in preschool and school settings. The literature on cluttering presents little in the way of an original program of therapy for cluttering. The author has not worked with so many clutterers that he is prepared to state exactly what such a program must involve. However, basic suggestions will be offered, to be amended on a client-to-client basis. The reader is also referred to Froeschels (1946), Weiss (1964, 1960), Bradford (1963), Luchsinger and Arnold (1965), and Daly (1986) for discussion and suggestions.

General approaches   To the extent needed, secure assistance for problems in reading, writing, and other education areas; medical attention may be needed for organic syndromes; counseling may be useful for behavioral problems; proper educational placement is important. Where outside resources are pooled, make every effort to maintain contact and collaborate with the other professionals.

Stage 1   Deal with any foundation problems in attending, responding to perceptual cues, auditory processing, auditory recall, retrieval, and so on. Luchsinger and Arnold (1965) have suggested direct borrowing of dysphasia therapy techniques where they will help foundation efforts. One wonders whether melodic intonation therapy (MIT) procedures would be an aid or an interference with its components of rhythm, stress, and melody. Basic language skills should be worked on, and many of the language-development programs can be utilized, in whole or parts. On a simple basis, the ELU approach discussed earlier in this text can be used and combined with various procedures cited in the next stage.

Stage 2   The most appropriate therapy approaches for cluttering dysfluency are usually those having a rate control core. The author has used syllable-timed speech, metronome sequences, and DAF therapy. Daly (1986) has commented on the value of Shames and Florance's (1980) stutter-free speech DAF approach, especially because of its structure and monitoring provisions. Monitoring usually requires a great deal of stress, regardless of the fluency program. Ability to monitor often needs more practice than with stutterers, and motivation or willingness to monitor can be a problem requiring attention. Overall, fluency therapy seems to require more structuring, and it is more often necessary to break skills acquisitions into substeps, to push harder, to work more frequently, and to pay continuous attention to reinforcement and penalty schedules.

Stage 3   As always, generalization, transfer, and maintenance are extremely important. It has seemed to the author that with clutterers, these goals have been more difficult than usual to achieve. Spontaneous generalization appears to occur less, and it is necessary to plan progressive transfer steps and check closely on them. In several clients, we have scheduled transfer and maintenance to include monthly booster sessions for six months after dismissal, and then to follow-up for two years after that time.

OTHER PROCEDURES

Many different procedures have been, and are, used to deal with stuttering. Stutterers have been treated by being asked to self-record their own dysfluencies (LaCroix 1973), by working with computer-managed programs (Williams 1983), and by various forms of intensive programs of therapy (Hasbrouck et al. 1987). Mowrer (1987) even reported on a stutterer who apparently developed his own program of therapy by developing a Japanese accent! It would be impossible to cover all aspects of the many therapy approaches that have been used. However, the author wants to comment on two aspects that seem worthy of attention—drug therapy and hypnosis. The drug therapy is included because of our growing awareness of neurologically related fluency problems, where medical intervention may involve various drugs. Hypnosis is included because we have in it an ancient technique that has struggled for acceptance, is formally used by a few in our field, and is approached or used in part by many more than are realized. Both areas, drugs and hypnosis, have been discussed previously in this book but appear to warrant a second review.

Drug Therapy

In the past stutterers have been given mulled wine, laudanum (a tincture of opium), blistering salves, and concocted substances better not described. In this century effects of substances such as metherdrine, chlopromazine, pentobarbitol, amphetamines, meprobamate, and other drugs have been evaluated. Meduna (1948, 1958) reported favorably on using carbon-dioxide inhalation with stuttering, where a 30 percent CO_2 mixture was inhaled several times a week. In spite of favorable reports, hard data were lacking, and up to half of the stutterers seemed to show no improvement. Kent (1961) was generally positive in her evaluations of CO_2 therapy, but data again were minimal and results variable.

In recent times, attention has focused on tranquilizing drugs. One of the early forms was reserpine, a derivative of raulwulfia. It seemed to reduce stuttering severity and stutterers' anxieties, but there were no particular gains in fluency. Reserpine can result in negative effects with depression-prone clients, cause allergic reactions, and exaggerate symptoms if there is a pretreatment tendency to have gastric problems. Meprobamate, a mild tranquilizer, has received varying reviews in terms of its value. Kent and Williams (1959) failed to find particular values in using meprobamate as part of a therapy program, but Maxwell and Paterson (1958) and DiCarlo, Katz, and Batkin (1959) reported various values in its use. Side effects can include drowsiness, ataxia, slurred speech, nausea, allergies, and heart palpitations. Other studies have included evaluations of depressant and stimulant barbiturates and chlorpromazine, but these studies are few and data are lacking. Overview summaries are available in Van Riper (1973), Bloodstein (1986), Lee (1983), and Ingham (1984).

One powerful tranquilizer that has received special attention is haloperidol. This drug has been a resource in treating serious psychotic disorders and in treating neuromotor tics and involuntary utterances occurring in Gilles de la Tourette syndrome. Haloperidol appears to reduce dopamine production of the midbrain substantia nigra and to facilitate production of acetylcholine. Dopamine, a neurotransmitter, is typically overabundant in schizoid disorders and is lacking in Parkinsonism syndromes. Acetylcholine, also a neurotransmitter, is a facilitating agent and stimulates neuron activity. Results of haloperidol use, again, have been variable. Quinn and Peachey (1975) had less than one-fourth of their stutterers achieve a significant reduction in stuttering, Andrews and Dozsa (1977) reported that about 40 percent of their sample achieved significant improvement, and Wells and Malcolm (1971) stated that 10 of 12 stutterers displayed significant improvement after four weeks of treatment. However, in the latter study four of the ten subjects declined further treatment, and those returning did not show additional significant reductions in stuttering. Side effects of haloperidol can include tardive dyskinesia, bronchopneumonia, impairment of mental and/or physical abilities,

mood swings, Parkinsonian motor behaviors, anorexia, cardiac problems, and so on.

The overall picture of drug therapy is one of mixed results. Many of the studies reviewed lacked objective data, test populations often were small, and long-term effects were not available. The differences among various drugs hinder comparisons. Comparisons of the same drug across different studies are complicated by variations in dosage strength and timing and by use or nonuse of other chemicals to minimize possible side effects. It is also appropriate to note that client opinions of drug effects and side effects were often not reported, and those opinions could be a factor to consider. Use of drugs requires medical prescription and supervision, a resource not easily available to many clinicians. Although the author has never been involved in a drug therapy program, he has worked with stutterers who for medical reasons were taking tranquilizers, antihypertensives, or antiepileptics. Most of the clients indicated they were less anxious about their speech and did not seem to "stutter as hard" as they did before taking the drug. However, no client reported a remission of stuttering or reduction to acceptable levels, and it was my subjective impression that reductions in dysfluency and reductions in motivation to progress in speech therapy tended to coincide. In general, pending more research information, it would seem that drug therapy is best considered on a special-case basis, and that we have not found the magic pill yet.

Hypnosis

Hypnosis, in general and particular, has a long and checkered history. Nearly all of us are familiar with fictional villains who hypnotize unsuspecting victims in order to commit or cause crimes. Many of us have watched stage hypnotists involve subjects in surprising activities that were impossible in nontrance states. Hypnosis, from the Greek *hypnos*, for sleep, involves putting the person into a directed conscious state in which the person is subject to the instructions and suggestions of the hypnotist. Visions/hallucinations can be induced, sensory responsiveness altered or blocked, perceptions altered, autonomic states changed, and attitudes varied. Exactly how conscious controls and reflex protection systems can be manipulated or bypassed is not clear, and we accept that persons vary in their susceptibility to hypnotic procedure. The principles of hypnosis are often used to a degree in deep relaxation therapy, alone or combined with desensitization, where suggestion and instruction are presented during altered mental and physical states. However, all control and volition are not surrendered to the therapist.

Hard data about the uses and values of hypnotherapy of stuttering are very sparse and often vague and incomplete. Moore (1946) described hypnosis efforts with 40 stutterers, 9 of whom did not respond, as a mode of inducing tension reduction in an overall SMT program. However,

Gottlober (1953) and Morley (1957) have concurred in noting that the fluency effects of hypnosis, which are generally of high degree, last only a short time after termination of the trance state. Restoration of dysfluencies usually occurs quickly, almost as if the fluency induction occurred without the awareness of conscious mechanisms that revert to what their feedback comparators regard as usual or typical speech, that is, stuttering. McCord (1955) reviewed hypnotherapy of stuttering and concluded that there is little support for its use to implant posthypnotic suggestions in order to cause fluency or inhibit stuttering. He felt use applications were more in the direction of emotional release and relaxation. Rousey (1961) suggested that hypnosis is more effective as an adjunct to therapy, not as a main or sole approach. Falck (1964) stated that hypnotherapy must consider each stutterer separately in terms of age, dysfluency development, and individual personal needs. He points out that hypnosis-only therapy is rarely successful and, further, that therapy should include information to the client, work on attitudes and fears, reinforcement of normal speech patterns, and minimization of factors causing or controlling stuttering.

There have over many years been occasional reports of hypnotherapy. Only a few of the more current ones are summarized here. Silber (1973) has utilized hypnosis with children (and adults) who stutter. He targets child self-confidence and self-esteem and the strengthening of areas where the child seems to be weak or vulnerable. Dempsey and Granich (1978) reported on a single-case use of hypnosis with a traumatic-stuttering syndrome in a war veteran. Suggestion therapy was used, and the authors reported good results (but not a cure). Lockhart and Robertson (1977) summarized therapy with 30 stutterers, ranging from hypnotherapy only (mild stutterers) to combined hypnosis and speech therapy. Speech therapy seemed to be of an easy-onset and light consonant contact form, while hypnosis concentrated on self-suggestion to reduce situation fears and on instructions to facilitate adoption of the speech controls. A less favorable evaluation of hypnotherapy has been presented by Van Riper (1973, 1971a, 1958a), who recounts personal experiences with having been hypnotized and of using hypnotism in various ways during therapy with other stutterers. He reported on different uses of hypnotism as part of SMT, finding most of the time that results were lacking or negative. The only success involved three clients who had posthypnotic suggestions implanted to stop avoidance behaviors or certain struggle reactions. Van Riper felt that hypnosis achieved nothing that, over time, he could not accomplish with a conscious client, and stated:

> We wanted to make our cases strong and free from us, not weak and dependent. So with some regret we discarded hypnotic therapy. (1973, p. 10)

In general, our profession has fiddled with hypnotherapy enough to

find it fascinating, but not enough to find out what it really can do. Lee (1983) has suggested that there is a need for "much further and more detailed research to discover the true extent and limitations of this technique" (p. 204). Ingham (1984) reviewed stutter hypnotherapy reports, from the past to the present time, and generally failed to find data to support claims of beneficial effect. However, he objected more to the lack of proper research than to the method, and he stated that it cannot move from its status as a "fringe treatment" associated with therapists outside the mainstream of clinical responsibility until there is better research. Finally, as done earlier, it is necessary to warn the clinician that some settings forbid the use of hypnosis, or would respond negatively to it, because of fears of child abuse or technique misuse.

GROUP THERAPY

Overview and Uses

"More often than not, group therapy for stuttering has been used to relieve shortages of time and personnel, rather than for its merits and qualitative aspects" (Shames & Egolf 1976, p. 156). Leith (1984a) observes that school environments foster the application of group therapy, but most of this occurs as individual therapy performed with a group of children. He defines group therapy as that in which group members receive therapy from, and provide therapy to, the rest of the group. It is not necessarily bad, in this writer's opinion, to use group therapy as a time-saving vehicle, as pointed out earlier. If five children can be seen individually for 30 minutes, twice weekly, that is five hours of time spent. On a group basis, all five could be seen for a one-hour session each week, three could be seen individually once a week for 30 minutes, and two could receive two such sessions per week—with one session "saved" per week for other purposes. Although great values lie in group interaction, simple group instruction is not poor therapy when used appropriately (if not, then our entire educational system is wrong!).

As a matter of fact, group therapy can be used in different ways in different stages of therapy, and it can also be a primary therapy vehicle. Use modes include motivation, instruction, socialization, transfer, skills learning, attitude change, expansion of individual therapy, and maintenance support. These modes can be reduced to one focus, or appear at appropriate times in the same group. Caughley (1961) reported favorably on using group therapy with children, indicating use of relaxation, role play, group discussion, and fluency procedures. It was advised that children needing individual attention not be withdrawn during part of the group session but be seen at another time. Withdrawal during group sessions, it was felt, distracted and frustrated the group itself. Wells (1987) recommends group therapy as an asset to motivation, in which children can see and identify and share with others who stutter. She also feels that group therapy offers unique opportunities for practicing transfer activities in a social setting. In a more psychosocial application Wakaba (1983) reported on use of group play therapy of stuttering with Japanese children. It was observed that initial anxiety and uncertainty in the group situation tended to be followed by occurrences of aggressive behavior. As aggression appeared, stuttering tended to fluctuate. Then, as cooperative relationships were established with other children in the group, stuttering and aggression decreased. Wakaba suggested that the appearance and release of aggression might be a significant factor in the development of fluency and of cooperative interaction with peers. The author has observed similar developments in working with older stutterers.

Other applications of group therapy have extended to fluency reinforcement, parent counseling, implementation of operant procedures, and the consideration of sociometric procedures and values in therapy. Rustin (1978) summarized intensive group therapy for adolescent stutterers (about 14 years of age). In group settings, the adolescents were taught relaxation procedures and slowed speech. Therapy was intensive and included role play, video recordings, and TO applications. The children worked together as a group, were paired to work together as "buddy teams", and received individual help as needed. Parents were invited to participate appropriately, and one-day refresher sessions were provided every six weeks, if needed. Rustin indicated that two refresher courses and individual follow-up by local clinicians were generally needed to stabilize results. Wells (1987) favors the use of group structures in counseling the parents of stutterers. Initially, the clinician selects topics and guides discussions, but parent needs will vary and group agendas will vary as time goes on. Early on the clinician functions as a teacher or information source about stuttering, speech development, and therapy. These areas usually need to be covered and are of value to the parents. However, in most cases, parents also need behavioral growth and change and emotional relief. Such activities may involve discussion, debate, role play, and interaction among group members (not just with the clinician). Clinical skills and planning and evaluation procedures are as important here as they are with the clients receiving therapy.

Behavior modification in group therapy is discussed by Leith and Uhlemann (1972), who have described a series of procedures designed to transfer operant techniques to a group setting, something generally lacking in group therapy of stuttering, and to use the group in a fluency-shaping role. Group members were trained to establish goals, understand behavioral modification, and to consequate the desirable or undesirable behaviors of each person in the group. Results varied depending on individual clients, but the process was an excellent example of how "structure" is, per se, rigid but can be adaptable and flexible. Leith has expanded and provided description of "shaping group" therapy (1984a, 1984b, 1982, 1979). The discussion is too extensive to go into here, but clinicians can find useful outlines, steps, and methods in the sources just referred to. Earlier, Egolf, Shames, and Seltzer (1971) had applied TO in a group setting as a part-time contingency. When TO was in use, it was highly effective; this serves as another examples of operant principles applied within a group format. Stromsta (1986) is a strong advocate of group therapy, if for no other reasons than those of effectiveness and efficiency. He points out that group interaction can be used to stimulate individual clients, challenge behaviors they display, and set examples for all to follow or strive for. In an earlier publication (1965) Stromsta described using group sociometrics as part of therapy. Providing examples, and winnowing among entries, the clinician helps the group assemble a list of questions. Any questions can occur, but examples are the following:

1. Who has the best/worst eye contact during stuttering and during general speech?
2. Who has slowed down rate most since our sessions started?
3. Who tries hardest to find exceptions when the group is attempting to agree on something?
4. Who talks most/least during sessions?
5. Who still tries most to hide stuttering?
6. Who has the most mechanical/natural speech pattern?

The clinician helps limit the questions to a reasonable number, administers them at set intervals, collects the unsigned forms, and summarizes and posts results for the entire group to review and discuss. Depending on group chemistry, questions can be general and soft or can become pressing and punitive for group members not behaving or performing in ways the others desire. Stromsta (1986) states that a group therapy value unavailable to individual therapy is the opportunity for stutterers to observe the good and bad attitudes and behaviors of other group members. Similarly, they can observe which behaviors and attitudes bring success and which result in failure or frustration. Such external comparisons can provide external references for self-evaluation and change.

Values and Limitations

Mention has been made of particular uses or applications of group therapy, and of some disadvantages. For best values, it is used in the gestalt sense that the whole is greater than the sum of its parts. There is a group dynamic, group interaction, and a group "personality." Many clinicians are not trained in group therapy methods, other than structured elements of how to rotate performance, count data, and prepare plans. In planning group therapy, there are some advantages and disadvantages that might be considered. Look first at the advantages:

1. The client finds that her or his problems are not unique, that others stutter, and others have similar feelings.
2. The group creates an ongoing psychosocial interaction situation, for ordinary social interactions, and for ones that can be created and developed deliberately.
3. The client can observe and experience tolerance for and acceptance of stuttering. Desensitization can be a major development of group therapy.
4. There is greater efficiency and effectiveness, saving time and energy.
5. The group is a safe place for a client to try out and practice new or revised behaviors.
6. Through observing other group members, a client can see alternative forms of performance and behavior.
7. Either generally, or by clinician instigation, clients function as therapists to each other, as well as to themselves.
8. The group, as an entity, can provide motivation, reward, and penalty. This can occur on a moment-to-moment basis and also as an overall "keep up with the group" pressure.

With reference to the last point, the author has often found out that group members would go to a lagging person and, outside of group meetings, work to bring him or her up to the general level of group performance. Of course, there are possible disadvantages to group therapy:

1. There may be incompatible personalities in a group, developing as a result of group interaction or having existed before the group was formed.
2. Individual stutterers may try to disappear into the group and escape the clinician's attention. Some may try to manipulate the group to gain sympathy, resist therapy, or serve other selfish needs.
3. In the bad-apple-in-the-barrel mode, one client can adversely affect the attitudes and cooperativeness of the whole group. Should it occur (more likely among adolescents), the clinician will need strength and skill to avoid losing the group or having to resort to the use of blunt adult authority.
4. There may be in-group struggles for dominance. This can be quite subtle and cognitive or overt and behavioral. Its effects are not necessarily negative, but they can be and the clinician must watch for that negativity.
5. The group may foster a group dependence, slowing individual development and distorting it to conform to group "requirement."
6. The pace of group progress may be too rapid or slow for specific individuals, pressure may be too great, or penalties too severe; and there may be other group aspects that can cause individual problems.
7. Group therapy requires skill, flexibility, perceptive insight, and constant awareness by the clinician of each person and of the whole group.
8. Group therapy reduces attention paid to individuals and may inhibit subtleties of individual expression.

Age Applications

There is no age limit on group formation, but planning and conduct will vary. Fawcus (1970) has suggested that school-age children be grouped approximately by age ranges of 7–11, 12–15, and 15 or more years of age. At the Group I level, the author prefers to hold group size to about three children. Very young children are not experienced in social behavior and require more direct and individual attention to guide behavior and build group structure. Emphasis is placed on social interaction experiences—sharing, turn taking, and building tolerance for disruption—and frustration resistance. Direct therapy can be used, with fluency patterns practiced and evaluated. In general, the greatest values appear to be in the area of interaction skills and in fostering generalization of fluency outside of individual therapy sessions. Guided parent observation of group sessions is useful as part of the environmental process, and parents can be moved in and out of a group once it has stabilized.

Group II applications tend to reflect the time efficiency aspects of group therapy because therapy occurs most often in school settings. My personal preference is to have no more than four or five children of this age range in a group. Children have learned, or are learning, the rules of group behavior, and so the clinician can concentrate more on group dynamics and interactions. However, time is often spent on direct-therapy procedures in the form of group instruction and practice. The Shames and Florance (1980) stutter-free program is a good example of structured therapy in this age range. However, self-analysis and desensitization goals can be worked for overtly, and SMT methods can be utilized. Role play, relaxation, avoidance reduction, and insight development can also be targeted.

Group III adolescents offer a full range of opportunities, and challenges, to the clinician. Today, my preference is five to seven Group III children because the group dynamics favor the clinician. Many clinicians have used group therapy at this age level as a focus for motivation, self-analysis, environmental evaluation, attitude formation, and ventilation of feelings. Symptom or fluency control is often acquired during individual sessions and then transferred for refinement and spread to group settings. Issues relative to out-clinic transfer and maintenance, and sharing of fear hierarchies, can be dealt with very well in group settings, especially through role play and behavior rehearsal. The author has not had opportunity to do so, but a number of school clinicians have reported values in a "permanent intermittent" group therapy program as part of the maintenance schedule. When clients reach the dismissal stage, the group meets on a monthly basis for the rest of the time the clients are in school. One clinician had a monthly support group into which all Group III stutterers funneled after dismissal, including clients from different groups, as well as some who had received only individual therapy previously or had transferred into school after receiving therapy elsewhere.

Section Summary

Group therapy can be used with the parents of stutterers, particularly at the preschool level, and this has been discussed previously.

Many other applications of group therapy exist, especially if the purpose is directed to specific or limited goals. The author has deliberately not attempted to discuss the more formal aspects of psychotherapy in groups, since this is a broad field of specialization in and of itself. However, the psychotherapeutic aspects of group therapy are constant, occur at every age level, and are one of its great values. In short, outside of Group I children, it seems that group therapy is the most valuable asset or procedure available to the clinician as she or he works with stuttering.

CHAPTER SUMMARY

This chapter is tangible proof of the view that one can never say everything about anything, that there always is something else to comment on. Each of the areas covered could alone have occupied a full chapter; indeed, some of the topics have been the subject of entire books. It is, perhaps, a reminder to the clinician that therapy is a multifaceted skill which we never stop learning about. Most of the topics lack adequate research, in the strictest sense, to justify their use with stutterers, much less to support some of the variations cited. However, within each decade accumulating evidence helps us sort out and structure procedures more adequately. Ten years from now the topic list for this chapter will have changed and, most certainly, the organization and application factors within areas will have been altered by clinicians who have used them, some of those clinicians being those of you now reading this summation.

CHAPTER SIXTEEN
TRANSFER AND
MAINTENANCE

OVERVIEW

Background

Most of us have experienced transfer and maintenance problems personally. In transfer we have experienced the terror and self-efficacy doubts attending a public music recital of piano pieces we zipped easily through in the practice room, or found that our first peripheral speech mechanism examination of a client did not run as smoothly or confidently as did our practice examinations of friends and classroom peers. On the maintenance side, probably all of us have failed to keep solemn resolves to lose weight, do assignments early, not sleep late on weekends, and so on. Over and over again, people struggle to transfer skills from learning to performance situations, and to maintain behavioral changes in the face of influences favoring the erosion and disruption of maintenance. Both of these factors, transfer and maintenance, are critical in therapy of stuttering. In addition, there are continuing problems with controversies over what to transfer, when to do it, and how to achieve it. Maintenance is similarly beset.

This author has stated previously that instating fluency in stutterers is a fairly easy process, one that can be accomplished by supportive personnel with a few weeks of training. However, normalizing and transferring this fluency is not simple. Costello (1980) has expressed the opinion that generalization and transfer, not establishment of fluency, is the hardest and most difficult task a clinician faces (p. 319). Shames and Egolf (1976), and many other clinicians reviewed in following sections, have expressed similar opinions. The problem is not new, but it has become more significant over the past 10–15 years. In his early training days, the author was instructed in procedures for step-by-step transfer during symptom therapy and how to construct a long-range and consistent maintenance program. When fluency therapy developed and attained popularity, there was a tendency by some to establish therapy and then dismiss the client with minimal or no maintenance follow-up. Since in-clinic elimination of stuttering is fairly simple in most cases, there was a high probability of relapse as quickly learned new behaviors crumbled under reality pressures and old habituations. This neglect was not inherent in FRT per se, and there were professionals who constructed careful designs to implement transfer and maintenance. Nevertheless, the 1980 Banff international conference on stuttering devoted its agenda totally to transfer and maintenance issues (Boberg 1981).

Although transfer and maintenance problems occur in SMT also, and in spite of the variance, it appears that such problems were exacerbated by certain of the claims and behaviors of some of the early fluency reinforcement programs. Shames and Florance (1982), while recognizing that SMT programs have their own problems with transfer and maintenance, stated that

> many of the newer therapies which emphasize fluency-inducing behavior focus primarily on tactics for initially changing the stutterer's speech in the clinic, with much less attention to transfer and maintenance. These therapeutic regimes can be seriously and severely criticized as being nothing less than laboratory exercises in fluency with little or no impact on the real problem. Any therapy program must involve transfer. (p. 212)

The structure of operant therapy has tended to reinforce transfer and maintenance problems. Careful attention to continuous reinforcement and contingency responses tend to result in gratifyingly rapid reduction in, or extinctions of, dysfluencies. This rapid establishment of fluency, in and of itself, can become a problem:

> Although responses that are acquired through continuous reinforcement have the fastest acquisition, they also have the most rapid extinction rate when reinforcement is withdrawn. (Shames and Egolf 1976, p.162)

Shames and Egolf suggest that it might be wiser to shift, progressively, from continuous to fixed-intermittent to variable-intermittent reinforcement. Reinforcement also can be done on an interval basis or ratio (one reinforcement for *X* number of correct responses) basis. A number of FRT programs have been structured in an intensive format where stutterers receive daily therapy over a period of weeks, and this rapid change and the artificial environments place special strain on transferring skills to real life and maintaining the effects. Intensive therapy programs, more so than conventional ones, require careful planning for transfer and maintenance, especially for Group II and Group III children. After "living with" therapy for a week or a month, many stutterers find the outside world too different, and relapses are very likely. Rustin (1978) reported that their intensive program involved clinician visits to each child's school to talk with the child's teachers, as well as plan for carryover support. Booster sessions were scheduled every six weeks (two sessions were the average for most clients), and stability of effects was monitored.

Definitions

Generalization, transfer, stabilization, maintenance, and other terms have been defined in a number of forms according to the backgrounds and purposes of those concerned. The following definitions will apply in subsequent discussions:

Transfer   when the occurrence of a response to one form of stimuli generalizes to include similar stimuli in other situations, as a result of planned efforts by those involved in therapy.

Generalization   see transfer; some clinicians define generalization and transfer differently.

Spontaneous Transfer   or spontaneous generalization; the transfer is unscheduled and may or may not include all response aspects desired; usually considered to be a progressive phenomenon.

Stabilization   when a newly learned behavior is emitted in the desired form, at the desired rate, under stipulated conditions. It may occur with similar or different criteria on in-clinic and out-clinic bases.

Maintenance   a stable transferred response that is under control of the client on an out-clinic basis and continues to meet, or improves on, the criteria initially established for transfer. It often includes psychosocial aspects of client adjustment. It can be redefined by the client, rather than the clinician, in personal terms.

Exactly what is to be transferred or maintained complicates definitions and applications. Therapy programs vary in what they intend to accomplish and, therefore, how success is to be measured. Communication does not involve fluency only, however it is defined. In preparing stutterers for communication, clinicians need to look at a spectrum of factors. Reference has already been made at various times to possible problems in articulation and voice among stutterers. Fifteen years ago, Perkins (1973a, 1973b) wrote of the need to focus special attention on general speech production of stutterers. Even subtler needs have been noted, research suggesting that stutterers can be deficient in turn-taking skills (measured by response latency, body movement, and eye contact) so that they tended to have a "conversational disrhythmia" that interfered with communication (Jensen, Markel & Beverung 1986). In addition to fluency and general speech production, other factors may need consideration.

Both SMT and FRT programs usually stress self-monitoring by the stutterer, partly because new skills are being learned and partly because it has been assumed that stutterers are deficient in self-monitoring (Van Riper 1982). A study by Burley and Morley (1987) explored this, and the suggestion was made by Klevans and Lynch (1977) that stutterers are so preoccupied with their own communication problems that they do not adequately attend to other speakers. Using the Snyder Self-Monitoring Scale they found that stutterer scores were significantly lower overall and significantly lower also in each of three subscale categories—acting, extraversion, and other-directedness. Successful transfer and maintenance typically requires self-monitoring for skill refinement and to minimize relapse possibilities.

An additional complication in evaluating transfer and maintenance success involves the fact that many stutterers still stutter after therapy is complete. In a paired-comparison study, Runyan and Adams (1978) asked speech and language pathology graduates to identify the stutterers from paired readings. The stutterers represented incomplete therapy and completed therapy from the following approaches: metronome, DAF, operant, precision fluency shaping, symptom modification, and "holistic" therapy. For the incomplete therapy group, and for all of the therapy modes named, sophisticated judges were able (statistical significance) to identify the stutterers. The design (paired comparisons, sophisticated judges) prevents fair comparison to real-life communication but raises issues that will be discussed further in the section on maintenance.

Since so many factors, some of them just reviewed, can affect how we assess transfer and maintenance efforts, the author wishes to stipulate what he feels transfer and maintenance should involve, with the age and problem severity, and concomitant problems of clients, varying the content and emphases of the stipulations. Shames and Florance (1980) raise seven or eight "tactical" questions relative to what should be considered in planning for transfer and maintenance, and I have referred to them in stating what I feel might be "tactical guidelines" for transfer and maintenance in therapy planning:

1. Therapy should routinely attempt to increase self-responsibility and self-reinforcement in the client in order to facilitate transfer and support maintenance.
2. Effective transfer requires that use of new skills occur in situations, with people, and during emotions associated with stuttering.
3. Where possible and feasible, environmental others should be recruited to participate in transfer and maintenance training, or at least to provide support when activities are implemented.
4. The degree of balance between external and internal support should evolve away from the clinician and to the client during therapy, and this should be

reflected in both transfer and maintenance. The initial balance and rate of change should be adjusted individually for each client.

5. Maintenance is an active process. Since maintaining the status quo requires effort to resist change, then maintaining changed and changing behavioral states cannot be passive.

6. It should be assumed that maintenance programs will require therapeutic intervention to prevent or correct relapse, or to stimulate continued progress. Finding (later) such preparation to have been unnecessary is far preferable (and rarer) than not having provided for it in the first place.

7. Scheduled measurement activities following therapy are a form of therapeutic intervention. However, simply dysfluency counts are not sufficient and measurement should include wider evaluations of fluency, naturalness of speech, and attitudes of the client. In addition, the clinician should be ready to provide more intervention if needed.

8. Strategic planning in therapy must consider speech and self-concept goals that are appropriate for each client. Failure to do this, replacing it with rigid goals for clients, invites posttransfer and maintenance instability. Negotiation and stimulation to change are appropriate clinical activities, but final goals either must represent an accord between the client and the clinician, or the client must be transferred to another clinician.

The final statement will stimulate some disagreement from clinicians on the issues of ethics or wisdom (who knows best, the client or the clinician?). This author would note the appropriateness of both points and has no objection with "subversion goals" of changing the client's goals and aspirations. However, as a bottom line, the author would argue that behavioral, lifestyle decisions must be made, not by the clinician, but by the person who will live with those decisions.

RELAPSE

The enemy of every therapy is relapse. Problems in transfer can and do occur, but the ultimate defeat for a clinician is to find that a dismissed client has regressed to a point where therapy again is required. Most of the time we define relapse as a return of undesired symptoms that therapy either had replaced or brought under control. There is a subtler form of relapse in which psychosocial behaviors that were encouraged, or coerced, by therapy fade so that the client fails to behave personally and socially as an adequate communicator might be expected. Enabling the stutterer to speak fluently on the telephone or to strangers, or to groups, may not be sufficient support to allow the client to go out and freely enter situations they avoided for years previously. Even if the fluency or symptom control would not break down, the stutterer can still behave like a stutterer. Owen (1981), at the Banff conference on maintenance and transfer (Boberg 1981), summarized studies of programs designed to secure "adult lifestyle" changes and stated that, over time, "not much more than

30% . . . will have persisted with the initial changes that they have achieved" (p. 33). Lifestyle changes can involve smoking, obesity, drinking, nail biting, and stuttering.

Why stutterers tend to relapse has been discussed extensively at conferences and the literature. Boberg, Howie, and Woods (1979) have suggested that stutterer relapse may relate to the persistence of small dysfluencies that pass in therapy, but they later "grow" to become major spasms after dismissal. They also suggest that cessation of monitoring may allow relapse, and that stutterers with heavy genetic and/or neurophsyiological fluency factors may create an "inevitable relapse" situation. Turning away from built-in or inevitable relapse factors (see earlier discussion about Cooper's 1987 article on chronic irreversible stuttering), Webster (1979) has stated that relapse is related to the adequacy of the therapy training, clinician competence, and whether the client "slips" in ability to evaluate production aspects of respiration, phonation, and articulation. While these all are valid concerns, Webster's list is far too simplistic. The factors that influence therapy success also operate in the maintenance of therapy effects.

Neaves (1966, 1970) reported on 165 stutterers, ages 8 to 17 years, of which 84 were rated as "successful" and 81 as "unsuccessful" after therapy. Success was defined as mild (1.5%SW or less) or no stuttering. The two groups were compared on about 13 separate categories or measures. Significant differences were found in measures of motor ability, intelligence, speech development, age of stuttering onset, family history, and social class. When measures of multiple elements were run, four factors seemed to stand out:

• Motor impairment.
• Speech development
• Age of stuttering onset
• Family history of stuttering

If a child presented only one of the factors listed, the success rate of therapy was 80 percent, dropping to 50 percent if any two of the factors operated. The therapy success rates dropped to 10 and to 5 percent respectively if three or all four factors occurred in the same child. What relevance these factors might have for maintenance is not clear, but certainly worth considering.

Sheehan (SFA 19) enumerated seven reasons for relapse, including false fluency, Jost's law, artificiality of new speaking modes, and occurrence of catastrophic stress. Over the years, this author has observed the factors listed by Sheehan, plus a few more:

1. False fluency. The client really is not fluent but, in response to suggestion and pressure, is persuaded into a false fluency. Rarely, one can observe a 'flight into fluency' where the client, to escape undesirable aspects of

therapy, is miraculously 'cured' and leaves therapy. In both types, relapse follows.

2. Self-efficacy doubts. Clients may overdepend on the clinician and the therapy program, rather than develop confidence in their own capacities. Some therapy programs, or clinicians, foster this dependency.

3. Weak establishment and transfer of new speaking modes. This may be a program fault that fails to achieve adequate criterion levels, or assumes spontaneous generation that does not occur. It also can be failure to monitor accurately the client's efforts at establishment and transfer.

4. Failure to develop or, more likely, to use self-monitoring adequately. It can also be clinician failure to monitor accurately the client's efforts at transfer.

5. Dissatisfaction of the client with the new speech mode. Initial acceptance may be persuaded or coerced by the clinician, or simply by the difference from stuttering. However, especially if the client fails to refine and normalize the speech mode, it may become less desirable as a goal to perpetuate.

6. Failure to eradicate social avoidance behaviors. Teaching a client prolonged speech, or pullouts, may not automatically eradicate years of psychosocial avoidance and covert behaviors. These behaviors can negate the values of speech fluency or control accomplishments and erode recently acquired capacities.

7. Boredom. Behaviors that have to be worked on and nurtured can become boring and lose their appeal.

8. Jost's law. When two approximately equal responses compete, the older response will, over time, tend to displace the new one. The less sure, firm, acceptable, and so on, the new response is, the sooner relapse will occur.

9. Catastrophes in health, family life, personal relationships, or directly in speech situations may overwhelm a fragile therapy construct.

10. Penalty of fluency. Many stutterers obtain values from dysfluency. Group I children may use it to manipulate parents, Group II children to avoid classroom activity, and Group III children to provide an alibi for social and vocational avoidances or failures. Some find the responsibilities and penalties of fluency just not rewarding enough to maintain.

11. Residual dysfluency that was not anticipated by the client or planned for by the clinician. This occurs particularly when there is some small regression early in postdismissal maintenance, and the client is not prepared for it.

12. Neurophysiological deficits in timing and coordination that respond to slower rate and simplified patterns during in-clinic establishment. However, as normalization of speech occurs, the neuromotor patterning cannot cope. Also, these deficits may be due to automatization as conscious controls habituate and move down to brain stem levels of function.

TRANSFER

General Considerations

Owen (1981) distinguishes between generalization and transfer, in that generalization is the process by which conditioned responses to certain stimuli occur after similar stimuli in separate situations. Transfer, on the other hand, occurs when behavior developed "under one set of circumstances is also manifesting itself under other circumstances" (p. 35). Distinctions will not be made here, but it is emphasized that transfer is not something that occurs later in therapy. It is a major goal of therapy from the time of therapy initiation (Wells 1987). At its simplest, transfer involves establishing a newly learned behavior and then planning for that behavior to occur on an out-clinic basis in the client's environment. However, beyond simplistic levels, there are other variables to consider. Transfer activities involve three forms of complexity and stress, which can be managed to varying degrees:

1. **Situation Stress**—refers to situation variables such as location, person(s) involved, and size of audience. The lowest stress usually is the clinician and the familiar therapy room. From there, therapy can move to another room, then another person is introduced, and so on.
2. **Message stress**—refers to two forms of stress. One is length and complexity of utterance (linguistic stress), a topic discussed previously. The other factor is message significance, varying from mundane "I am fine" to requests, response to important questions, emotional issues, and so on.
3. **Response stress**—refers to the response of the environment to the speaker. Low stress would be the attentive and responsive listener (clinician), moving to less attentive, distracted listeners. Disruption elements can also figure into response stress.

Shames (1975) states that carryover work requires clinician awareness of the out-clinic speech and life aspects of the client. Carryover planning can include, but not be limited to, size of the audience, specific person or persons involved, competitiveness of talking, speed and time pressure, topics involved, emotional weight of situation, probable audience reactions, and so on. Wells (1987) recommended that transfer should develop at each ability level, and not wait until the skill has reached conversational levels of function. Fiedler and Standop (1983) also make the point that transfer should be gradual, not dramatic. Further, creating situations that simulate reality are important. They recommend that outsiders be brought in regularly so that the client becomes used to variations in the numbers and personalities of people. Carryover then moves to "therapeutic excursions" where the client and clinician go to places that are appropriate for the client. This can be difficult at times, but it can be arranged.

Clinician Applications

There has been a steady growth in the literature about transfer and maintenance, and many programs now make it an integral part of therapy. Ryan (1974) described a six-location program of 23 steps to achieve transfer. Locales involved change of therapy room, increases in audience, and speech at home, at school, on the telephone, and with strangers. The first four situations required criterion fluency during one minute of reading and four minutes of conversation, in each, and the last two required five minutes of conversation at criterion fluency level. Maintenance involved periodic performance with criterion fluency for three minutes each in reading, monologue, and conversation. The best time factor reported was 36 minutes of criterion fluency over a period of 15 weeks. In general, the foregoing appears to be rather mechanical in nature, and limited.

One transfer method often used has been that of overlearning, as exemplified by Hanna and Owen (1977). Overlearning is the modern jargon for what older clinicians call drill. By whatever name, the procedure has neurological validity. In theory, consciously voluntary motor acts involve major cortical participation on an elective process of selecting one particular motor pattern from a number of possible variations. As a particular motor pattern is repeated, it is assumed to develop representation or storage at subcortical levels (basal ganglia to cerebellum) so that a stimulus, instead of triggering a review and selection process, triggers a programmed (overlearned) set of motor responses. This may or may not be a correct analysis. If it is, some clinicians have commented that overlearning will increase the importance of desensitization, avoidance reduction, and attitude change—because of the possible limbic (emotional) effects on motor behaviors that have a subcortical, as opposed to cortical, predominance. That is, as we stop paying conscious attention to motor acts, they become more easily disrupted by emotional reactions. This concept is completely speculative, but it could be a possible factor in relapse as consciously learned skills habituate and recede from overt monitoring and control.

Among many other approaches to transfer, Adams (1980) has utilized the fear hierarchy structure development, drawing upon parents if a client is too young to participate adequately in development. Transfer then procedes on a step-by-step basis. Adams notes that some children spontaneously generalize, while others are slow to do so. One approach he uses in such cases is progressive role play. At first the clinician verbally recreates a situation while the child, with eyes closed, visualizes it. In the second step, the child speaks a message created by the clinician, and continues to develop responsibility until ready for actual role playing. Another method recommended by Adams is the familiar one of including parents or significant others in therapy, by stages, and training them to become substitute clinicians at home.

Guitar (1984) has outlined a fluency-shaping program for children who stutter. He states that before transfer is developed, the child not only should be fluent, but the fluent speech should sound essentially normal. He suggests the training of parents to be models of slow and easy speech and to function in a tangible reinforcement program. Nagging, interrupting parents must be rechanneled, or transfer should start and develop in other situations first, such as with playmates or teachers. Guitar advises a step hierarchy of transfer, with pass criteria at each step until the child can demonstrate fluency in nearly all situations. I think I disagree with Guitar's proviso that transfer should not occur until speech is fluent and normal sounding, but I otherwise endorse his plan. In a more technologically complex method, Strang and Meyers (1987a, 1987b; Meyers and Strang 1987) have utilized a computer-assisted program to help parents and family members deal with stuttering (also used to train student clinicians). The auditor listens to a computer-vocalized "child" stutter and then selects a response to the dysfluencies. An operator enters their response, and the vocoder replies or responds with a fluency level keyed to auditor response. Poor auditor responses result in continued and/or intensified vocoder stuttering, while the reverse is true for appropriate responses. Such programs could be developed where maintenance clients could develop problem solutions on their own, calling the clinician in only when stuck, or to review a series of practice efforts. Other individual transfer programs will be cited as this section reviews age group considerations.

Transfer Problems

The previous sections have commented on and enumerated general problems in transfer and maintenance, as well as factors contributing to relapse. Looking specifically at transfer, one can consider a number of obstacles. A consistent problem in transfer is that of client fears concerning using new therapy methods and feelings of inadequacy (Adams 1983; Shames and Florance 1980). Overall, the things that can bedevil transfer efforts include, but are not restricted to, the following:

1. The client actually does not understand clearly what is to be done and/or how it is to be performed.
2. Inadequate practice and refinement has occurred on an in-clinic basis.
3. Too much is attempted for transfer, at one time, instead of smaller steps.
4. The client has been prepared inadequately in self-monitoring and self-evaluation.
5. A fall-back or safety net behavior has not been practiced for use if disaster strikes.
6. The client does not trust or have faith in therapy effects.
7. The client lacks faith in his or her own ability.
8. Personal and situational anxieties have not been or are not dealt with.
9. Client motivation to transfer is low. This can be for many reasons and must be explored.
10. Boredom with the whole control effort sets in.
11. Occurrence of personal traumas, outside of speech, disrupt concentration and commitment.
12. Significant others in the environment are not responsive to therapy or may even be opposed to it.

13. Client realizes how fluency demands and dysfluency loss may change her or his lifestyle.
14. The client misuses therapy-taught procedures.
15. There is a poor relationship with clinician.
16. There is poor follow-up by clinician, leaving client alone.
17. There is failure to evaluate successes/failures of transfer efforts.
19. There is failure to adapt or revise transfer activities on the basis of evaluations that were performed.
20. Therapy resulted in fluency that was inadequately normal in the outside world.

Group I Transfer

Transfer with preschool children often occurs in the form of spontaneous generalization and there frequently is the expectation that, except for minor fluctuations, a formal transfer program is not required (Ryan 1971; Martin, Kuhl & Haroldson 1972; Costello 1980). However, it is not wise or safe to assume that all Group I children will fit this pattern. Wall and Myers (1984) anticipate spontaneous transfer among Group I stutterers, but they are prepared if it occurs imperfectly. Family members are brought into therapy, other clinicians and clients are recruited, and accompanied out-clinic activities are developed. With older children, hierarchy development is used. With each step or phase of performance, once it is stable, it is useful to bring other persons into the therapy room to hear (and reinforce) the client's performance. Children can be rehearsed in small performances for in-home consumption, and parents can be alerted to make time for them. When circumstances are favorable, the client can be rehearsed, for instance, to teach "easy speech" at home to parents, siblings, or playmates.

Therapy programs that involve parents during in-clinic sessions will aid in transfer. An approximate sequence might be the following:

1. Clinician models and instructs; child performs; parent observes (out of room or apart from work group).
2. Child performs separately; clinician reinforces; parent sits in group but does not participate verbally.
3. Child performs and parent performs; clinician stimulates and reinforces each, separately.
4. Clinician stimulates, parent repeats stimulus; child performs; parent reinforces, clinician reinforces.
5. Parent stimulates; child performs; parent reinforces; clinician repeats sequence afterwards.
6. Parent and child exchange stimulating, performing, and reinforcing; clinician moderates.
7. Parent and child have one or two 5–15-minute "therapy sessions" at home each day, following clinician's plan.

The clinician can plan for specific out-clinic situations where acquired skills are to be used. Times such as story telling, meals, bedtime, and so on, can be organized. Parents can be trained in "easy speech" patterns and time intervals set up daily where only that pattern is to be used. Parents also can be counseled and guided in general speech modeling, controlling speech disruptors, and making appropriate responses if fluency breaks occur. Data collection and observation by parents will help the clinician keep track of transfer effectiveness, and it will cue the parents to maintain their side of transfer support.

It should not be assumed that all parents and home situations favor transfer activities. Wall and Myers (1984) make a wise departure from rigid insistence that home therapy must always occur, and they note that some home environments will be negative. In such instances, the clinician can try stronger counseling and manipulation of the environment, to try to lessen problems. Basal fluency reinforcement, discussed under desensitization, can be inserted as a major goal as the child's fluency progresses. Behavior rehearsal and role play can be used effectively also. However, it can be anticipated that therapy overall will take longer, transfer will be slower, and more individual problems will have to be solved.

Group II Transfer

Many Group II children receive therapy in school settings or, at least, must transfer therapy effects to school environments. Therapy may be fluency, symptom, or a mixture. Self-monitoring becomes more important, since parents often are not available and teachers lack the time/familiarity to do it. Some clinicians have questioned the ability of children to function effectively in self-monitoring, and it is true that mature skills may be incomplete. However, Silverman and Williams (1972) evaluated 38 stutterers (third through sixth grades) in their abilities to estimate stuttering severity. A seven-inch rule was used to create a seven-point ordinal scale, and each child picked the ruler length that best represented her or his stuttering severity. Of the 38 children, 30 had self-ratings that correlated significantly with actual dysfluency analyses. Other self-monitoring skills can be taught or approximated so that clients can become more self-sufficient in transfer.

Schools create unique opportunities, and problems, in transfer. One of the problems may be the frequency and duration of therapy sessions—too few and too short. Williams (SFA 19), writing of transfer for Group II stutterers, states that two 15-minute individual therapy sessions each week is "professionaly irresponsible." He argues that "two to three individual sessions per week, each for 30–40 minutes is a minimal requirement" (p.31) and that additional clinician time must be spent with school personnel and the parents. If clinician schedules cannot adapt to client needs, then the child should be referred to a therapy source that can adapt.

Williams is correct in his feelings about what constitutes proper therapy, although not totally realistic in his recommendations. Other clinicians may not be available, and schedule elasticity is limited. However, the clinician can often exercise ingenuity in grouping and scheduling stutterers, and even in mixing different problem types in order to increase available time.

The classroom is a natural arena for transfer practice, and school personnel are potential participants in assignments. Both (situations and persons) may occupy points on a hierarchy list. Wall and Myers (1984) stress the value and importance of classroom performance for Group II and Group III children, spending therapy time on rehearsal, discussion, role play, and live practice. Backup options in case of difficulty are discussed and practiced in therapy, so that the child receives practice in evaluation and problem solving. Group therapy is particularly amenable to these types of rehearsal and role-play activities. Children can be afraid of in-school transfer because their revised speech pattern, fluency or symptom, is "different" and they fear the attention of classmates and school staff. Stuttering may be a daily pain and frustration, but it is what the child and environment are used to, and many children resist departing from their familiar image. They also may be unsure of school staff reactions, fearing that adults will misconstrue their efforts. Williams (SFA 19) has pointed out that teachers and school administrators often tend to speak less to or with stuttering children. Oddly enough, the reason is not that they dislike stuttering so much (they are "used to" children with problems). Their reluctance apparently stems from guilt feelings over having caused the child to stutter by calling on, or talking with, them. Williams also makes several points about supposedly noncooperative classroom teachers. Many teachers reported that clinicians would come to them, without prior notice, when they were intent on other things. Often, the clinician attitude was of the "you will do this" type, of the specialist to ancillary personnel. Many resented being asked to subtract time from 30–40 children to devote it to one child and to make judgments they were not trained to make. An example Williams used was that of one teacher who was ordered to ask the child only questions that could be answered with three words, followed in the next week by questions requiring five-word answers. Williams gives advice and suggestions for keeping teachers informed, enlisting them as allies (not support personnel), becoming informed about classroom procedures and activities, and encouraging teachers to suggest ways in which they can help the child transfer speech. With appropriate information, courtesy and diplomacy, school personnel can become valuable parts of the whole transfer program. Then, lessons can be practiced in therapy, group sessions can rehearse classroom situations, and feedback from teachers can be solicited.

The home is not neglected in Group II, but time restraints suggests the clinician devote effort to where it will be most effective and controllable. Home assignments can be given, utilizing skills already stabilized in therapy. If parent conferences can be scheduled, home cooperation and feedback can usually be developed. If feasible, parent attendance at some therapy sessions can be arranged. There will be some degree of spontaneous transfer among younger Group II children, especially if the clinician can reach into the environment and minimize fluency disruption factors. Older Group II clients will tend to present transfer needs similar to those among Group III children.

Group III Transfer

Adolescents in Group III will present problems discussed earlier, and so these will only be indicated here. Stuttering patterns are usually more severe, have more struggle, and avoidance behaviors have proliferated and become more habituated. There also may be more resistance to adult direction in transfer, plus a greater fear of looking/sounding different before their peers. On the plus side, transfer can be approached more cognitively, direct desensitization procedures utilized, and the fear hierarchy developed fully and used. Boberg (SFA 19) describes transfer procedures, in an intensive therapy program, with adolescents and adults. Initial steps involve recorded conversations with clinic staff persons, and then move to the client conducting "opinion surveys" about stuttering (directed at strangers). The next step is general conversation with strangers, followed by telephone and shopping assignments. The final transfer assignment is a "for real" job interview with a prospective employer, or one in the area of the client's interest. About halfway through the transfer sequence, the client is to develop a ten-situation list of problem situations, and this semihierarchy is worked on. Boberg notes that transfer work is physically and emotionally exhausting, and clients should not be overloaded or pushed too fast.

One can follow preset patterns, such as the one described by Boberg, or simply establish parameters around which different situations can be arranged.

1. Construction and use of a fear hierarchy, as a transfer point itself, and also to check intended transfer activities.
2. Progressively increasing client responsibility in monitoring, evaluating, and consequating behaviors.
3. Progressively increasing client responsibility in planning and scheduling transfer activities, preparing for maintenance after dismissal.
4. Role play and behavior rehearsal.
5. Major attention paid to motivation, attitudes, and feelings.

It sometimes is difficult to effect transfer into home settings, since adolescents often have a love-hate relationship with home and parents. Daly

(1987) reported on the use of a home VCR unit, with one adolescent and one adult, to replay in-clinic therapy experiences at home. These were used to reinforce self-confident images of fluency control and to alter the perceptions of significant others in the client's environment. Many clinicians will not have access to videotaping facilities, but audiotapes can be made. By planning with the client, recordings can be prepared that demonstrate progress and open the way for further home activity. Specific home situations or persons can be explored and role played to rehearse transfer activities and develop solutions for anticipated problems.

MAINTENANCE

General Considerations

Successful planning for transfer, and effective transfer, does not mean that the transfer plan then becomes a maintenance plan, or that maintenance will be stable. As noted early in this chapter, relapse rates range from vexing to catastrophic in stuttering. However, attention paid to maintenance has, until very recent times, been quite variable. Hanna and Owen (1977) have suggested that schedules and performance criteria, coupled with contingency contracting, are valuable in maintenance, and that booster workshop sessions can be used. However, Boberg, Howie, and Woods (1979) reviewed maintenance programs (at the time) and concluded that we generally lack programs that have been designed and evaluated according to standard criteria. Adams (1980) has stated that, for a long time, clinicians took a passive role in maintenance. At times it was assumed that transfer procedures were sufficient to prepare the client for dismissal. Some clinicians set up maintenance guidelines but, after that, it was up to the client or the environment to carry activities out, change behaviors, contact the clinician, and so on.

Part of the maintenance problem has ranged about the issue of when dismissal occurs, what it implies in terms of speech performance, and also what is implied in terms of future clinician involvement. For Group I clients, points at issue are few; but older stutterers present the questions, in full. Stromsta (1986) argues against the semantic connotations of "therapy termination," stating that the stutterer must be prepared for future occurrence of dysfluencies and be ready to serve as her or his own clinician when the need arises. Cooper (1984) disagrees with therapy dismissal when a client reaches a certain preset fluency criterion, but begins withdrawal when the clients "experience and maintain the feeling of control outside the clinic situation without the clinician's assistance" (p. 27). However, some clinicians set criteria. For instance, Wall and Myers (1984) suggest a dismissal criterion of 4 percent, or less, stuttererd words (Ryan 1978), and Webster (1979) proposed a 3 percent or less average for all types of fluency breaks. When therapy achieves and holds the criterion level for two or three months, maintenance stops. This assumes that there are no speech or situation avoidances. For six months the child is seen bimonthly, and then he or she is seen every six months for about two years. Parents may contact the client at any time. It would appear that Cooper, and Wall and Myers, arrive at the same place via different routes through the semantic differential—one stressing dysfluency counts and the other emphasizes the client having a "feeling of control."

In general, maintenance has become a long-term concept. Guitar (1984) states that most children require a long-term contract program if fluency is to stabilize and endure. Clinical judgment will vary the frequency and form of clinical contacts, but he projected that a year or more of follow-up contacts would be typical. If fluency turns out to be rather fragile, more detailed contacts and possible booster work on fluency may be needed. Cooper (1984) argues that clients will vary in how much time and energy they are willing to expend on maintenance. He feels that clinicians are mandated to confirm the willingness, explore it with the client, and avoid setting up unrealistic demands the client will not meet. In reviewing the literature, this author found 18–24 months to be the most frequently cited duration for maintenance programs.

What we are trying to maintain, and "what else" is supposed to happen to speech during maintenance also has been a point of controversy. Shames (1981) has called Van Riperian symptom therapy a "reasoning of resignation" because the maintenance program provides for stuttering to occur after in-clinic therapy is completed: "Relapse is built into his therapy in such a way that it isn't even called a relapse" (p. 236). Shames would have a telling point if it were not for the fact that so many FRT programs did not have pass dismissal criteria of so many SW/M or such-and-such a %SW figure. Further, many of these programs have been reported on favorably when maintenance follow-up recorded slippage to "only" *X, Y,* or *X* %SW. Since, typically, both therapy approaches have posttherapy dysfluency results, it seems inappropriate to condemn the one to praise the other.

The variability of therapy results is illustrated vividly in two stutterers' autobiographies, referred to a number of times in chapters past. Both Murray (1980) and Carlisle (1985) describe and discuss therapies that, individually, covered decades of the authors' times. Both individuals considered themselves to be stutterers as of the time they wrote their books about stuttering, but both seemed to feel that they (not stuttering) were in control of their speech. Dalton (1983a) has pointed out that tolerance of fluency failure is seen by many clinicians as being essential, and an alternative to a return to avoidance mechanisms. She stresses that therapy should develop the self-responsibility of the client, and not an overreliance on the clinician. The author would add that it also may not be wise to lead the stutterer to anticipate fluent normalcy when past history and present odds are against its occurrence. Perkins (1980b), in discussing transfer and maintenance concerns, used the joke about the drunk searching for his car keys under a streetlight, where he had not lost them, because it was too dark to search where he had lost them. The point raised was whether we were measuring (arguing about) what needed measuring, or whether we were using what we knew enough about as the measure—that is, do measure what we know rather than what needs to be measured? Is the proper criterion SW/M, %SW, severity scales, the normalcy character of speech, the satisfaction of the speaker, or other factors? Whatever the measure or measures, it is apparent that in many instances maintenance involves the continued occurrence of dysfluencies (SFA 1987, #21), nontypical speech patterns, and timing characteristics that deviate from normal.

Group I Maintenance

It has been suggested by some that Group I children do not need maintenance because of spontaneous generalization. There is enough truth in this suggestion to make it dangerous if the result is a general decision not to plan for maintenance. An excellent example of foresight is presented by Riley and Riley (1984). They use transfer activities in twice-daily practice home assignments of capacities learned in the clinic. Maintenance was not planned because none of the children in the test sample required it within one year of dismissal. However, parents and teachers were contacted by telephone every six months for two years following termination of therapy. The author approves of the Rileys' monitoring, and predismissal preparation, but would prefer a more structured maintenance program to avoid a parent saying at one six-month checkpoint, "Oh yes, he's been having trouble for the last couple of months. Do you think we should be concerned?"

Culp (1984), in her preschool fluency program, presents another example of routine planning for maintenance needs. She works to transfer from fluency in play settings to fluency during disruption, to practice in home settings. When the child is 95 percent adequate over six to eight weeks in therapy sessions and home assignments, therapy drops to biweekly sessions. When criterion measures again hold for six to eight weeks, session frequency drops to once a month. After two months of criterion performance, the client is retested by a new clinician and, if performance is adequate, discharged. A recheck is made three months later and repeated (for research purposes) two years later. Procedures in the Riley and the Culp programs use transfer to lead into maintenance generalization, but they are careful to provide follow-up contacts or checks to assure that progress has been stabilized.

Group I Maintenance Steps

A thorough transfer program is the core of maintenance in the future for Group I children and all other age and severity groups. If transfer has not been encouraged and planned, then maintenance has little chance for success if spontaneous transfer does not do the job. Several guidelines can be suggested that should be useful when planning maintenance with Group I children.

1. Implement step-by-step transfer strategies throughout therapy.
2. Involve parents or significant others in therapy sessions and make home practice part of the transfer program.
3. In parent counseling, prepare parents for maintenance. Discuss expected fluency fluctuations and how to respond with speech modeling, pressure reduction, and evaluation.
4. When fluency goals have been reached and are stable (70–90 percent consistency) for at least six consecutive therapy sessions, reduce the frequency of therapy sessions by half. Replace the dropped in-clinic sessions with two 15-minute home sessions per week. The in-home sessions are to be basic practice in fluency reinforcement, and not to solve problems or take on new issues.
5. Orient in-clinic sessions toward increasing tolerance for fluency disruptions, and work as needed on further desensitization and behavioral alternatives.
6. When fluency has been stable for six to eight clinic sessions (and home reports are positive), reduce clinic sessions by half again (usually biweekly sessions). The home therapy continues, but only during the "off" week of clinic therapy.
7. When fluency has been stable for six clinic sessions (and home reports are positive), drop to three monthly sessions and eliminate formal home sessions. At special times model and encourage easy speech patterns (for example, bedtime stories). Clinic sessions are booster activities, problem solving, and planning with the parents for maintenance.
8. For the next three months, each month, have the parent monitor the child's speech during three 5-minute talking periods each day for three consecutive days. The parent is to call the clinic and report on the 45-minute sample.
9. Six months later, the parent (reminded by clinician) is to perform another three-day sampling program and report to the clinician. If all is well, scheduled contacts will be terminated.

The author has been careful not to stipulate what criteria of fluency or normalcy should be set, expecting individual clinicians to do this. The sequence of steps can be shortened or lengthened as needs indicate, and the sequence should fit with any packaged or individually prepared program.

Group II Maintenance

Children at the lower age level of Group II will often display spontaneous fluency transfer, simplifying maintenance. However, as the children mature, "controlled fluency or acceptable stuttering are probably more realistic goals" (SFA 16, 1980, p. 62). Group II children often are worked with in school settings, and the previous maintenance comments about school personnel apply here. In private therapy settings, most of the nine-point sequence just described for Group I can be adapted for the lower range of Group II ages, while Group III maintenance suggestions will have general application to older Group II children. One of the factors to be dealt with more often in Group II maintenance is the idea contained in the quote just cited—that maintenance may not be fluent-normal. Often, the product shows evidence of fluency control efforts and/or is marked by variable occurrences of stuttering.

Williams (SFA 19) states that if the child understands what must be done to speak well, understands that improvement is progressive, and understands that "goofs" or fluency breaks will occur, then the child is ready to cope with most problems that occur. The author would endorse the foregoing but add to it that the child should also understand what he or she can do if the breaks occur. Williams advocates having the school-age child develop evaluation and planning capacities for maintenance. As these developments occur, therapy drops to biweekly or triweekly sessions focused on further planning and on problem solving. He suggests that such sessions, even for 15 minutes, can continue for one to two years, with values for the child. Also, during this prolonged period, the clinician can check with teachers and other school personnel as to how the child is performing.

In school settings, Group II therapy and transfer need to reach out to the classroom and to school personnel, as noted earlier. Also, maintenance should reach out to the school environment. Transfer activities in the later stages of therapy can focus on specific classes and be used as progressive steps in informing and "training" significant school personnel about stuttering. As therapy shifts to maintenance stages, these persons can be enlisted to function as monitors, evaluators, and speech models. In school or nonschool settings, fear hierarchies can be used more extensively and are particularly applicable to discrete situations and persons in the school. For the same reasons, role play and behavior rehearsal are useful during maintenance as school problems are evaluated and behavioral options explored. Overall, to plan for Group II maintenance the sequences from Group I and Group III can be borrowed and merged as needed.

Group III Maintenance

The Group III stutterer is moving fully in adult stuttering forms of dysfluency, avoidance behaviors, and attitudes. The results of therapy frequently tend to leave a residuum of dysfluency, and relapse probabilities are greater. In referring to adolescent and adult stuttering, the statement has been made that most of the stutterers will not retain fluency always, "but will have small temporary relapses and exhibit stuttering from time to time." (SFA 16, 1980, p.46). In the most recent SFA publication (21, 1987), a self-guide for adolescent stutterers, the emphasis spread across several chapters is that there is no "cure" for stuttering. While more or less total fluency can occur, and even not relapse, cures are beyond our capacities or ethics to promise.

A significant factor in maintenance stability and the possibilities for future improvement may rest less on the fluency or symptom techniques, more on the attitude and adjustment factors of the client. Evesham and Huddleston (1983) have reported on a carefully designed program to establish and maintain fluency, combining various elements of conversational rate control and prolonged speech during an intensive residential program. Therapy then went to weekly group sessions (ten), biweekly sessions (four), and monthly meetings (six). As fluency was established elements of Fransella's (1972) adaptations of personal construct therapy were used to change client attitudes and feelings. Out-clinic transfer practice was initially accompanied by clinicians, then alone or with other stutterers. Group sessions were used to role play, evaluate, and plan. During the maintenance phase, skills refinement, problem solving, and attitude sharing were stressed. The authors reported that posttherapy fluency, assessed for 18 months with some clients, was stable and that the stutterers functioned well as communicators. Subsequently, Evesham and Fransella (1985) compared two groups of stutterers, both of whom received and responded well to fluency reinforcement therapy. One group received more or less standard treatment in refining, transferring, and maintaining their new fluency skills. The second group worked through a personal construct program to help them revise their self-concepts and reconstrue their images to those of fluent persons. During a two-year follow-up period, the construct program group showed a significantly lower occurrence of relapse than did those following standard fluency reinforcement techniques, in spite of the fact that design factors inserted some construct elements into the technique group and altered it from "typical" fluency reinforcement groups. Had this been avoidable, the authors agreed, relapse differences would have been even greater. This significance of psychosocial pressures is emphasized by Rose and McFarlane's (1981) single-case study, where the client, after receiving conversational rate control therapy, charted his fluency/dysfluency each day for about five months after dismissal from therapy. They reported that continued practice on the fluency techniques made the greatest contribution to fluency increases, while situational pressures were most related to dysfluency increases.

The continued-practice aspect of maintenance has been emphasized by Peins, McGeough, and Lee (1984), where they feel the out-clinic design of their double tape recorder therapy program is particularly applicable to maintenance needs. A mixture of personal and practice aspects of maintenance, with emphasis on the former, has been developed recently by Johnson (1987), who presents a maintenance structure termed the ten commandments, which is for self-help by severe or hard-core stutterers. These commandments seem particularly applicable to Group III and adult stutterers. The recommendations cover objective self-analysis, rational thinking, change of philosophy about life, avoiding anticipation, and developing spontaneity and facilitating commitment while reducing procrastination. Other suggestions include physical and mental health procedures, stress on personal independence, and self-talk to maintain a good balance in life. In a poignant comment, Johnson urges the stutterer to avoid the "guru complex," stating that Sheehan, Van Riper, Webster, Schwartz, and other notable clinicians cannot change the stutterer—only the stutterer can do this. Finally, Johnson recommends MAP (acronym for monitoring, action, performance) in which the stutterer takes over and maintains the role of being her or his own therapist. In an interesting application, Johnson suggests that the discussion between the client and clinician, about the commandments, be recorded and the tape cassette given to the stutterer for future replays after dismissal.

The author's preference for Group III therapy is to have each client scheduled individually and also in group therapy. If this is not feasible early in therapy, then I prefer to develop group work later in therapy or, as a last resort, develop a maintenance support group after therapy is terminated. Carlisle (1985) states that stutterers do not like to work in groups, and that this dislike is the reason self-help groups are difficult to form and often fade away. His statement is difficult to verify, but it probably has overtones of truth to it. My experiences with groups resembles Carlisle's comment. Under clinician control and during active therapy, the groups function well. When they convert into support groups during maintenance, especially if they become client run, a measured group life expectancy is usually involved. On the average, most maintenance support groups have an 18-month lifespan, which is not an unprofitable time period and may be a measure of the time lapse before clients no longer feel the need of, or profit from, such groups. In the following sequences, group activity is assumed, but it is not necessary.

1. Individual therapy sessions, through transfer activities, progressively prepare the client for maintenance independence. The fear hierarchy becomes focal in moving progressively from level to level of difficulty. Group sessions draw from members' transfer work, fear hierarchies, and individual problems. Role play and rehearsal, cross-evaluation, and response alternatives can be stressed.

2. When fluency criteria have been stable for 10–12 sessions, an individual client drops to biweekly individual and weekly group sessions. Clients can vary in their schedules, and those on reduced schedules become incentive or goal models for those lagging behind.

3. When biweekly individual sessions have been stable for six consecutive sessions, drop to monthly individual sessions. Group sessions remain weekly

for one more month, and then drop to biweekly for the next two months. Out-of-phase clients can, if needed, receive increased individual sessions.

4. After the third month, terminate individual sessions, with renewal options at the discretion of the client. With the group, establish a frequency schedule to cover six months of group sessions. The clinician remains as group moderator and stimulus, but provides wide latitude for group self-governance and activity.

During the final step, the relapse possibilities are greatest and the clinician will watch the speech and behavior of each client. In particular, early drop-outs and those who stop talking in group sessions can be contacted individually to determine if renewed work is needed (or will be accepted).

Aids to maintenance of Group III stutterers vary with the environment, the clients, and the possibilities of group interaction. The following items are some, but not all, factors that can be considered in preparing for and carrying out maintenance programs:

1. **Altering Response to Stimuli**—identification of stimuli most likely to precipitate stuttering, and deliberately practicing and rehearsing alternate responses. Slowing rate, relaxing, easy speech, initiation of monitoring procedures, establishment of eye contact, use of preparatory sets, and so on, are ways in which responses can be varied. In a similar vein, the occurrences of dysfluency can be used as a stimulus to trigger monitoring, fluency or symptom controls, and other behavioral changes.

2. **Self-Monitoring**—in three applications. The first application is to let the occurrence of dysfluencies become a cue for the client to revert to close monitoring of speech patterns and the environment. The second application is to let predesignated factors operate as cues for pushing the "monitor button." These factors could include specific situations or auditors, feelings of stress, or indicative changes in speech production characteristics. The third application is scheduled monitoring for purposes of self-review. The schedule might be daily, weekly, or monthly, and it can be arranged in various ways, with the purpose of alerting the client to the status of his or her speech.

3. **Consequation**—desired behaviors should produce rewards, and negative behaviors should produce penalties. People vary in how they respond to both aspects. Group I and Group II children more often can be subjected to external control of reward and penalty, but this is more difficult to arrange for Group III adolescents. When self-consequation is involved, there is a question of whether or not the person will regard it seriously and actually view rewards as "rewarding" and penalties as penalizing, since they have made the choices themselves.

4. **Self-Instruction**—this can vary from pep talks to oneself to self-suggestions for relaxation or other behavioral instructions. Instruction can extend its definition also to cover learning more about stuttering and about one's own particular behaviors.

5. **Therapy Review**—during maintenance, and cuts across other areas. Involves selecting elements of past therapy and recreating them for practice purposes. Since the client is usually applying only the most advanced therapy procedures at the time of dismissal, therapy review might involve procedures learned in earlier stages. For instance, extra slow rate, whisper

speech, cancellations, or faking and pullouts might be reviewed. Such activities fight habituation slippage, careless monitoring, and erosion of the client's feelings of self-efficacy.

6. **Relaxation Practice**—review if used earlier in therapy, or taught as maintenance-stage procedure. The cumulative accretions of tension and anxiety can be reduced, and specific relaxation procedures and self-suggestion can be practiced.

7. **Fluency Practice**—whether for FRT or SMT clients. Find fluent-speech situations (reading aloud, talking alone, talking to animals, and so on) where, literally, fluency or controls can be practiced and expanded.

8. **Improve General Speech Abilities**—rate, vocabulary, articulation, phonation, prosody, and so on. Become a better speaker and improve the self-image as a speaker.

9. **Redefine the Fear Hierarchy**—on a periodic basis. This reinforces feelings of self-efficacy as the list is shortened and helps monitor any resurgences of situation fears or avoidance behaviors. It also challenges the stutterers to add items that, originally, were never on the list because they were completely outside the person's range of typical or possible behaviors.

10. **Record Keeping**—tiresome and usually will be dropped if made too demanding. Depending on the client, arrange some type of schedule where there will be a periodic summary of targeted behaviors. If performed faithfully, record keeping provides early warning of regression while the client, alone, can deal with it.

11. **Support Groups**—previously discussed. Local groups can be formed, or the client may join groups such as the National Stuttering Project or the National Council on Stuttering. In these groups, stutterers edit a newsletter and sponsor meetings and workshops about various topics in stuttering.

12. **Aiding and Abetting**—having the stutterer arrange for persons in the environment to monitor specified behaviors and call attention to lapses or errors. Penalties, given or paid or peformed, to/for the monitors can be established. These helpers also, like the client, can become bored with monitoring, so it is wise to rotate them often, alter their listening tasks, and so on.

CHAPTER SUMMARY

The beginning of this chapter emphasized the importance of transfer and maintenance, and the dangers of relapse, in therapy of stuttering. Only in Group I, and partially in Group II, can we reasonably anticipate spontaneous transfer to occur and result in stable fluency or symptom control behavior. At all times, it is wiser to assume that planned transfer and maintenance is required. In the face of this, it is embarrassing to admit that our areas of least knowledge, weakest practice, and fewest benchmark research studies include transfer and maintenance. On the brighter side, our attention finally is focusing on them and it is hoped that the coming decade will see better delineation of useful procedures, reliable criteria, definitions of normal speech and, above all, reduced levels of relapse prevalence.

REFERENCES
AND
BIBLIOGRAPHY

ADAMCZYK, B. (1959). Use of instruments for the production of artificial feedback in the treatment of stuttering. *Folia Phoniatrica* 11:216–18.

ADAMS, M. R. (1984a). Stuttering theory, research, and therapy: A five-year retrospective and look ahead. *Journal of Fluency Disorders* 9:103–13.

ADAMS, M. R. (1984b). The differential assessment and direct treatment of stutterers. In J. Costello (ed.), *Speech Disorders in Children: Recent Advances.* San Diego: College-Hill Press.

ADAMS, M. R. (1983). Learning from negative outcomes in stuttering therapy: I. Getting off on the wrong foot. *Journal of Fluency Disorders* 8:147–53.

ADAMS, M. R. (1982). A case report on the use of flooding in stuttering therapy. *Journal of Fluency Disorders* 7:343–54.

ADAMS, M. R. (1980). The young stutterer: Diagnosis, treatment, and assessment of progress. In W. H. Perkins (ed.), *Strategies in Stuttering Therapy.* Seminars in Speech, Language, and Hearing. New York: Thieme-Stratton.

ADAMS, M. R. (1978). Stuttering theory, research, and therapy: The present and the future. *Journal of Fluency Disorders* 3:139–47.

ADAMS, M. R. (1977). A clinical strategy for differentiating the normally nonfluent child and the incipient stutterer. *Journal of Fluency Disorders* 2:141–48.

ADAMS, M. R. (1972). The use of reciprocal inhibition procedures in the treatment of stuttering. *Journal of Communication Disorders* 5:59–66.

ADAMS, M. R. (1969). Psychological differences between stutterers and non-stutterers: A review of the experimental literature. *Journal of Communication Disorders* 2:163–70.

ADAMS, M. R., & P. HAYDEN (1976). The ability of stutterers and non-stutterers to initiate and terminate phonation during production of an isolated vowel. *Journal of Speech and Hearing Research* 19:290–96.

ADAMS, M. R., & J. HOTCHKISS (1973). Some reflections and responses of stutterers to a miniaturized metronome and metronome conditioning therapy: Three case reports. *Behavior Therapy* 4:565–69.

ADAMS, M. R., J. LEWIS & T. E. BESOZZI (1973). The effect of reduced reading rate on stuttering frequency. *Journal of Speech and Hearing Research* 16:671–75.

ADAMS, M. R., & W. H. MOORE (1972). The effects of auditory masking on the anxiety level, frequency of disfluency, and selected vocal characteristics of stutterers. *Journal of Speech and Hearing Research* 15:572–78.

ADAMS, M. R., & G. POPELKA (1971). The influence of "time out" on stutterers and their disfluency. *Behavior Therapy* 2:734–39.

ADAMS, M. R., & P. RAMIG (1980). Vocal characteristics of normal speakers and stutterers during choral reading. *Journal of Speech and Hearing Research* 23:457–69.

ADAMS, M. R., & R. REIS (1974). Influence of the onset of phonation on the frequency of stuttering: A replication and reevaluation. *Journal of Speech and Hearing Research* 17:752–53.

ADAMS, M. R., & R. REIS (1971). The influence of the onset of phonation on the frequency of stuttering. *Journal of Speech and Hearing Research* 14:639–44.

ADAMS, M. R., S. RIEMENSCHNEIDER, D. METZ & E. CONTURE (1974). Voice onset and articulatory constriction requirements in a speech segment and their relation to the amount of stuttering adaptation. *Journal of Fluency Disorders* 1:23–29.

ADAMS, M. R., & C. RUNYAN (1981). Stuttering and fluency: Exclusive events or points on a continuum? *Journal of Fluency Disorders* 6:197–218.

ADAMS, M. R., C. RUNYAN & A. R. MALLARD (1975). Airflow characteristics of the speech of stutterers and nonstutterers. *Journal of Fluency Disorders* 1:4–12.

ADAMS, M. R., R. L. SEARS & P. R. RAMIG (1982). Vocal changes in stutterers and nonstutterers during monotoned speech. *Journal of Fluency Disorders* 7:21–35.

AINSWORTH, S. (1975). *Stuttering: What It Is and What to Do about It.* Lincoln, Nebr.: Cliff Notes.

AINSWORTH, S., & J. F. GRUSS (1981). *If Your Child Stutters: A Guide for Parents.* Memphis: Speech Foundation of America, no. 11.

ALLAN, F. E., & C. L. WILLIAMS (1974). Interaction patterns of families containing a stuttering sibling. *Australian Journal of Human Disorders of Communication* 2:32–40.

AMMONS, R. & W. JOHNSON (1944). Studies in the psychology of stuttering: 18, the construction and application of a test of attitudes toward stuttering, *Journal of Speech Disorders* 9:39–49.

ANDREWS, G. (1974). The etiology of stuttering. *Australian Journal of Human Communication Disorders* 2:8–12.

ANDREWS, G. (1973). Stuttering therapy: How simple can an effective treatment programme become? *Australian Journal of Human Communication Disorders* 2:44–46.

ANDREWS, G., A. CRAIG, A. FEYER, S. HODDINOTT, P. HOWIE & M. NEILSON (1983). Stuttering: A review of research findings and theories circa 1982. *Journal of Speech and Hearing Disorders* 48:226–46.

ANDREWS, G., & J. CUTLER (1974). Stuttering therapy: The relation between changes in symptom levels and attitudes. *Journal of Speech and Hearing Disorders* 39:309–11.

ANDREWS, G., & M. DOZSA (1977). Haloperidol and the treatment of stuttering. *Journal of Fluency Disorders* 2:217–24.

ANDREWS, G., & M. HARRIS (1964). *The Syndrome of Stuttering.* Clinics in Developmental Medicine, no. 17. London: William Heinemann Medical Books.

ANDREWS, G., M. HARRIS, R. GARSIDE & D. KAY (1964). The inhibition of stuttering by syllable-timed speech. In G. Andrews & M. Harris (eds.), *The Syndrome of Stuttering.* Clinics in Developmental Medicine, no. 17. London: William Heinemann Medical Books.

ANDREWS, G., P. M. HOWIE, M. DOZSA & B. E. GUITAR (1982). Stuttering speech pattern characteristics under fluency inducing conditions. *Journal of Speech and Hearing Research* 25:208–15.

ANDREWS, G., & R. INGHAM (1972). Stuttering: An evaluation of follow-up procedures for syllable-timed speech/token system therapy. *Journal of Communication Disorders* 5:307–19.

ANDREWS, G., & S. TANNER (1982a). Stuttering treatment: An attempt to replicate the regulated breathing method. *Journal of Speech and Hearing Disorders* 47:138–40.

ANDREWS, G., & S. TANNER (1982b). Stuttering: The results of 5 days treatment with the airflow technique. *Journal of Speech and Hearing Disorders* 42:427–29.

ANDRONICO, M. P., & I. BLAKE (1971). The application of filial therapy to young children with stuttering problems. *Journal of Speech and Hearing Disorders* 36:377–81.

ATKINSON, C. J. (1958). Adaptation to delayed sidetone. *Journal of Speech and Hearing Research* 18:386–91.

AVARI, D. N., & O. BLOODSTEIN (1974). Adjacency and prediction in school-age stutterers. *Journal of Speech and Hearing Research* 17:33–40.

AZRIN, N., R. JONES & B. FLYE (1968). A synchronization effect and its application to stuttering by a portable apparatus. *Journal of Applied Behavioral Analysis* 1:283–95.

AZRIN, N. H., & R. G. NUNN (1974). A rapid method of eliminating stuttering by a regulated breathing approach. *Behavioral Research and Therapy* 12:279–86.

AZRIN, N. H., R. G. NUNN & S. FRANTZ (1979). Comparison of regulated breathing versus abbreviated desensitization on reported stuttering episodes. *Journal of Speech and Hearing Disorders* 44:331–39.

BACHRACH, D. L. (1964). Sex differences in reactions to delayed auditory feedback. *Perceptual and Motor Skills* 19:81–82.

BAR, A. (1973). Increasing fluency in young stutterers vs. decreasing stuttering: A clinical approach. *Journal of Communication Disorders* 6:247–58.

BAR, A. (1971). The shaping of fluency, not the modification of stuttering. *Journal of Communication Disorders* 4:1–8.

BARBARA, D. A. (1965a). *New Directions in Stuttering: Theory and Practice.* Springfield, Ill.: Charles C. Thomas.

BARBARA, D. A. (1965b). *Questions and Answers on Stuttering.* Springfield, Ill.: Charles C. Thomas.

BARBARA, D. A. (1962). *The Psychotherapy of Stuttering.* Springfield, Ill.: Charles C. Thomas.

BARBARA, D. A. (1954). *Stuttering: A Psychodynamic Approach to Its Understanding and Treatment.* New York: Julian Press.

BARBER, V. (1940). Studies in the psychology of stuttering: XVI. Rhythm as a distraction in stuttering. *Journal of Speech Disorders* 5:29–42.

BARBER, V. (1939). Studies in the psychology of stuttering: XV. Chorus reading as distraction in stuttering. *Journal of Speech Disorders* 4:371–83.

BEAUMONT, J., & B. FOSS (1957). Individual differences in reacting to delayed auditory feedback. *British Journal of Psychology* 48:85–89.

BEECH, R., & F. FRANSELLA (1969). Explanation of the rhythm effect in stuttering. In B. Gary & G. England (eds.), *Stuttering and the Conditioning Therapies.* Monterey, Calif.: Monterey Institute of Speech and Hearing.

BEECH, R., & F. FRANSELLA (1968). *Research and Experiment in Stuttering.* London: Pergamon Press.

BERECZ, J. M. (1973). The treatment of stuttering through precision punishment and cognitive arousal. *Journal of Speech and Hearing Disorders* 38:256–67.

BERLIN, S., & L. BERLIN (1964). Acceptability of stuttering and control patterns. *Journal of Speech and Hearing Disorders* 29:436–41.

BERNSTEIN, N. (1981). Are there constraints on childhood disfluency? *Journal of Fluency Disorders* 6:341–50.

BERRY, M. F. (1938). A common denominator in twinning and stuttering. *Journal of Speech Disorders* 3:51–57.

BERRY, R. C., & F. H. SILVERMAN (1972). Equality of intervals on the Lewis-Sherman scale of stuttering severity. *Journal of Speech and Hearing Research* 15:185–88.

BERWICK, N. H. (1955). Stuttering in response to photographs of selected listeners. In W. Johnson & R. Leutenegger (eds.), *Stuttering in Children and Adults.* Minneapolis: University of Minnesota Press.

BESOZZI, T. E., & M. R. ADAMS (1969). The influence of prosody on stuttering adaptation. *Journal of Speech and Hearing Research* 12:818–24.

BIGGS, B., & J. SHEEHAN (1969). Punishment or distraction? Operant stuttering revisited. *Journal of Abnormal Psychology* 74:256–62.

BLACK, J. W. (1951). The effect of sidetone delay upon vocal rate and intensity. *Journal of Speech and Hearing Disorders* 16:50–56.

BLANKENSHIP, J. (1964). Stuttering in normal speech. *Journal of Speech and Hearing Research* 7:95–96.

BLOOD, G. W., & S. B. HOOD (1978). Elementary school-aged stutterers' disfluencies during oral reading and spontaneous speech. *Journal of Fluency Disorders* 3:155–65.

BLOOD, G. W., & R. SEIDER (1981). The concomitant problems of young stutterers. *Journal of Speech and Hearing Disorders* 46:31–33.

BLOODSTEIN, O. (1986). Semantics and beliefs. In G. H. Shames & H. Rubin (eds.), *Stuttering Then and Now*. Columbus, Ohio: Charles E. Merrill.

BLOODSTEIN, O. (1979). *Speech Pathology: An Introduction*. Boston: Houghton-Mifflin.

BLOODSTEIN, O. (1975). Stuttering as tension and fragmentation. In J. Eisenson (ed.), *Stuttering: A Second Symposium*. New York: Harper & Row.

BLOODSTEIN, O. (1974). The rules of early stuttering. *Journal of Speech and Hearing Disorders* 39:379–94.

BLOODSTEIN, O. (1969). *A Handbook on Stuttering*. Chicago: National Easter Seal Society for Crippled Children and Adults.

BLOODSTEIN, O. (1961a). The development of stuttering: III. Theoretical and clinical implications. *Journal of Speech and Hearing Disorders* 26:67–82.

BLOODSTEIN, O. (1961b). Stuttering in the families of adopted stutterers. *Journal of Speech and Hearing Disorders* 26:395–96.

BLOODSTEIN, O. (1960a). The development of stuttering: I. Changes in nine basic features. *Journal of Speech and Hearing Disorders* 25:219–37.

BLOODSTEIN, O. (1960b). The development of stuttering: II. Developmental phases. *Journal of Speech and Hearing Disorders* 25:366–76.

BLOODSTEIN, O. (1958). Stuttering as an anticipatory struggle reaction. In J. Eisenson (ed.), *Stuttering: A Symposium*. New York: Harper.

BLOODSTEIN, O. (1950). A rating scale of conditions under which stuttering is reduced or absent. *Journal of Speech and Hearing Disorders* 15:29–36.

BLOODSTEIN, O. (1949). Conditions under which stuttering is reduced or absent: A review of literature. *Journal of Speech and Hearing Disorders* 14:295–302.

BLOODSTEIN, O., & B.F. GANTWERK (1967). Grammatical function in relation to stuttering in young children. *Journal of Speech and Hearing Research* 10:786–89.

BLOODSTEIN, O., & M. GROSSMAN (1981). Early stutterings: Some aspects of their form and distribution. *Journal of Speech and Hearing Research* 24:298–302.

BLUEMEL, C. S. (1960). Concepts of stammering: A century in review. *Journal of Speech and Hearing Disorders* 25:24–32.

BLUEMEL, C. S. (1957). *The Riddle of Stuttering*. Danville, Ill.: The Interstate.

BLUEMEL, C. S. (1935). *Stammering and Allied Disorders*, New York: Macmillan.

BLUEMEL, C. S. (1932). Primary and secondary stammering. *Quarterly Journal of Speech* 18:187–200.

BOBERG, E. (1981). *Maintenance of Fluency*. New York: Elsevier.

BOBERG, E. (1980). Intensive adult therapy program. In W. H. Perkins (ed.), *Strategies in Stuttering Therapy*. Seminars in Speech, Language, and Hearing. New York: Thieme-Stratton.

BOBERG, E., P. HOWIE & L. WOODS (1979). Maintenance of fluency: A review. *Journal of Fluency Disorders* 4:93–116.

BOBERG, E., Behavioral transfer and maintenance programs for adolescent and adult stutterers. In *Stuttering Therapy, Transfer and Maintenance*. Memphis: Speech Foundation of America, no. 19.

BOEHMLER, R. M. (1958). Listener responses to non-fluencies. *Journal of Speech and Hearing Research* 1:132–41.

BOLAND, J. L. (1953). A comparison of stutterers and non-stutterers on several measures of anxiety. *Speech Monographs* 20:144.

BOLAND, J. L. (1951). Type of birth as related to stuttering. *Journal of Speech and Hearing Disorders* 16:320–26.

BONIN, B., P. RAMIG & T. PRESCOTT (1985). Performance differences between stuttering and nonstuttering subjects on a sound fusion task. *Journal of Fluency Disorders* 10:291–300.

BOOME, E. J., & M. A. RICHARDSON (1939). *The Nature and Treatment of Stammering*. London: Methuen.

BOUDREAU, L. A., & C. L. JEFFREY (1973). Stuttering treated by desensitization. *Journal of Behavior Therapy and Experimental Psychiatry* 4:209–12.

BOURDON, K. H., & D. SILBER (1970). Perceived parental behavior among stutterers and non-stutterers. *Journal of Abnormal Psychology* 75:93–97.

BRADFORD, D. (1963). Studies in tachyphemia: VII. A framework of therapeusis for articulation therapy with tachyphemia and/or general language disability. *Logos* 6:59–65.

BRADY, J. P. (1973). Metronome-conditioned relaxation: A new behavioral procedure. *British Journal of Psychiatry* 122:729–30.

BRADY, J. P. (1971). Metronome-conditioned speech retraining for stuttering. *Behavior Therapy* 2:129–50.

BRADY, J. P. (1968). A behavioral approach to the treatment of stuttering. *American Journal of Psychiatry* 125:843–48.

BRADY, J. P., & C. N. BRADY (1972). Behavior therapy of stuttering. *Folia Phoniatrica* 24:355–59.

BRADY, W., & D. HALL (1976). The prevalence of stuttering among school-age children. *Language, Speech, and Hearing Services in Schools* 7:75–81.

BRANDON, S., & M. HARRIS (1967). Stammering—an experimental treatment programme using syllable-timed speech. *British Journal of Disorders of Communication* 2:64–68.

BRAYTON, E. R., & E. G. CONTURE (1978). Effects of noise and rhythmic stimulation on the speech of stutterers. *Journal of Speech and Hearing Research* 21:25–34.

BROKAW, S.P., S. SINGH & J. W. BLACK (1966). The duration of speech in conditions of delayed sidetone. *Speech Monographs* 33:452–55.

BROWN, J. K. (1985). Dysarthria in children: Neurologic perspective. In J. K. Darley (ed.), *Speech and Language Evaluation in Neurology: Childhood Disorders*. New York: Grune & Stratton.

BROWN, S. (1938). Stuttering with relation to word accent and word position. *Journal of Abnormal and Social Psychology* 33:112–20.

BROWN, S. (1937). The influence of grammatical function on the incidence of stuttering. *Journal of Speech Disorders* 2:207–15.

BRUNDAGE, S. B., & N. B. RATNER (1987). Three predictors of stuttering frequency. Paper presented at convention of the American Speech and Hearing Association, New Orleans.

BRUTTEN, E. J. & B. B. GRAY (1961). Effect of a word cue removal on adaptation and adjacency: A clinical paradigm. *Journal of Speech and Hearing Disorders* 26:385–89.

BRUTTEN, G. J. (1986). Two-factor behavior theory and therapy. In G.H. Shames & H. Rubin (eds.), *Stuttering Then and Now*. Columbus, Ohio: Charles E. Merrill.

BRUTTEN, G. J. (1980). The effect of punishment on a factor I stuttering behavior. *Journal of Fluency Disorders* 5:77–85.

BRUTTEN, G. J. (1963). Palmar sweat investigation of disfluency and expectancy adaptation. *Journal of Speech and Hearing Research* 6:40–48.

BRUTTEN, G. J., & M. N. HEGDE (1984) Stuttering: A clinical related overview. In S. Dickson (ed.), *Communication Disorders: Remedial Principles and Practices*. 2d ed. Dallas: Scott, Foresman.

BRUTTEN, G. J., & D. J. SHOEMAKER (1967). *The Modification of Stuttering*. Englewood Cliffs, N.J.: Prentice Hall.

BRYNGELSON, B. (1966). *Clinical Group Therapy for Problem People: A Practical Treatise for Stutterers and Normal Speakers*. Minneapolis: T. S. Denison.

BRYNGELSON, B. (1935). Sidedness as an etiological factor in stuttering. *Journal of Genetic Psychology* 47:205–17.

BRYNGELSON, B., M. CHAPMAN & O. HANSEN (1944). *Know Yourself: A Guide for Those Who Stutter*. Minneapolis: Burgess Publishing.

BRYNGELSON, B., & B. RUTHERFORD (1937). Comparative study of laterality of stutterers and non-stutterers. *Journal of Speech Disorders* 2:15–16.

BURGRAFF, R. I. (1974). The efficacy of systematic desensitization via imagery as a therapeutic technique with stutterers. *British Journal of Disorders of Communication* 9:134–39.

BURKE, B. D. (1975). Susceptibility to delayed auditory feedback and dependence on auditory or oral sensory feedback. *Journal of Communication Disorders* 8:75–96.

BURKE, B. D. (1975). Variables affecting stutterers' initial reactions to delayed auditory feedback. *Journal of Communication Disorders* 8:141–55.

BURLEY, P. M., & R. MORLEY (1987). Self-monitoring processes in stutterers. *Journal of Fluency Disorders* 12:71–78.

BURR, H. G., & J. M. MULLENDORE (1960.). Recent investigations on tranquilizers and stuttering. *Journal of Speech and Hearing Disorders* 25:33–38.

BUTANY, V., & E. PERSED (1982). Is stuttering a contraindication to psychotherapy? *Canadian Journal of Psychiatry* 27:330–31.

CANTER, G. J. (1971). Observations on neurogenic stuttering: A contribution to differential diagnosis. *British Journal of Disorders of Communication* 6:139–43.

CANTRELL, J., R. E. HAM & D. FUCCI (1984). Further evaluation of self and peer judgments of speech during delayed auditory feedback. *Journal of Fluency Disorders* 9:125–29.

CARLISLE, J. A. (1985). *Tangled Tongue: Living with a Stutterer*. Toronto: University of Toronto Press.

CAUGHLEY, N. (1961). Group therapy in the speech clinic: The pros and cons. *New Zealand Speech Therapist Journal* 16:24–27.

CECCONI, C. P., S. B. HOOD & R. K. TUCKER (1977). Influence of reading level difficulty on the disfluencies of normal children. *Journal of Speech and Hearing Research* 20:475–84.

CHAPMAN, M. E. (1959). *Self Inventory: Group Therapy for Those Who Stutter*. Minneapolis: Burgess.

CHASE, R. A. (1958). Effect of delayed auditory feedback on the repetition of speech sounds. *Journal of Speech and Hearing Disorders* 23:583–90.

CHASE, R. A., S. SUTTON, D. FIRST & J. ZUBIN (1961). A developmental study of changes in behavior under delayed auditory feedback. *Journal of Genetic Psychology* 99:101–12.

CHASE, R. A., S. SUTTON & I. RAPIN (1961). Sensory influences on motor performances. *Journal of Auditory Research* 3:212–23.

CHEASMAN, C. (1983). Therapy for adults: An evaluation of current techniques for establishing fluency. In P. Dalton (ed.), *Approaches to the Treatment of Stuttering*. London: Croom Helm.

CHERRY, E. C. (1957). *On Human Communication*. Cambridge, Mass.: MIT Press.

CHERRY, E. C. (1953). Some experiments on the recognition of speech, with one and two ears. *Journal of the Acoustical Society of America* 25:975–79.

CHERRY, E. C., & B. SAYERS (1956). Experiments upon the total inhibition of stammering by external control, and some clinical results. *Journal of Psychosomatic Research* 1:233–46.

CHERRY, E. C., B. M. SAYERS & P. MARLAND (1955). Experiments on the complete suppression of stammering. *Nature* 176:874–75.

CIMORELL-STRONG, J. M., H. R. GILBERT & J. V. FRICK (1983). Dichotic speech perception: A comparison between stuttering and non-stuttering children. *Journal of Fluency Disorders* 8:77–91.

CODE, C., & D. MULLER (1980). Comments on "The Long Term Use of an Automatically Triggered Auditory Feedback Masking Device in the Treatment of Stammering." *British Journal of Disorders of Communication* 14:212–29.

COHEN, E. (1953). A comparison of oral and spontaneous speech of stutterers with special reference to the adaptation and consistency effects. *Speech Monographs* 20:144–45.

COHEN, L. R., P. F. THOMPSON, R. W. RUPPEL & R. P. FLAHERTY (1974). Assertive training: An adjunct to fluency shaping. *Journal of Fluency Disorders* 1:10–25.

COLCORD, R. D., & M. R. ADAMS (1979). Voicing duration and vocal SPL changes associated with stuttering reduction during singing. *Journal of Speech and Hearing Research* 22:468–79.

COMMODORE, R. W., & E. B. COOPER (1978). Communicative stress and stuttering frequency during normal, whispered, and articulation-without-phonation speech modes. *Journal of Fluency Disorders* 3:1–12.

CONTURE, E. G. (1982). *Stuttering*. Englewood Cliffs, N.J.: Prentice Hall.

CONTURE, E. G. (1974). Some effects of noise on the speaking behavior of stutterers. *Journal of Speech and Hearing Research* 17:714–23.

CONTURE, E. G., & E. V. NAERSSEN (1977). Reading abilities of school-age stutterers. *Journal of Fluency Disorders* 2:295–300.

COOPER, E. B. (1987). The chronic perseverative stuttering syndrome: Incurable stuttering. *Journal of Fluency Disorders* 12:381–89.

COOPER, E. B. (1984). Personalized fluency control therapy: A status report. In. M. Peins (ed.), *Contemporary Approaches in Stuttering Therapy*. Boston: Little, Brown.

COOPER, E. B. (1982). A disfluency descriptor digest for clinical use. *Journal of Fluency Disorders* 2:355–58.

COOPER, E. B. (1979). *Understanding Stuttering.* Chicago: National Easter Seal Society.

COOPER, E. B (1977). Controversies about stuttering therapy. *Journal of Fluency Disorders* 2:75–86.

COOPER, E. B. (1976). *Personalized Fluency Control Therapy: An Integrated Behaviour and Relationship Therapy for Stutterers.* Austin, Tex.: Learning Concepts.

COOPER, E. B. (1971a). Integrating behavior therapy and traditional insight treatment procedures with stutterers. *Journal of Communication Disorders* 4:40–43.

COOPER, E. B. (1971b). Reflections on conceptualizing the stuttering therapy process from a single theoretical framework. *Journal of Speech and Hearing Disorders* 36:471–75.

COOPER, E. B. (1971c). Structuring counseling for the parent of the stuttering child. *Journal of the American Speech and Hearing Association* 1:17–22.

COOPER, E. B. (1965). Structuring therapy for the therapist and stuttering child. *Journal of Speech and Hearing Disorders* 30:75–78.

COOPER, E. B., B. B. CADY & C. J. ROBBINS (1970). The effect of the verbal stimulus words *wrong, right* and *tree* on the disfluency rates of stutterers and nonstutterers. *Journal of Speech and Hearing Research* 13:239–44.

COOPER, E. B., & C. S. COOPER (1985). Clinician attitudes toward stuttering: A decade of change (1973–1983). *Journal of Fluency Disorders* 10:19–33.

COOPER, E. B., & C. S. COOPER (1980). *Personalized Fluency Control Therapy: IEP Forms.* Hingham, Mass.: Teaching Resources.

COOPER, E. B., & C. S. COOPER (1976). *Personalized Fluency Control Therapy Kit.* Hingham, Mass.: Teaching Resources.

COOPER, M. H., & G. D. ALLEN (1977). Timing control accuracy in normal speakers and stutterers. *Journal of Speech and Hearing Research* 20:55–71.

COPPA, A., & A. BAR (1974). Use of questions to elicit adaptation in the spontaneous speech of stutterers and non-stutterers. *Folia Phoniatrica* 26:378–88.

CORIAT, I. H. (1943). The psychoanalytic concept of stammering. *Nervous Child* 2:167–71.

CORCORAN, J. A. (1980). Effects of neutral and positive stimuli on stuttering: "Calling attention to stuttering." *Journal of Fluency Disorders* 5:99–114.

COSTELLO, J. M. (1983). Current behavior treatments for children. In D. Prins & R. J. Ingham (eds.), *Treatment of Stuttering in Early Childhood: Methods and Issues.* San Diego: College-Hill Press.

COSTELLO, J. M. (1981). Pretreatment assessment of stuttering in young children. *Communicative Disorders: An Audio Journal for Continuing Education.* New York: Grune & Stratton.

COSTELLO, J. M. (1980). Operant conditioning and the treatment of stuttering. In W. H. Perkins (ed.), *Strategies in Stuttering Therapy.* Seminars in Speech, Language, and Hearing. New York: Thieme-Stratton.

COSTELLO, J. M. (1977). Programmed instruction. *Journal of Speech and Hearing Disorders* 43:3–28.

COSTELLO, J. M. (1975). The establishment of fluency with time-out procedures: Three case studies. *Journal of Speech and Hearing Disorders* 40:216–31.

COX, N. J., & K. K. KIDD (1983). Can recovery from stuttering be considered a genetically milder subtype of stuttering? *Behavior Genetics* 13:129–39.

COX, N. J., R. A. SEIDER & K. K. KIDD (1984). Some environmental factors and hypotheses for stuttering in families with several stutterers. *Journal of Speech and Hearing Research* 27:543–48.

CROSS, D. E., & H. L. LUPER (1983). Relation between finger reaction time and voice reaction time in stuttering and nonstuttering children and adults. *Journal of Speech and Hearing Research* 26:356–61.

CROSS, D. E., & H. L. LUPER (1979). Voice reaction time of stuttering and nonstuttering children and adults. *Journal of Fluency Disorders* 4:59–77.

CROSS, D. E., & P. OLSON (1987). Interaction between jaw kinematics and voice onset for stutterers and nonstutterers in a VR task. *Journal of Fluency Disorders* 12:367–80.

CROWE, T. A., & E. B. COOPER (1977). Parental attitudes toward and knowledge of stuttering. *Journal of Communication Disorders* 10:343–57.

CRYSTAL, D. (1980). *Introduction to Language Pathology*. Baltimore: University Park Press.

CULATTA, R. A. (1977). The acquisition of the label "stuttering" by primary level school children. *Journal of Fluency Disorders* 2:29–34.

CULATTA, R. A. (1976). Fluency: The other side of the coin. *Asha* 18:795–99.

CULATTA, R., J. BADER, A. McCASLIN & N. THOMASON (1985). Primary-school stutterers: Have attitudes changed? *Journal of Fluency Disorders* 10:87–91.

CULLEN, J. K., N. FARGO, R. A. CHASE & P. BAKER (1968). The development of auditory feedback monitoring: I. Delayed auditory feedback studies on infant cry. *Journal of Speech and Hearing Research* 11:85–93.

CULLER, M., & F. FREEMAN (1984). Stuttering: The six blind men revisited. *Journal of Fluency Disorders* 19:25–30.

CULLINAN, W. L. (1963). Stability of consistency measures in stuttering. *Journal of Speech and Hearing Research* 6:134–38.

CULP, D. M. (1984). The preschool fluency development program. In M. Peins (ed.), *Contemporary Approaches in Stuttering Therapy*. Boston: Little, Brown.

CURLEE, R. F. (1985). Disorders of fluency. In P. H. Skinner & R. L. Shelton (eds.), *Speech, Language, and Hearing: Normal Processes and Disorders*. 2d ed. New York: John Wiley.

CURLEE, R. F. (1984). Stuttering disorders: An overview. In J. M. Costello (ed.), *Speech Disorders in Children*. San Diego: College-Hill Press.

CURLEE, R. F. (1980). A case selection strategy for young disfluent children. In W. H. Perkins (ed.), *Strategies in Stuttering Therapy*. Seminars in Speech, Language, and Hearing. New York: Thieme-Stratton.

CURLEE, R. F., & W. H. PERKINS (1973). Effectiveness of a DAF conditioning program for adolescent and adult stutterers. *Behavioral Research and Therapy* 1:395–401.

CURLEE, R. F., & W. H. PERKINS (1969). Conversational rate-control therapy for stuttering. *Journal of Speech and Hearing Disorders* 34:245–50.

CURRY, F. K. W., & H. H. GREGORY (1969). The performance of stutterers on dichotic listening tasks thought to reflect cerebral dominance. *Journal of Speech and Hearing Research* 12:73–82.

CURRY, N. E. (1974). Dramatic play as a curricular tool. In D. Spouseller (ed.), *Play as a Learning Medium*. Washington, D.C.: National Association for the Education of Young Children.

DALALI, I. D., & J. G. SHEETS (1974). Stuttering and assertion training. *Journal of Communication Disorders* 7:97–111.

DALTON, P. (1983a). Maintenance of change towards the integration of behavioral and psychological procedures. In P. Dalton (ed.), *Approaches to the Treatment of Stuttering*. London: Croom Helm.

DALTON, P. (1983b). *Approaches to the Treatment of Stuttering*. London: Croom Helm.

DALTON, P. (1983c). Psychological approaches to the treatment of stuttering. In P. Dalton (ed.), *Approaches to the Treatment of Stuttering*. London: Croom Helm.

DALTON, P. (1983d). Major issues for the therapist. In P. Dalton (ed.), *Approaches to the Treatment of Stuttering*. London: Croom Helm.

DALTON, P., & W. J. HARDCASTLE (1977). *Disorders of Fluency and Their Effects on Communication*. London: Edward Arnold.

DALY, D. A. (1987). Use of the home VCR to facilitate transfer of fluency. *Journal of Fluency Disorders* 12:103–106.

DALY, D. A. (1986). The clutterer. In K. O. St. Louis (ed.), *The Atypical Stutterer*. New York: Academic Press.

DALY, D. A., & E. B. COOPER (1967). Rate of stuttering adaptation under two electroshock conditions. *Behavior Research and Therapy* 5:49–54.

DALY, D., & M. KIMBARROW (1978). Stuttering as operant behavior. Effects of the verbal stimuli "wrong," "right," and "tree" on the disfluency rates of school-age stutterers. *Journal of Speech and Hearing Research* 21:589–97.

DANILOFF, R., G. SCHUCKERS & L. FETH (1980). *The Physiology of Speech and Hearing*. Englewood Cliffs, N. J.: Prentice Hall.

DANZGER, M., & H. HALPERN (1973). Relation of stuttering to word abstraction, part of speech, word length, and word frequency. *Perceptual and Motor Skills* 37:959–62.

DARLEY, F. L. (1964). *Diagnosis and Appraisal of Communication Disorders*. Englewood Cliffs, N. J.: Prentice Hall.

DARLEY, F. L., A. E. ARONSON & J. R. BROWN (1975). *Motor Speech Disorders*. Philadelphia: W. B. Saunders.

DEHIRSCH, K. (1970). Stuttering and cluttering. *Folia Phoniatrica* 22:311–24.

DELL, C. W. (1980). *Treating the School Age Stutterer: A Guide for Clinicians*. Memphis: Speech Foundation of America.

DEMPSEY, G. L., & GRANICH, M. (1978). Hypno-behavioral therapy in the case of a traumatic stutterer: A case study. *International Journal of Clinical and Experimental Hypnosis* 26:125–33.

DERAZNE, J. (1966). Speech pathology in the U.S.S.R. In R. Rieber & R. Brubaker (eds.), *Speech Pathology*. Amsterdam: North-Holland.

DEVORE, J. E., M. S. NANDUR & W. H. MANNING (1984). Projective drawings and children who stutter. *Journal of Fluency Disorders* 9:217–26.

DEWAR, A., A. D. DEWAR, & J. F. K. ANTHONY (1976). The effect of auditory feedback masking on concomitant movements of stuttering. *British Journal of Disorders of Communication* 11:95–102.

DEWAR, A., A. D. DEWAR, W. T. S. AUSTIN & H. M. BRASH (1979). The long term use of an automatically triggered auditory feedback masking device in the treatment of stammering. *British Journal of Disorders of Communication* 14:219–30.

DEWAR, A., A. D. DEWAR & H. E. BARNES (1976). Automatic triggering of auditory feedback masking in stammering and stuttering. *British Journal of Disorders of Communication* 11:19–26.

DiCARLO, L., J. KATZ & S. BATKIN (1959). An exploratory investigation of the effect of meprobamate on stuttering behavior. *Journal of Nervous and Mental Diseases* 128:558–61.

DIEDRICH, W. M. (1984). Cluttering: Its diagnosis. In H. Winitz (ed.), *Treating Articulation Disorders: For Clinicians by Clinicians*. Baltimore: University Park Press.

DIJK, M. B. V. (1973). "Distraction" in the treatment of stuttering. In Y. Lebrun & R. Hoops (eds.), *Neurolinguistic Approaches to Stuttering*. The Hague: Mouton.

DOLLARD, J., & N. E. MILLER (1950). *Personality and Psychotherapy*. New York: McGraw-Hill.

DOPHEIDE, B. (1987). Competencies expected of beginning clinicians working with children who stutter. *Journal of Fluency Disorders* 12:157–66.

DUMKE, H. D., G. HEESE, W. KROKER & L. SIEMS (1963). The symptomatology of clutterers. *Folia Phoniatrica* 15:155–69.

DUNCAN, M. H. (1949). Home adjustment of stutterers vs. nonstutterers. *Journal of Speech and Hearing Disorders* 14:255–59.

DUNLAP, K. (1942). The technique of negative practice. *American Journal of Psychology* 55:270–76.

DUNLAP, K. (1932). *Habits: Their Making and Unmaking*. New York: Liveright.

EGLAND, G. O. (1970). *Speech and Language Problems: A Guide for the Classroom Teacher*. Englewood Cliffs, N.J.: Prentice Hall.

EGOLF, D. B., G. H. SHAMES & J. J. BLIND (1971). The combined use of operant procedures and theoretical concepts in the treatment of an adult female stutterer. *Journal of Speech and Hearing Disorders* 36:414–21.

EGOLF, D. B., G. H. SHAMES, P. R. JOHNSON & A. KASPRISIN-BURRELLI (1972). The use of parent-child interaction patterns in therapy for young stutterers. *Journal of Speech and Hearing Disorders* 37:222–32.

EGOLF, D. B., G. H. SHAMES & H. N. SELTZER (1971). The effects of time-out on the fluency of stutterers in group therapy. *Journal of Communication Disorders* 4:111–18.

EISENSON, J. (1975a). Stuttering as perseverative behavior. In J. Eisenson (ed.), *Stuttering: A Second Symposium*. New York: Harper & Row.

EISENSON, J. (ed). (1975b). *Stuttering: A Second Symposium*. New York: Harper & Row.

EISENSON, J. (1958). *Stuttering: A Symposium*. New York: Harper & Row.

EISENSON, J., & C. WELLS (1942). A study of the influence of communicative responsibility in a choral speech situation for stutterers. *Journal of Speech Disorders* 7:259–63.

EISENSON, J., & C. N. WINSLOW (1938). The perseverating tendency in stutterers in a perceptual function. *Journal of Speech Disorders* 3:195–98.

ELDRIDGE, M., & B. K. RANK (1970). *A History of the Treatment of Speech Disorders.* Edinburgh: E. & S. Livingstone, 1968.

EMERICK, L. L. (1970). *Therapy for Young Stutterers,* Danville, Ill.: The Interstate.

EMERICK, L. L. (1963). A clinical observation of the "final" stuttering. *Journal of Speech and Hearing Disorders* 28:194–95.

EMERICK, L. L., & C. E. HAMRE (eds.) (1972). *An Analysis of Stuttering: Selected Readings.* Danville, Ill.: The Interstate.

EMERICK, L. L., & J. T. HATTEN (1979). *Diagnosis and Evaluation in Speech Pathology.* 2d ed. Englewood Cliffs, N. J.: Prentice Hall.

EMERICK, L. L., & E. B. HOOD (1974). *The Client-Clinician Relationship.* Springfield, Ill.: Charles C. Thomas.

ENDERBY, P. E., & R. PHILIPP (1986). Speech and language handicap: Towards knowing the size of the problem. *British Journal of Disorders of Communication* 21:151–65.

ERICKSON, R. L. (1969). Assessing communication attitudes among stutterers. *Journal of Speech and Hearing Research* 12:711–24.

EVESHAM, M., & F. FRANSELLA (1985). Stuttering relapse: The effect of a combined speech and psychological reconstruction programme. *British Journal of Disorders of Communication* 20:237–48.

EVESHAM, M., & A. HUDDLESTON (1983). Teaching stutterers the skill of fluent speech as a preliminary to the study of relapse. *British Journal of Disorders of Communication* 18:31–38.

FAIRBANKS, G. (1954). Systematic research in experimental phonetics: 1. A theory of the speech mechanism as a servosystem. *Journal of Speech and Hearing Disorders* 19:133–39.

FAIRBANKS, G., & N. GUTTMAN (1958). Effects of delayed auditory feedback upon articulation. *Journal of Speech and Hearing Research* 1:12–22.

FALCK, F. J. (1969). *Stuttering: Learned and Unlearned.* Springfield, Ill.: Charles C. Thomas.

FALCK, F. J. (1964). Stuttering and hypnosis. *International Journal of Clinical and Experimental Hypnosis* 12:67–74.

FALCK, F. J., P. S. LAWLER & A. YONOVITZ (1985). Effects of stuttering on fundamental frequency. *Journal of Fluency Disorders* 10:123–35.

FALKOWSKI, G. L., A. M. GUILFORD & J. SANDLER (1982). Effectiveness of a modified version of airflow therapy: Case studies. *Journal of Speech and Hearing Disorders* 47:160–64.

FAWCUS, M. (1970). Intensive treatment and group therapy for the child and adult stammerer. *British Journal of Communication Disorders* 5:59–65.

FENICHEL, O. (1945). *The Psychoanalytic Theory of Neurosis.* New York: W.W. Norton.

FIEDLER, P. A., & R. STANDOP (1983). *Stuttering: Integrating Theory and Practice* (translated by S. R. Silverman). Rockville, Md.: Aspen Systems.

FINKELSTEIN, P., & S. E. WEISBERGER (1954). The motor proficiency of stutterers. *Journal of Speech and Hearing Disorders* 19:52–58.

FITZGERALD, H. E., P. A. COOKE & J. R. GREINER (1984). Speech and bimanual hand organization in adult stutterers and nonstutterers. *Journal of Fluency Disorders* 9:51–65.

FLANAGAN, B. (1986). Operant stuttering update. In G. H. Shames & H. Rubin (eds.), *Stuttering Then and Now.* Columbus, Ohio: Charles E. Merrill.

FLANAGAN, B., I. GOLDIAMOND & N. AZRIN (1958). Operant stuttering: The control of stuttering behavior through response-contingent consequences. *Journal of the Experimental Analysis of Behavior* 1:173–77.

FLETCHER, S. G. (1972). Time-by-count measurement of diadochokokinetic syllable rate. *Journal of Speech and Hearing Research* 15:763–70.

FLORANCE, C. L., & G. H. SHAMES (1980). Stuttering treatment: Issues in transfer and maintenance. In W. H. Perkins (ed.), *Strategies in Stuttering Therapy.* Seminars in Speech, Language, and Hearing. New York: Thieme-Stratton.

FORTE, M., & I. M. SCHLESINGER (1972). Stuttering as a function of time of expectation. *Journal of Communication Disorders* 5:347–58.

FOWLIE, G. M., & E. B. COOPER (1978). Traits attributed to stuttering and non-stuttering children by their mothers. *Journal of Fluency Disorders* 3:233–46.

FOX, D. R. (1966). Electroencephalographic analysis during stuttering and non-stuttering. *Journal of Speech and Hearing Research* 9:488–97.

FRANSELLA, F. (1981). "Nature babling to herself." In H. Bonarius, R. Holland & S. Rosenberg (eds.), *Personal Construct Psychology: Recent Advances in Theory and Practice.* London: Macmillan.

FRANSELLA, F. (1975). Personal construct theory applied to stuttering and measurement of change. *Australian Journal of Human Communication Disorders* 3:6–18.

FRANSELLA, F. (1974a). George Kelly's personal construct theory. *Australian Journal of Human Communication Disorders* 2:62–70.

FRANSELLA, F. (1974b). Personal construct theory applied to stuttering and measurement of change. *Australian Journal of Human Communication Disorders* 2:70–75.

FRANSELLA, F. (1974c). The therapeutic or reconstruction process. *Australian Journal of Human Communication Disorders* 2:76–85.

FRANSELLA, F. (1972). *Personal Change and Reconstruction: Research on a Treatment of Stuttering.* New York: Academic Press.

FRANSELLA, F. (1971). The "rhythm effect" in stuttering as a function of predictability of utterance. *Behavioral Research Therapy.* 9:265–71.

FRANSELLA, F. (1970). Stuttering: Not a symptom but a way of life. *British Journal of Disorders of Communication* 5:22–29.

FRANSELLA, F. (1968). Self-concepts and the stutterer. *British Journal of Psychiatry* 114:1531–35.

FRANSELLA, F., & H. R. BEECH (1965). An experimental analysis of the effect of rhythm on the speech of stutterers. *Behavioral Research and Therapy* 3:195–201.

FRASER, J., & W. H. PERKINS (1987). *Do You Stutter? A Guide for Teens.* Memphis: Speech Foundation of America, no. 21.

FREUND, H. (1966). *Psychotherapy and the Problem of Stuttering.* Springfield, Ill.: Charles C. Thomas.

FREUND, H. (1953). Psychopathological aspects of stuttering. *American Journal of Psychotherapy* 7:689–701.

FRICK, J. V. (1965). Evaluation of motor planning techniques for the treatment of stuttering. Grant no. 32-48-0720-5003. Washington, D.C.: United States Department of Health, Education and Welfare, United States Office of Education, Division of Handicapped Children and Youth.

FRIEDMAN, G. M. (1955). A test of attitude toward stuttering. In W. Johnson (ed.), *Stuttering in Children and Adults.* Minneapolis: University of Minnesota Press, 1955.

FRIEL, J. P. (ed.) (1965). *Dorland's Illustrated Medical Dictionary.* 25th ed. Philadelphia: W. B. Saunders.

FROESCHELS, E. (1962). A survey of European literature in speech and voice pathology. *Journal of the American Speech and Hearing Association* 4:172–81.

FROESCHELS, E. (1952a). Chewing methods as therapy. *Archives of Otolaryngology* 56:427–34.

FROESCHELS, E. (1952b). *Dysarthric Speech.* Magnolia, Mass.: Expression Company.

FROESCHELS, E. (1950). A technique for stutterers—"ventriloquism." *Journal of Speech and Hearing Disorders* 15:336–37.

FROESCHELS, E. (1946). Cluttering. *Journal of Speech Disorders* 11:31–36.

FROESCHELS, E., & A. JELLINEK (1941). *The Practice of Voice and Speech Therapy.* Boston: Expression Company.

FUCCI, D., L. PETROSINO, P. GORMAN & D. HARRIS (1985). Vibrotactile magnitude production scaling: A method for studying sensory-perceptual responses of stutterers and fluent speakers. *Journal of Fluency Disorders* 10:69–75.

GALLOWAY, H. F. (1974). Stuttering and the myth of therapeutic singing. *Journal of Music Therapy* 11:202–207.

GARBEE, F. E. (1985). The speech-language pathologist as a member of the educational team. In R. J. van Hattum (ed.), *Organization of Speech-Language Services in Schools: A Manual* San Diego: College-Hill Press.

GARBER, S. F., & R. R. MARTIN (1977). Effects of noise and increased vocal intensity on stuttering. *Journal of Speech and Hearing Research* 20:233–40.

GARBER, S. F., & R. R. MARTIN (1974). The effects of white noise on the frequency of stuttering. *Journal of Speech and Hearing Research* 17:73–79.

GAUTHERON, B., A. LIORZOU, C. EVEN & B. VALLANCIEU (1972). The role of the larynx in stuttering. In Y. Lebrun & R. Hoops (eds.), *Neurolinguistic Approaches to Stuttering.* Proceedings of the International Symposium on Stuttering. The Hague: Mouton.

GENDELMAN, E. G. (1977). Confrontation in the treatment of stuttering. *Journal of Speech and Hearing Disorders* 42:85–89.

GERSTMAN, H. L. (1983). The concatenation of stuttering to negative behavioral events: A clinical insight. *Journal of Fluency Disorders* 8:168–74.

GIFFORD, M. (1940). *Correcting Nervous Speech Disorders.* New York: Prentice Hall.

GILDSTON, P. (1967). Stutterers' self-acceptance and perceived parental acceptance. *Journal of Abnormal Psychology* 72:59–64.

GILLESPIE, S. K., & E. B. COOPER (1973). Prevalence of speech problems in junior and senior high schools. *Journal of Speech and Hearing Research* 16:739–43.

GLADSTEIN, K. L., R. A. SEIDER & K. K. KIDD (1981). Analysis of the sibship patterns of stutterers. *Journal of Speech and Hearing Research* 24:460–62.

GLAUBER, I. P. (1958). The psychoanalysis of stuttering. In J. Eisenson (ed.) *Stuttering: A Symposium.* New York: Harper & Row.

GOLDIAMOND, I. (1967). Supplementary statement to operant analysis and control of fluent and non-fluent verbal behavior. United States Department of Health, Education and Welfare, Public Health Services, no. M. H. 0887-03.

GOLDIAMOND, I. (1965). Stuttering and fluency as manipulable operant response classes. In L. Krasner & L .P. Ullman (eds.), *Research in Behavior Modification.* New York: Holt, Rinehart & Winston.

GOLDIAMOND, I. (1960). *Effects of delayed feedback upon the temporal development of fluent and blocked speech communication.* Carbondale, Ill.: Southern Illinois University, TR-2 on AFCRC Contract AF 19(604)6127.

GOLDIAMOND, I., C. J. ATKINSON & R. C. BILGER (1962). Stabilization of behavior and prolonged exposure to D.A.F. *Science* 135:437–38.

GOLDMAN-EISLER, F. (1958). The predictability of words in context and the length of pauses in speech. *Language and Speech* 1:266–81.

GOLDMAN, R., & G. H. SHAMES (1964). Comparisons of the goals that parents of stutterers and parents of nonstutterers set for their children. *Journal of Speech and Hearing Disorders* 29:381–89.

GOLDSMITH, L. (1973). Dramatic play in group stuttering therapy. In Y. Lebrun & R. Hoops (eds.), *Neurolinguistic Approaches to Stuttering.* The Hague: Mouton.

GORAJ, J. J. (1974). Stuttering therapy as crisis intervention. *British Journal of Disorders of Communication* 9:51–57.

GORDON, P. (1985). *The relationship of language to the development and treatment of stuttering in preschool children.* Fort Lauderdale, Fla.: FLASHA CEU workshop.

GORDON, P., H.L . LUPER & H. A. PETERSON (1986). The effects of syntactic complexity on the occurrence of disfluencies in 5-year-old nonstutterers. *Journal of Fluency Disorders* 11:151–64.

GOSS, A. E. (1956). Stuttering behavior and anxiety as a function of experimental training. *Journal of Speech and Hearing Disorders* 21:343–51.

GOSS, A. E. (1952). Stuttering behavior and anxiety as a function of the duration of stimulus words. *Journal of Abnormal and Social Psychology.* 47:38–50.

GOTTLOBER, A. B. (1953). *Understanding Stuttering.* New York: Grune & Stratton.

GRAY, B. B., & E. J. BRUTTEN (1965). The relationship between anxiety, fatigue, and spontaneous recovery. *Behavioral Research and Therapy* 2:251–59.

GRAY, B. B., & E. ENGLAND (1972). Some effects of anxiety deconditioning upon stuttering. *Journal of Speech and Hearing Research* 15:114–22.

GRAY, B. B., & E. ENGLAND (1969). *Stuttering and the Conditioning Therapies.* Monterey, Calif.: Monterey Institute of Speech and Hearing.

GRAY, B. B., & J. L. KARMEN (1967). The relationship between non-verbal anxiety and stuttering adaptation. *Journal of Communication Disorders* 1:141–51.

GRAY, M. (1940). The "X" family: A clinical and laboratory study of a "stuttering" family. *Journal of Speech Disorders* 5:343–48.

GREGORY, H. H. (ed.) (1986). *Stuttering Therapy: Prevention and Intervention with Children.* Memphis, Tenn.: Speech Foundation of America, no. 20.

GREGORY, H. H. (ed.) (1979). *Controversies about Stuttering Therapy.* Baltimore: University Park Press.

GREGORY, H. H. (1973). *Stuttering: Differential Evaluation and Therapy.* Indianapolis: Bobbs-Merrill.

GREGORY, H. H. (1968). *Learning Theory and Stuttering Therapy*. Evanston, Ill.: Northwestern University Press.

GREGORY, H. H., & D. HILL (1984). Stuttering therapy for children. In W. H. Perkins (ed.), *Current Therapy of Communication Disorders, Stuttering Disorders*. New York: Thieme-Stratton.

GREGORY, H. H., & D. HILL (1980). Stuttering therapy for children. In W. H. Perkins (ed.), *Strategies in Stuttering Therapy*. Seminars in Speech, Language, and Hearing. New York: Thieme-Stratton.

GREGORY, J. F., T. SHANAHAN & H. WALBERG (1985). A descriptive analysis of high school seniors with speech disabilities. *Journal of Communication Disorders* 18:295–304.

GREINER, J. R., H. E. FITZGERALD, P. A. COOKE & S. D. DJURDJIC (1985). Assessment of sensitivity to interpersonal stress in stutterers and nonstutterers. *Journal of Communication Disorders* 18:215–25.

GRONHOVD, K. D. (1977). A comparison of the fluent and reading rates of stutterers and nonstutterers. *Journal of Fluency Disorders* 2:247–52.

GRONHOVD, K. D., & A. A. ZENNER (1982). Anxiety in stutterers: Rationale and procedures for management. In N. J. Lass (ed.), *Speech and Language Advances in Basic Research and Practice*. New York: Academic Press.

GRUBER, L. (1971). The use of the portable voice masker in stuttering therapy. *Journal of Speech and Hearing Disorders* 36:287–89.

GRUBER, L., & R. L. POWELL (1974). Responses of stuttering and nonstuttering children to a dichotic listening task. *Perceptual and Motor Skills* 28:203–204.

GUERNEY, B., JR. (1964). Filial therapy: Description and rationale. *Journal of Consulting Psychology* 28:303–10.

GUITAR, B. (1984). Indirect treatment of stuttering. In J. Costello (ed.), *Speech Disorders in Children: Recent Advances*. San Diego: College-Hill Press.

GUITAR, B. (1976). Pretreatment factors associated with the outcome of stuttering therapy. *Journal of Speech and Hearing Research* 19:590–600.

GUITAR, B. (1975). Reduction of stuttering frequency using analog electromyographic feedback. *Journal of Speech and Hearing Research* 18:672–85.

GUITAR, B., & C. BASS (1978). Stuttering therapy: The relation between attitude change and long-term outcome. *Journal of Speech and Hearing Disorders* 43:393–400.

GUITAR, B., & S. GRIMS (1977). Developing a scale to assess communication attitudes in children who stutter. Atlanta: Annual convention of the American Speech, Language, and Hearing Association.

GUITAR, B., & T. PETERS (eds.) (1980). Comparison of stuttering modification and fluency shaping therapies. In *Stuttering: An Integration of Contemporary Theories*. Memphis: Speech Foundation of America, no. 16.

HALL, P. K. (1977). The occurrence of disfluencies in language disordered school-age children. *Journal of Speech and Hearing Disorders* 42:364–69.

HAM, R. E. (1988). Unison speech and rate control therapy. *Journal of Fluency Disorders*. In press.

HAM, R. E. (1986). *Techniques of Stuttering Therapy*. Englewood Cliffs, N. J.: Prentice Hall.

HAM, R. E., J. CANTRELL & D. FUCCI, (1984). Experience and motivation in two types of speech during delayed auditory feedback. *Journal of Fluency Disorders* 9:3–10.

HAM, R. E., D. FUCCI & J. CANTRELL (1984a). The effects of temporal delay and frequency alterations on the speaking rates of children. *Bulletin of the Psychonomic Society* 22:418–20.

HAM, R. E., D. FUCCI & J. CANTRELL (1984b). Residual effects on speech after exposure to delayed auditory feedback. *Perceptual and Motor Skills* 59:61–62.

HAM, R. E., & A. HOLBROOK (1986). Oral/manual reaction times and delayed auditory feedback disturbances among normally speaking females. *Journal of Fluency Disorders* 11:117–29.

HAM, R. E., & M. D. STEER (1967). Certain effects of alterations in auditory feedback. *Folia Phoniatrica* 19:53–62.

HAMRE, C. E. (1972). A comment on the possible organicity of stuttering. *British Journal of Disorders of Communication* 7:148–50.

HAMRE, C. E., & M. E. WINGATE (1973). Stuttering consistency in varied contexts. *Journal of Speech and Hearing Research* 16:238–47.

HAMRE, C. E., & M. E. WINGATE (1967). Pyknolepsy and stuttering. *Quarterly Journal of Speech* 53:374–77.

HANLEY, J. M. (1986). Speech motor processes and stuttering in children: A theoretical and clinical perspective. In H. H. Gregory (ed.), *Stuttering Therapy: Prevention and Intervention with Children.* Memphis: Speech Foundation of America, no. 20.

HANNA, R., & N. OWEN (1977). Facilitating transfer and maintenance of fluency in stuttering therapy. *Journal of Speech and Hearing Disorders* 42:65–76.

HANNA, R., F. WILFING & B. MCNEILL (1975). A biofeedback treatment for stuttering. *Journal of Speech and Hearing Disorders* 40:27–73.

HANNAHM, E. P., & J. G. GARDNER (1968). A note of syntactic relationships in nonfluency. *Journal of Speech and Hearing Research* 11:853–60.

HANNLEY, M. & M. F. DORMAN (1982). Some observations on auditory function and stuttering. *Journal of Fluency Disorders* 7:93–108.

HAROLDSON, S. K., R. MARTIN & C. D. STARR (1968). Time-out as a punishment for stuttering. *Journal of Speech and Hearing Research* 11:560–66.

HARRIS, R. D. (1977). The speech pathologist as counselor. *Australian Journal of Human Communication Disorders* 5:72–78.

HASBROUCK, J. M., J. DOHERTY, M. A. MEHLMANN, R. NELSON, B. RANDLE & R. WHITAKER (1987). Intensive stuttering therapy in a public school setting. *Language, Speech, and Hearing Services in School* 18:330–43.

HAYDEN, P. A., M. R. ADAMS & N. JORDAHL (1982). The effects of pacing and masking on stutterers' and nonstutterers' speech initiation times. *Journal of Fluency Disorders* 7:9–19.

HAYNES, W. O., & S. B. HOOD (1977). Language and disfluency variables in normal speaking children from discrete chronological age groups. *Journal of Fluency Disorders* 2:57–74.

HEALEY, E. C., & M.R. ADAMS (1981). Rate reduction strategies used by normally fluent and stuttering children and adults. *Journal of Fluency Disorders* 6:1–14.

HEALEY, E. C., A. R. MALLARD III & M. R. ADAMS (1976). Factors contributing to the reduction of stuttering during singing. *Journal of Speech and Hearing Research* 19:475–80.

HELMREICH, H. G., & O. BLOODSTEIN (1973). The grammatical factor in childhood disfluency in relation to the continuity hypothesis. *Journal of Speech and Hearing Research* 16:731–38.

HELPS, R., & P. DALTON (1979). The effectiveness of an intensive group speech therapy programme for adult stammerers. *British Journal of Disorders of Communication* 14:17–30.

HENDEL, O., & O. BLOODSTEIN (1973). Consistency in relation to intersubject congruity in the loci of stuttering. *Journal of Communication Disorders* 6:37–43.

HIGGINS, R. L., M. B. FRISCH, & D. SMITH (1983). A comparison of role-played and neutral responses to identical circumstances. *Behavior Therapy* 14:159–69.

HILL, H. (1944a). Stuttering I: A critical review and evaluation of biochemical evaluations. *Journal of Speech Disorders* 9:245–61.

HILL, H. (1944b). Stuttering II: A review and integration of physiological data. *Journal of Speech Disorders* 9:289–324.

HIXON, T. J. (1973). Respiratory function in speech. In F. J. Minifie, T. J. Hixon & F. Williams (eds.), *Normal Aspects of Speech, Hearing and Language.* Englewood Cliffs, N. J.: Prentice Hall.

HOERR, N. L., & A. OSOL (eds.) (1956). *Blakiston's New Gould Medical Dictionary.* New York: McGraw-Hill.

HOLBROOK, A, & R. E. HAM (1988). Speaker self-confidence and performance during delayed auditory feedback. Tallahassee, Fla.: Florida State University, unpublished research.

HOLGATE, D. (1967). Comments on the electronic metronome in the treatment of stuttering. *Journal of the Australian College of Speech Therapists* 17:67–68.

HOLLIDAY, A. (1959). Effect of meprobamate on stuttering. *Northwest Medicine* 58:837–41.

HOLLINGSWORTH, H. L. (1939). Chewing as a technique of relaxation. *Science* 90:385–87.

HOLZ, W., & N. AZRIN (1966). Operant behavior. In W. Honig (ed.), *Operant Behavior: Areas of Research and Application.* New York: Appleton-Century-Crofts.

HOMZIE, M. J., & J. S. LINDSAY (1984). Language and the young stutterer: A new look at old theories and findings. *Brain and Language* 22:232–52.

HONIG, P. (1947). The stutterer acts it out. *Journal of Speech and Hearing Disorders* 12:105–9.

HOOD, S. B. (1978). The assessment of fluency disorders. In S. Singh & J. Lynch (eds.), *Diagnostic Procedures in Hearing, Language, and Speech.* Baltimore: University Park Press.

HOOD, S. B. (1974). Clinical assessment of the moment of stuttering. *Journal of Fluency Disorders* 1:22–34.

HOOD, S. B. (1973). Integration of directive and non-directive therapies for adults who stutter. *Ohio Journal of Speech and Hearing* 8:28–35.

HOROWITZ, M. W. (1965). Fluency: An appraisal and a research approach. *Journal of Communication* 15:4–13.

HORSLEY, I. A., & C. T. FITZGIBBON (1987). Stuttering children: Investigation of a stereotype. *British Journal of Disorders of Communication* 22:19–35.

HOWIE, P. M. (1981a). Concordance for stuttering in monozygotic and dyzygotic twin pairs. *Journal of Speech and Hearing Research* 24:317–21.

HOWIE, P. M. (1981b). Intrapair similarity in frequency of disfluency in monozygotic and dyzygotic twin pairs containing stutterers. *Behavioral Genetics* 1:227–38.

HOWIE, P. M. (1976). The identification of genetic components in speech disorders. *Australian Journal of Human Communication Disorders* 4:155–63.

HULL, C. L. (1951). *Essentials of Behavior.* New Haven: Yale University Press.

HUTCHINSON, J. M. (1983). Diagnosis of fluency disorders. In I. J. Meitus & B. Weinberg (eds.), *Diagnosis in Speech-Language Pathology.* Baltimore: University Park Press.

HUTCHINSON, J. M. (1976). A review of rhythmic pacing as a treatment strategy for stuttering. *Rehabilitation Literature* 37:297–303.

HUTCHINSON, J. M., & K. W. BURKE (1973). An investigation of the effects of temporal alterations in the auditory feedback upon stutterers and clutterers. *Journal of Communication Disorders* 6:193–205.

HUTCHINSON, J. M., & B. M. NAVARRE (1977). The effect of metronome pacing on selected aerodynamic patterns of stuttered speech. *Journal of Fluency Disorders* 2:189–204.

HUTCHINSON, J. M., & R. I. RINGEL (1975). The effect of oral sensory deprivation on stuttering behavior. *Journal of Communication Disorders* 8:249–58.

ICKES, W. K., & PIERCE, S. (1973). The stuttering moment: A plethysmographic study. *Journal of Communication Disorders* 6:155–64.

INGHAM, R. J. (1984). *Stuttering and Behavior Therapy.* San Diego: College-Hill Press.

INGHAM, R. J. (1982). The effects of self-evaluation training on maintenance and generalization during stuttering treatment. *Journal of Speech and Hearing Disorders* 47:271–80.

INGHAM, R. J. (1980). Modification of maintenance and generalization during stuttering treatment. *Journal of Speech and Hearing Research* 23:732–45.

INGHAM, R. J. (1979a). Evaluation and maintenance in stuttering treatment: A search for ecstasy with nothing but agony. In E. Boberg (ed.), *The Maintenance of Fluency.* New York: Elsevier North-Holland.

INGHAM, R. J. (1979b). Comment on "Stuttering therapy: The relation between attitude change and long-term outcome." *Journal of Speech and Hearing Disorders* 44:397–403.

INGHAM, R. J., (1979c). A further evaluation of the speech of stutterers during chorus and non-chorus reading situations. *Journal of Speech and Hearing Research* 22:784–93.

INGHAM, R. J. (1975a). Operant methodology in stuttering therapy. In J. Eisenson (ed.), *Stuttering: A Second Symposium.* New York: Harper & Row.

INGHAM, R. J. (1975b). A comparison of covert and overt assessment procedures in stuttering therapy outcome evaluation. *Journal of Speech and Hearing Research* 18:346–54.

INGHAM, R. J., & G. ANDREWS (1973a). Details of a token economy stuttering therapy programme for adults. *Australian Journal of Human Communication Disorders* 1:13–17.

INGHAM, R. J., & G. ANDREWS (1973b). An analysis of a token economy in stuttering therapy. *Journal of Applied Behavioral Analysis* 6:219–29.

INGHAM, R. J., & G. ANDREWS (1971). Stuttering: The quality of fluency after treatment. *Journal of Communication Disorders* 4:279–88.

INGHAM, R. J., & P. J. CARROLL (1977). Listener judgment of differences in stutterers' non-stuttered speech during chorus- and nonchorus-reading conditions. *Journal of Speech and Hearing Research* 20:293–302.

IRVING, R. W., & M. W. WEBB (1961). Teaching esophageal speech to a preoperative severe stutterer. *Annals of Otology, Rhinology and Laryngology* 70:1069–79.

IRWIN, A. (1980). *Successful Treatment of Stuttering.* New York: Walker and Company.

IRWIN, A. (1972). The treatment and results of "easy stammering." *British Journal of Disorders of Communication* 7:151–56.

JACOBSON, E. (1938). *Progressive Relaxation.* Chicago: University of Chicago Press.

JACOBSON, M. (1978). *Developmental Neurobiology.* New York: Plenum Press.

JAMES, D. O. (1977). *Play Therapy: An Overview.* Oceanside, N.Y.: Dabor Science Publications.

JAMES, J. E. (1983). Parameters of the influence of self-initiated time-out from speaking on stuttering. *Journal of Communication Disorders* 16:123–32.

JAMES, J. E. (1981). Punishment of stuttering: Contingency and stimulus parameters. *Journal of Communication Disorders* 14:375–86.

JAMES, J. E. (1976). The influence of duration on the effects of time-out from speaking. *Journal of Speech and Hearing Research* 19:206–15.

JANSSEN, P., F. KRAAIMAAT & S. VAN DER MEULEN (1983). Reading ability and disfluency in stuttering and nonstuttering elementary school children. *Journal of Fluency Disorders* 8:39–53.

JANSSEN, P., G. WIENEKE & E. VAANE (1983). Variability in the initiation of articulatory movements in the speech of stutterers and normal speakers. *Journal of Fluency Disorders* 8:341–58.

JENSEN, P. J., N. N. MARKEL & J. W. BEVERUNG (1986). Evidence of conversational disrhythmia in stutterers. *Journal of Fluency Disorders* 11:183–200.

JOHNS, D. (1978). *Clinical Management of Neurogenic Communicative Disorders.* Boston: Little, Brown.

JOHNSON, G. F. (1987). Ten commandments for long-term maintenance of acceptable self-help skills for persons who are hard-core stutterers. *Journal of Fluency Disorders* 12:9–18.

JOHNSON, L. J. (1980). Facilitating parental involvement in therapy of the disfluent child. In W. H. Perkins (ed.), *Strategies in Stuttering Therapy.* Seminars in Speech, Language, and Hearing. New York: Thieme-Stratton.

JOHNSON, W. (1961). *Stuttering and What You Can Do about It.* Danville, Ill.: The Interstate.

JOHNSON, W. (1959). The six men and the stuttering elephant, ETC. *Review of General Semantics* 16:419–33.

JOHNSON, W. (1955). A study of the onset and development of stuttering. In W. Johnson (ed.), *Stuttering in Children and Adults.* Minneapolis: University of Minnesota Press.

JOHNSON, W. (1946). *People in Quandaries.* New York: Harper & Row.

JOHNSON, W., R. M. BOHMLER, W. G. DAHLSTROM, F. L. DARLEY, L. D. GOODSTEIN, J. A. KOOLS, J. N. NEELLEY, W. F. PRATHER, D. SHERMAN, C. G. THURMAN, W. D. TROTTER, D. WILLIAMS & M. A. YOUNG (1959). *The Onset of Stuttering.* Minneapolis: University of Minnesota Press.

JOHNSON, W., F. L. DARLEY & D. C. SPRIESTERSBACH (1963). *Diagnostic Methods in Speech Pathology.* New York: Harper & Row.

JOHNSON, W., & J. R. KNOTT (1937). Studies in the psychology of stuttering: I. The distribution of moments of stuttering in successive readings of the same material. *Journal of Speech Disorders* 2:17–19.

JOHNSON, W., & L. ROSEN (1937). Studies in the psychology of stuttering: VII. Effect of certain changes in speech patterns upon frequency of stuttering. *Journal of Speech Disorders* 2:105–109.

JOHNSTON, J., & SCHERY, T. (1976). The use of grammatical morphemes by children with communication disorders. In E. Morehead & A. Morehead (eds.), *Normal and Deficient Child Language.* Baltimore: University Park Press.

JONAS, G. (1977). *Stuttering: The Disorder of Many Theories.* New York: Farrar, Strauss and Giroux.

JONES, H. G. (1969). Behavior therapy and stuttering: The need for a multifarious approach to a multiplex problem. In B. B. Gray & E. England (eds.), *Stuttering and the Conditioning Therapies.* Monterey, Calif.: Monterey Institute for Speech and Hearing.

JONES, R. J., & N. H. AZRIN (1969). Behavioral engineering: Stuttering as a function of stimulus duration during speech synchronization. *Journal of Applied Behavioral Analysis* 2:223–29.

JUDD, D. (1983). *King George VI, 1895–1952.* New York: Franklin Watts.

KASSIN, K., & B. BJERKAN (1982). Critical words and the locus of stuttering in speech. *Journal of Fluency Disorders* 7:433–46.

KALLEN, B. (1979). Errors in the differentiation of the central nervous system. In N. C. Myrianthopoulos & D. Bergsma (eds.), *Recent Advances in the Developmental Biology of Central Nervous System Malformations.* New York: Alan R. Liss.

KASPRISIN-BURRELLI, A. T., E. B. EGOLF & G. H. SHAMES (1972). A comparison of parental verbal behavior with stuttering and non-stuttering children. *Journal of Communication Disorders* 5:335–46.

KASTEIN, S. (1947). The chewing method of treating stuttering. *Journal of Communication Disorders* 12:195–98.

KELLY, G. A. (1955). *The Psychology of Personal Constructs.* New York: W. W. Norton.

KELLY, T. L., & M. D. STEER (1949). Revised concept of rate. *Journal of Speech and Hearing Disorders* 14:222–26.

KELSO, J. A. S., B. TULLER & K. S. HARRIS (1983). A "dynamic pattern" perspective on the control and coordination of movement. In P. F. MacNeilage (ed.), *The Production of Speech.* New York: Springler-Verlag.

KENT, L. R. (1961). Carbon dioxide therapy and medical treatment for stuttering. *Journal of Speech and Hearing Disorders* 26:268–72.

KENT, L. R., & D. E. WILLIAMS (1959). Use of meprobamate as an adjunct to stuttering therapy. *Journal of Speech and Hearing Disorders* 24:64–70.

KIDD, K. K. (1983). Recent progress on the genetics of stuttering. In C. L. Ludlow & J. A. Cooper (eds.), *Genetic Aspects of Speech and Language.* New York: Academic Press.

KIDD, K. K. (1980). Genetic models of stuttering. *Journal of Fluency Disorders* 5:187–202.

KIDD, K. K. (1977). A genetic perspective on stuttering. *Journal of Fluency Disorders* 2:259–69.

KIDD, K. K., R. C. HEIMBUCH & M. A. RECORDS (1981). Vertical transmission of susceptibility to stuttering with sex-modified expression. *Proceedings of the National Academy of Science* 78:606–10.

KIDD, K. K., R. C. HEIMBUCH, M. A. RECORDS, G. OEHLERT & R.L. WEBSTER (1980). Familial stuttering patterns are not related to one measure of severity. *Journal of Speech and Hearing Research* 23:539–45.

KIDD, K. K., J. R. KIDD & M. A. RECORDS (1978). The possible causes of the sex ratio in stuttering and its implications. *Journal of Fluency Disorders* 3:13–23.

KIMBARROW, M. J., & D. A. DALY (1980). Influence of stuttering therapy on clinicians' disfluencies: Effects of client model. *Journal of Fluency Disorders* 5:321–30.

KINSTLER, D. B. (1961). Covert and overt maternal rejection in stuttering. *Journal of Speech and Hearing Disorders* 26:145–56.

KIRK, L. (1977). Stuttering and quasi-stuttering in Ga. *Journal of Communication Disorders* 10:109–26.

KLEVANS, D. R., & G. P. LYNCH (1977). Group training in communication skills for adults who stutter: A suggested program. *Journal of Fluency Disorders* 2:11–20.

KLINE, M. L., & C. W. STARKWEATHER (1979). Receptive and expressive language performance in young stutterers. *Journal of the American Speech and Hearing Association* (convention abstracts) 21:797.

KLINGBEIL, G. M. (1939). The historical background of the modern speech clinics. Reprinted in L. L. Emerick & C. E. Hamre (eds.), *An Analysis of Stuttering, Selected Readings.* Danville, Ill.: The Interstate, 1972.

KLINGER, H. (1987). Effects of pseudostuttering on normal speakers' self-ratings of beauty. *Journal of Communication Disorders* 20:353–58.

KODMAN, F. (1961). Controlled reading rate under delayed speech feedback. *Journal of Auditory Research* 1:186–93.

KONDAS, O. (1968). Experiment of the shadowing method with children stammerers. *Psychologica* 19:109–16.

KONDAS, O. (1967). The treatment of stammering in children by the shadowing method. *Behavior Research and Therapy* 5:325–29.

KORZYBSKI, A. (1933). *Science and Sanity: An Introduction to Non-Aristotelian Systems and General Semantics.* New York: International Non-Aristotelian Library Publishing.

KOWAL, S., D. C. O'CONNELL & E. F. SABIN (1975). Development of temporal patterning and vocal hesitations in spontaneous narrations. *Journal of Psycholinguistic Research* 4:195–207.

KUFFLER, S. W., J. G. NICHOLLS & A. R. MARTIN (1984). *From Neurons to Brain.* Sunderland, Mass.: Senauer Associates.

KUHR, A. & L. RUSTIN (1985). The maintenance of fluency after intensive in-patient therapy: Long-term follow-up. *Journal of Fluency Disorders* 10:229–36.

LACROIX, Z. E. (1973). Management of disfluent speech through self-recording procedures. *Journal of Speech and Hearing Disorders* 38:272–74.

LADOUCEUR, R., C. COTE, G. LEBLOND & L. BOUCHARD (1982). Evaluation of regulated-breathing method and awareness training in the treatment of stuttering. *Journal of Speech and Hearing Disorders* 47:422–26.

LADOUCEUR, R., & L. SAINT-LAURENT (1986). Stuttering: A multidimensional treatment and evaluation package. *Journal of Fluency Disorders* 11:93–103.

LANGLOIS, A., L. L. HANRAHAN & L. L. INOUYE (1986). A comparison of interactions between stuttering children, nonstuttering children, and their mothers. *Journal of Fluency Disorders* 11:263–73.

LANGOVA, J., & M. MORAVEK (1964). Some results of experimental examinations among stutterers and clutterers. *Folia Phoniatrica* 16:290–96.

LANYON, R. I. (1969). Behavior changes in stuttering through systematic desensitization. *Journal of Speech and Hearing Disorders* 34:253–60.

LANYON, R. I. (1968). Some characteristics of nonfluency in normal speakers and stutterers. *Journal of Abnormal Psychology* 73:550–55.

LAY, T. (1982a). Nonspecific elements in therapy with stutterers. *Journal of Fluency Disorders* 2:479–86.

LAY, T. (1982b). Stuttering: Training the therapist. *Journal of Fluency Disorders* 7:63–69.

LEE, B. S. (1950a). Some effects of sidetone delay. *Journal of the American Speech Association* 22:639–40.

LEE, B. S. (1950b). Effects of delayed speech feedback. *Journal of the American Speech Association* 22:824–26.

LEE, B. S., W. E. MCGOUGH & M. PEINS (1973). A new method for stutter therapy. *Folia Phoniatrica* 25:186–95.

LEE, J. (1976). Applications of Martin Schwartz's airflow technique in the treatment of stuttering. *Journal of Speech and Hearing Disorders* 41:133–34.

LEE, R. (1983). Adjuncts of speech therapy. In P. Dalton (ed.), *Approaches to the Treatment of Stuttering.* London: Croom Helm.

LEITENBERG, H. (1965). Is time-out positive reinforcement an aversive event? *Psychological Bulletin* 64:428–41.

LEITH, W. R. (1984a). *Handbook of Stuttering Therapy for the School Clinician.* San Diego: College-Hill Press.

LEITH, W. R. (1984b). *Handbook of Clinical Methods in Communication Disorders.* San Diego: College-Hill Press.

LEITH, W. R. (1982). The shaping group: A group treatment procedure for the speech/language clinician. *Communicative Disorders* 8:103–15.

LEITH, W. R. (1979). The shaping group: Habituating new behaviors in the stutterer. In N. J. Lass (ed.), *Speech and Language: Advances in Basic Research and Practice.* vol. 2. New York: Academic Press.

LEITH, W. R. (1971). Clinical training in stuttering therapy: A survey. *Journal of the American Speech Association* 13:6–8.

LEITH, W. R., & C. C. CHMIEL (1980). Delayed auditory feedback and stuttering: Theoretical and clinical implications. In N. J. Lass (ed.), *Speech and Language: Advances in Basic Research and Practice.* New York: Academic Press.

LEITH, W. R., & M. R. UHLEMANN (1972). The shaping group approach to stuttering. *Comparative Group Studies* 3:175–99.

LEMERT, E., & C. VAN RIPER (1958). The use of psychodrama in the treatment of speech defects. In C. F. Diehl (ed.), *A Compendium of Research and Theory on Stuttering.* Springfield, Ill.: Charles C. Thomas.

LEWIS, D., & D. SHERMAN (1951). Measuring the severity of stuttering. *Journal of Speech and Hearing Disorders* 16:320–26.

LOCKHART, M. S., & A. W. ROBERTSON (1977). Hypnosis and speech therapy as a combined therapeutic approach to the problem of stammering. *British Journal of Disorders of Communication* 12:97–108.

LOVE, W. R. (1955). The effect of pentobarbitol sodium (nembutal) and amphetamine sulfate (benzedrine) on the severity of stuttering. In W. Johnson (ed.), *Stuttering in Children and Adults*. Minneapolis: University of Minnesota Press.

LUCHSINGER, R., & G. ARNOLD (1965). *Voice-Speech-Language. Clinical Communicology: Its Physiology*. Belmont, Calif.: Wadsworth.

LUND, R. D. (1978). *Development and Plasticity of the Brain*. New York: Oxford University Press.

LUPER, H. L. (1974). Transfer and maintenance. In H. Luper (ed.) *Therapy for Stutterers*. Memphis: Speech Foundation of America, no. 10.

LUPER, H. L., & R. L. MULDER (1964). *Stuttering Therapy for Children*. Englewood Cliffs, N.J.: Prentice Hall.

MACCLAY, H., & E.I. OSGOOD (1959). Hesitation phenomena is spontaneous English speech. *Word* 15:19–44.

MACCULLOCH, M. J., R. EATON & E. LONG (1970). The long-term effect of auditory masking on young stutterers. *British Journal of Disorders of Communication* 5:165–73.

MACKAY, D. G. (1968). Metamorphosis of a critical interval: Age-linked changes in the delay in auditory feedback that produces maximum disruption of speech. *Journal of the Acoustical Society of America* 43:811–21.

MAHAFFEY, R., & C. P. STROMSTA (1965). The effects of auditory feedback as a function of frequency, intensity, time, and sex. *De Theripia Vocis et Loquelles* 2:233–35.

MANNING, K., & A. SHARP (1977). *Structuring Play in the Early Years at School*. London: R. MacLehose and Company.

MARAIST, J. A., & C. HUTTON (1957). Effects of auditory masking upon the speech of stutterers. *Journal of Speech and Hearing Disorders* 22:385–89.

MARLAND, P. M. (1957). "Shadowing"—a contribution to the treatment of stammering. *Folia Phoniatrica* 9:242–45.

MARTIN, R. R. (1962). Stuttering and perseveration in children. *Journal of Speech and Hearing Research* 5:332–39.

MARTIN, R. R., & S. K. HAROLDSON (1981). Stuttering identification: Standard definition and moment of stuttering. *Journal of Speech and Hearing Research* 24:59–63.

MARTIN, R. R., & S. K. HAROLDSON (1979). Effects of five experimental treatments on stuttering. *Journal of Speech and Hearing Research* 22:132–46.

MARTIN, R. R., & S. K. HAROLDSON (1971). Time-out as a punishment for stuttering during conversation. *Journal of Communication Disorders* 4:15–19.

MARTIN, R. R., & S. K. HAROLDSON (1969a). The effects of two treatment procedures on stuttering. *Journal of Communication Disorders* 2:115–25.

MARTIN, R. R., & S. K. HAROLDSON (1969b). The effects of stuttering on problem solving. *Folia Phoniatrica* 21:442–48.

MARTIN, R. R., S. K. HAROLDSON & P. KUHL (1972). Disfluencies of young children in two speaking situations. *Journal of Speech and Hearing Research* 15:831–36.

MARTIN, R. R., P. KUHL & S. K. HAROLDSON (1972). An experimental treatment with two preschool stuttering children. *Journal of Speech and Hearing Research* 15:743–52.

MARTIN, R. R., & G. M. SIEGEL (1966a). The effects of response contingent shock on stuttering. *Journal of Speech and Hearing Research* 9:340–52.

MARTIN, R. R., & G. M. SIEGEL (1966b). The effects of simultaneously punishing stuttering and rewarding fluency. *Journal of Speech and Hearing Research* 9:466–75.

MARTIN, R. R., G. M. SIEGEL, L. J. JOHNSON & S. K. HAROLDSON (1984). Sidetone amplification and stuttering. *Journal of Speech and Hearing Research* 27:518–27.

MARZOLLO, J., & J. LLOYD (1972). *Learning through Play*. New York: Harper & Row.

MAXWELL, D. L. (1982). Cognitive and behavioral self-control strategies: Applications for the clinical management of adult stutterers. *Journal of Fluency Disorders* 7:403–32.

MAXWELL, R., & J. PATERSON (1958). Meprobamate in the treatment of stuttering. *British Medical Journal* 179:873–74.

MCCORD, H. (1955). Hypnotherapy and stuttering. *Journal of Clinical and Experimental Hypnosis* 3:210–14.

MCDONALD, E. (1964). *Articulation Testing and Treatment: A Sensory-Motor Approach*. Pittsburgh: Stanwix House.

MCFARLANE, S. C., & D. PRINS (1978). Natural response time of stutterers and nonstutterers in selected oral motor tasks. *Journal of Speech and Hearing Research* 21:768–78.

McIntyre, M. E., F. H. Silverman & W. D. Trotter (1974). Transcendental meditation and stuttering: A preliminary report. *Perceptual and Motor Skills* 39:294.

Meduna, L. J. (1958). *Carbon Dioxide Therapy.* 2d. ed. Springfield, Ill.: Charles C. Thomas.

Meduna, L. J. (1948). Alteration of neurotic patterns by use of CO_2 inhalations. *Journal of Nervous and Mental Disorders* 108:373–79.

Meltzer, H. (1944). Personality differences between stuttering and nonstuttering children as indicated by the Rorschach test. *Journal of Psychology* 17:39–59.

Merits-Patterson, R., & C. G. Reed (1981). Differences in the speech of language delayed children. *Journal of Speech and Hearing Research* 24:55–58.

Metz, D. E., E. G. Conture & R. H. Colton (1976). Temporal relations between the respiratory and laryngeal systems prior to stuttered disfluencies. Paper presented at annual convention of the American Speech and Hearing Association.

Meyer, V., & J. Comley (1969). A preliminary report on the treatment of stammer by the use of rhythmic stimulation. In B. B. Gray & F. England (eds.), *Stuttering and the Conditioning Therapies.* Monterey, Calif.: Monterey Institute for Speech and Hearing.

Meyer, V., & J. M. M. Mair (1963). A new technique to control stammering. *Behavioral Research and Therapy* 1:251–54.

Meyers, S. C., & F. Freeman (1985a). Mother and child speech rates as a variable in stuttering and disfluency. *Journal of Speech and Hearing Research* 28:436–44.

Meyers, S. C., & F. Freeman (1985b). Interruptions as a variable in stuttering and disfluency. *Journal of Speech and Hearing Research* 28:428–35.

Meyers, S. C., & F. J. Freeman (1985c). Are mothers of stutterers different? An investigation of social-communicative interaction. *Journal of Fluency Disorders* 10:193–209.

Meyers, S. C., & Strang, H. R. (1987). Microcomputer simulation training for student clinicians intervening with young stutterers. Paper presented at Voice I/O Systems Application Conference. Alexandria, Va.

Miller, S. (1982). Airflow therapy programs: Facts and/or fancy. *Journal of Fluency Disorders* 7:187–202.

Mohr, E. (1951). Chewing therapy in stuttering. In D. A. Weiss & H. H. Beebe (eds.), The Chewing Approach in Speech and Voice Therapy. New York: S. Karper.

Moleski, R., & D. J. Tosi (1976). Comparative psychotherapy: Rational-emotive therapy versus systematic desensitization in the treatment of stuttering. *Journal of Consulting and Clinical Psychology* 44:309–11.

Moncur, J. (1955). Symptoms of maladjustment differentiating young stutterers from nonstutterers. *Child Development* 26:91–96.

Moore, M., & N. Nystul (1979). Parent-child attitudes and communication processes in families with stutterers and families with non-stutterers. *British Journal of Disorders of Communication* 14:173–80.

Moore, W. E. (1946). Hypnosis in a system of therapy for stuttering. *Journal of Speech and Hearing Disorders* 11:117–22.

Moore, W. E., G. Soderberg & D. Powell (1952). Relations of stuttering in spontaneous speech to speech content and verbal output. *Journal of Speech and Hearing Disorders* 17:371–76.

Moore, W. H., Jr. (1986). Hemispheric alpha asymmetries of stutterers and nonstutterers for the recall and recognition of words and connected reading passages: Some relationships to severity of stuttering. *Journal of Fluency Disorders* 11:71–89.

Moore, W. H., Jr., & W. D. Haynes (1980). Alpha hemispheric asymmetry and stuttering: Some support for a segmentation dysfunction hypothesis. *Journal of Speech and Hearing Research* 23:229–47.

Moore, W. H., Jr., & M. K. Lang (1977). Alpha asymmetry over the right and left hemispheres of stutterers and control subjects preceding massed oral readings: A preliminary investigation. *Perceptual and Motor Skills* 44:223–30.

Moore, W. H., Jr., & L. C. Lorendo (1980). Hemispheric alpha asymmetries of stuttering males and nonstuttering males and females for words of high and low imagery. *Journal of Fluency Disorders* 5:11–26.

Moore, W. H., Jr., & S. I. Ritterman (1973). The effects of response contingent punishment upon the frequency of stuttered verbal behavior. *Behavioral Research and Therapy* 11:43–48.

Morley, M. (1957). *The Development and Disorders of Speech in Childhood.* Edinburgh: E. & S. Livingstone.

MOWRER, D. E. (1987). Reported use of a Japanese accent to promote fluency. *Journal of Fluency Disorders* 12:19–39.

MOWRER, D. E. (1979). *Fluent Speech*. Columbus, Ohio: Charles E. Merrill.

MOWRER, D. E. (1978). Effect of audience reaction upon fluency rates of six stutterers. *Journal of Fluency Disorders* 3:192–203.

MOWRER, D. E. (1977). *Methods of Modifying Speech Behaviors*. Columbus, Ohio: Charles E. Merrill.

MURPHY, A. T. (1977). Authenticity and creativity in stuttering theory and therapy. In R. W. Riebner (ed.), *The Problem of Stuttering*. New York: Elsevier.

MURRAY, E. (1932). Dysintegration of breathing and eye movements in stuttering during silent reading and reasoning. *Psychology Monographs* 43:218–75.

MURRAY, F. P., with S. G. EDWARDS (1980). *A Stutterer's Story*. Danville, Ill.: The Interstate.

MYSAK, E. D. (1966). *Speech Pathology and Feedback Theory*. Springfield, Ill.: Charles C. Thomas.

MYSAK, E. D. (1960). Servo theory and stuttering. *Journal of Speech and Hearing Disorders* 25:188–95.

NAYLOR, R. V. (1953). A comparative study of methods of estimating the severity of stuttering. *Journal of Speech and Hearing Disorders* 18:30–37.

NEAVES, A. I. (1970). To establish a basis for prognosis in stammering. *British Journal of Disorders of Communication* 5:46–58.

NEAVES, A. I. (1966). Prognosis in stammering. In *Speech Pathology Diagnosis: Theory and Practice*. Report of the National Conference of the College of Speech Therapists. Edinburgh: E. & S. Livingstone.

NEELLEY, J. N., & R. J. TIMMONS (1967). Adaptation and consistency in the disfluent speech of young stutterers and nonstutterers. *Journal of Speech and Hearing Research* 10:250–56.

NEIDECKER, E. A. (1987). *School Programs in Speech-Language: Organization and Management*. 2d ed. Englewood Cliffs, N.J.: Prentice Hall.

NELSON, L. A. (1986). Language formulation related to disfluency and stuttering. In H. H. Gregory (ed.), *Stuttering Therapy: Prevention and Intervention with Children*. Memphis: Speech Foundation of America, no. 20.

NEWMAN, P., R. CHANNELL & M. L. PALMER (1986). A comparative study of the independence of unilateral ocular motor control in stutterers and nonstutterers. *Journal of Fluency Disorders* 11:105–16.

NITTROUER, S., & C. CHENEY (1984). Operant techniques used in stuttering therapy: A review. *Journal of Fluency Disorders* 7:169–90.

NUTTALL, E. C., & T. M. SCHEIDEL (1965). Stutterers' estimates of normal apprehensiveness toward speaking. *Speech Monographs* 32:455–57.

OP'THOF, J., & I. C. UYS (1974). A clinical delineation of tachyphemia (cluttering): A case of dominant inheritance. *South African Medical Journal* 48:1624–28.

ORTON, S. T. (1927). Studies in stuttering. *Archives of Neurology and Psychiatry* 18:671–72.

OST, L-G., G. GOTESTAM & M. LENNERT (1976). A controlled study of two behavioral methods in the treatment of stuttering. *Behavior Therapy* 7:587–92.

OVERSTAKE, C. P. (1979). *Stuttering: A New Look at an Old Problem Based on Neurophysiological Aspects*. Springfield, Ill.: Charles C. Thomas.

OWEN, N. (1981). Facilitating maintenance of behavior change. In E. Boberg (ed.), *Maintenance of Fluency*. New York: Elsevier.

PATTIE, F. A., & B. B. KNIGHT (1944). Why does the speech of stutterers improve in chorus reading? *Journal of Abnormal and Social Psychology* 39:362–67.

PEARL, S. Z., & J. E. BERNTHAL (1980). The effects of grammatical complexity upon disfluency behavior of nonstuttering preschool children. *Journal of Fluency Disorders* 5:55–68.

PEINS, M. (1984). *Contemporary Approaches in Stuttering Therapy*. Boston: Little, Brown.

PEINS, M., B. S. LEE & W. E. McGOUGH (1970). A tape-recorded therapy method for stutterers: A case report. *Journal of Speech and Hearing Disorders* 35:188–93.

PEINS, M., W. E. McGOUGH & B. S. LEE (1984). Double tape recorder therapy for stutterers. In M. Peins (ed.), *Contemporary Approaches in Stuttering Therapy*. Boston: Little, Brown.

PEINS, M., W. E. McGOUGH & B. S. LEE (1972a). Tape recorder therapy for the rehabilitation of the stuttering handicapped. *Language, Speech, and Hearing Services in Schools* 3:30–35.

PEINS, M., W. E. McGOUGH & B. S. LEE (1972b). Evaluation of a tape-recorded method of stuttering therapy: Improvement in a speaking task. *Journal of Speech and Hearing Research* 15:364–71.

PERKINS, W. H. (1986). Functions and malfunctions of theories and therapies. *Journal of the American Speech, Language and Hearing Association* 28:31–33.

PERKINS, W. H. (1984). Stuttering as a categorical event: Barking up the wrong tree—reply to Wingate. *Journal of Speech and Hearing Disorders* 49:431–33.

PERKINS, W. H. (1983). Learning from negative outcomes in stuttering therapy: II. An epiphany of failures. *Journal of Fluency Disorders* 8:155–60.

PERKINS, W. H. (1980a). Disorders of speech flow. In T. J. Hixon, L. D. Shriberg & J. H. Saxman (eds.), *Introduction to Communication Disorders*. Englewood Cliffs, N.J.: Prentice Hall.

PERKINS, W. H. (1980b). Measurement and maintenance of fluency. In E. Boberg (ed.), *Maintenance of Fluency*. New York: Elsevier.

PERKINS, W. H. (1978). *Human Perspectives in Speech and Language Disorders*. St. Louis: C. V. Mosby.

PERKINS, W. H. (1977). *Speech Pathology: An Applied Behavioral Science*. 2d ed. St. Louis: C. V. Mosby.

PERKINS, W. H. (1975). Articulatory rate in the evaluation of stuttering treatments. *Journal of Speech and Hearing Disorders* 20:277–78.

PERKINS, W. H. (1973a). Replacement of stuttering with normal speech: I. Rationale. *Journal of Speech and Hearing Disorders* 38:283–94.

PERKINS, W. H. (1973b). Replacement of stuttering with normal speech: II. Clinical procedures. *Journal of Speech and Hearing Disorders* 38:295–303.

PERKINS, W. H. (1971). *Speech Pathology: An Applied Behavioral Science*. St. Louis: C. V. Mosby.

PERKINS, W. H., J. BELL, L. JOHNSON & J. STOCKS (1979). Phone rate and the effective planning-time hypothesis of stuttering. *Journal of Speech and Hearing Research* 22:747–55.

PERKINS, W. H., J. RUDAS, L. JOHNSON, W. B. MICHAEL & R. F. CURLEE (1974). Replacement of stuttering with normal speech: III. Clinical effectiveness. *Journal of Speech and Hearing Disorders* 39:416–28.

PEROZZI, J. A. (1970). Phonetic skills (sound-mindedness) of stuttering children. *Journal of Communication Disorders* 3:207–10.

PETERS, H. F. M., & W. HULSTIJN (1984). Stuttering and anxiety: The difference between stutterers and nonstutterers in verbal apprehension and physiologic arousal during the adaptation of speech and non-speech tasks. *Journal of Fluency Disorders* 9:67–84.

PETERSON, H. A. (1969). Affective meanings of words as rated by stuttering and nonstuttering readers. *Journal of Speech and Hearing Disorders* 2:337–43.

PORFERT, A., & D. ROSENFIELD (1978). Prevalence of stuttering. *Journal of Neurology, Neurosurgery and Psychiatry* 41:954–56.

PORTER, H. K. (1939). Studies in the psychology of stuttering: XIV. Stuttering phenomena in relation to size and personnel of audience. *Journal of Speech Disorders* 4:323–33.

PRINS, D. (1972). Personality, stuttering severity, and age. *Journal of Speech and Hearing Research* 15:128–54.

PRINS, D., & R. J. INGHAM (1983). *Treatment of Stuttering in Early Childhood: Methods and Issues*. San Diego: College-Hill Press.

PRINS, D., & M. MILLER (1973). Personality, improvement, and regression in stuttering therapy. *Journal of Speech and Hearing Research* 16:685–90.

PROSEK, R. A., & C. M. RUNYAN (1983). Effects of segment and pause manipulations on the identification of treated stutterers. *Journal of Speech and Hearing Research* 26:510–16.

PRUTTING, C. A., & D. M. KIRCHNER (1987). A clinical appraisal of the pragmatic aspects of language. *Journal of Speech and Hearing Disorders* 52:105–19.

PURPURA, D. P. (1977). Factors contributing to abnormal neuronal development in the cerebral cortex of the human infant. In S. R. Berenberg (ed.), *Brain: Fetal and Infant*. The Hague: Martinus Nijhoff.

QUARRINGTON, B. (1974). The parents of stuttering children: The literature re-examined. *Canadian Psychiatric Association Journal* 19:103–10.

QUARRINGTON, B. (1965). Stuttering as a function of the information value and sentence position of words. *Journal of Abnormal Psychology* 70:221–24.

QUARRINGTON, B. (1959). Measures of stuttering adaptation. *Journal of Speech and Hearing Research* 2:105–12.

QUARRINGTON, B., J. CONWAY & N. SIEGEL (1962). An experimental study of some properties of stuttered words. *Journal of Speech and Hearing Research* 5:387–94.

QUESAL, R. W., & K. H. SHANK (1978). Stutterers and others: A comparison of communication attitudes. *Journal of Fluency Disorders* 3:247–52.

QUINN, P. T. (1972). Stuttering: Cerebral dominance and the dichotic word test. *Medical Journal of Australia* 2:639–93.

QUINN, P. T., & E. PEACHEY (1975). Haloperidol in the treatment of stuttering. *British Journal of Psychiatry* 123:247–48.

QUIST, R. W., & R. R. MARTIN, (1967). The effect of response contingent verbal punishment on stuttering. *Journal of Speech and Hearing Research* 10:795–800.

RAGSDALE, J. D. (1976). Relationship between hesitation phenomena, anxiety, and self-control in normal communication situations. *Language and Speech* 19:257–65.

RAGSDALE, J. D., & J. K. ASHBY (1982). Speech-language pathologists' connotations of stuttering. *Journal of Speech and Hearing Research* 25:75–80.

RAKIC, P. (1975). Cell migration and neuronal ectopias in the brain. In N. C. Myrianthopoulos & D. Bergsma (eds.), *Morphogenesis and Malformation of Face and Brain*. New York: Alan R. Liss.

RAMIG, P. R., & M. L. WALLACE (1987). Indirect and combined direct-indirect therapy in a dysfluent child. *Journal of Fluency Disorders* 12:41–49.

RAMON Y CAJAL, S. (1960). *Studies on Vertebrate Neurogenesis*. Springfield, Ill.: Charles C. Thomas.

REED, C. G., & J. B. LINGWALL (1980). Conditioned stimulus effects on stuttering. *Journal of Speech and Hearing Research* 23:336–43.

RENTSCHLER, G. J. (1984). Effects of subgrouping in stuttering research. *Journal of Fluency Disorders* 9:307–11.

RHODES, R. (1973). Stuttering. In J. W. Wing & G. F. Holloway (eds.), *An Appraisal of Speech Pathology and Audiology*. Springfield, Ill.: Charles C. Thomas.

RIEBER, R. W. (1977). *The Problem of Stuttering: Theory and Therapy*. New York: Elsevier.

RIEBER, R. W. (1963). Stuttering and self-concept. *Journal of Psychology* 55:304–34.

RIEBER, R. W., S. BRESKIN & J. JAFFE (1972). Pause time and phonation time in stuttering and cluttering. *Journal of Psycholinguistic Research* 1:149–54.

RIEBER, R. W. & J. WOLLOCK (1977). The historical roots of the theory and therapy of stuttering. *Journal of Communication Disorders* 10:3–24.

RILEY, G. D. (1981). *Stuttering Prediction Instrument*. Tigard, Ore.: C. C. Publications.

RILEY, G. D. (1980). *Stuttering Severity Instrument*. Tigard, Ore.: C. C. Publications.

RILEY, G. D. (1972). A stuttering severity instrument for children and adults. *Journal of Speech and Hearing Disorders* 37:314–22.

RILEY, G. D., & J. RILEY (1986). Oral motor discoordination among children who stutter. *Journal of Fluency Disorders* 11:335–44.

RILEY, G. D., & J. RILEY (1984). A component model for treating stuttering in children. In M. Peins (ed.), *Contemporary Approaches in Stuttering Therapy*. Boston: Little, Brown.

RILEY, G. D., & J. RILEY (1983). Evaluation as a basis for intervention. In D. Prins & R. J. Ingham (eds.), *Treatment of Stuttering in Early Childhood: Methods and Issues*. San Diego: College-Hill Press.

RILEY, G. D., & J. RILEY (1980). Motoric and linguistic variables among children who stutter. *Journal of Speech and Hearing Disorders* 45:504–14.

RILEY, G. D., & J. RILEY (1979). A component model for diagnosing and treating children who stutter. *Journal of Fluency Disorders* 4:279–93.

ROBINSON, G. M. (1972). The delayed auditory feedback effect as a function of speech rate. *Journal of Experimental Psychology* 95:1–5.

ROMAN, K. G. (1963). Studies in tachyphemia: VI. The interrelationship of graphologic and oral aspects of language behavior. *Logos* 6:41–58.

ROSE, J. & McFARLANE, N. (1981). A personal project to examine the variation of fluency over 150 days. *British Journal of Disorders of Communication*. 16:11–18.

ROSENBERGER, P. B., J. A. WHEELDEN & M. KALOTKIN (1976). The effect of haloperidol on stuttering. *American Journal of Psychiatry* 13:331–34.

ROTH, F. P., & D. M. CLARK (1987). Symbolic play and social participation abilities of language-impaired and normally developing children. *Journal of Speech and Hearing Disorders* 52:17–29.

ROTHMAN, I. (1969). Practical rhythmic desensitization for stuttering with description of a new electronic pacer used for stuttering, insomnia, and anxiety. *Journal of the American Osteopathic Association* 68:573–77.

ROUSEY, C. L. (1961). Hypnosis in speech pathology and audiology. *Journal of Speech and Hearing Disorders* 26:258–62.

RUBIN, H. (1986). Cognitive therapy. In G. H. Shames & H. Rubin (eds.), *Stuttering Then and Now.* Columbus, Ohio: Charles E. Merrill.

RUBIN, H., & R. CULATTA (1986). A point of view about fluency. In G. H. Shames & H. Rubin (eds.), *Stuttering Then and Now.* Columbus, Ohio: Charles E. Merrill.

RUNYAN, C. M., & M. R. ADAMS (1978). Perceptual study of the speech of successfully therapeutized stutterers. *Journal of Fluency Disorders* 3:25–39.

RUNYAN, C. M., & D. C. BONIFANT (1981). A perceptual comparison: All-voiced versus typical reading passage read by children. *Journal of Fluency Disorders* 6:247–55.

RUNYAN, C. M., & S. E. RUNYAN (1986). Fluency rules therapy program for young children in the public schools. *Language, Speech, and Hearing Services in Schools* 17:276–84.

RUSTIN, L. (1978). An intensive group programme for adolescent stammerers. *British Journal of Disorders of Communication* 13:85–92.

RUSTIN, L., & F. COOK (1983). Intervention procedures for the disfluent child. In P. Dalton (ed.), *Approaches to the Treatment of Stuttering.* London: Croom Helm.

RUTISHAUSER, U., R. BRACKENBURY, J. P. THIERY & G. M. EDELMAN (1979). Surface molecules involved in interactions among neural cells during development. In N. C. Myrianthopoulos & D. Bergsma (eds.), *Recent Advances in Developmental Biology of Central Nervous System Malformations.* New York: Alan R. Liss.

RYAN, B. P. (1984). Treatment of stuttering in school children. In W. H. Perkins (ed.), *Current Therapy of Communication Disorders, Stuttering Disorders.* New York: Thieme-Stratton.

RYAN, B. P. (1979). Stuttering therapy in a framework of operant conditioning and programmed learning. In H. H. Gregory (ed.), *Controversies about Stuttering Therapy.* Baltimore: University Park Press.

RYAN, B. P. (1978). An illustration of operant conditioning therapy for stuttering. In *Conditioning in Stuttering Therapy.* Memphis: Speech Foundation of America, no. 7.

RYAN, B. P. (1974). *Programmed Therapy for Stuttering in Children and Adults.* Springfield, Ill.: Charles C. Thomas.

RYAN, B. P. (1971). Operant procedures applied to stuttering therapy for children. *Journal of Speech and Hearing Disorders* 36:264–80.

RYAN, B. P., & B. V. K. RYAN (1983). Programmed stuttering therapy for children: Comparisons of four establishment programs. *Journal of Fluency Disorders* 8:291–321.

RYAN, B. P., & B. VAN KIRK (1974). The establishment, transfer, and maintenance of fluent speech in 50 stutterers using delayed auditory feedback and operant procedures. *Journal of Speech and Hearing Disorders* 39:3–10.

RYAN, B. P., & B. VAN KIRK (1971). *Programmed Conditioning for Fluency.* Monterey, Calif.: Behavioral Sciences Institute.

SANTOSTEFANO, S. (1960). Anxiety and hostility in stuttering. *Journal of Speech and Hearing Research* 3:337–47.

SAPORA, A. V., & E. D. MITCHELL (1961). *The Theory of Play and Recreation.* New York: Ronald Press.

SCHILLING, V. A. (1960). X-ray kymographic investigation of the diaphragmatic action of stutterers. *Folia Phoniatrica* 12:145–53.

SCHINDLER, M. (1955). A study of educational adjustments of stuttering and nonstuttering children. In W. Johnson & R. Leutenegger (eds.), *Stuttering in Children and Adults.* Minneapolis: University of Minnesota Press.

SCHLESINGER, I. M., M. FORTE, B. FRIED & R. MELKMAN (1965). Stuttering, information load, and response strength. *Journal of Speech and Hearing Disorders* 30:32–36.

SCHLESINGER, I. M., R. MELKMAN & R. LEVY (1966). Word length and frequency as determinants of stuttering. *Bulletin of the Psychonomic Society* 6:255–56.

SCHLOSS, P. J., C. A. ESPIN, M.A. SMOTH & D. R. SUFFOLK (1987). Developing assertiveness during employment interviews with young adults who stutter. *Journal of Speech and Hearing Disorders* 52:30–36.

SCHWARTZ, M. F. (1976). *Stuttering Solved.* New York: McGraw-Hill.

SCHWARTZ, M. F. (1974). The core of the stuttering block. *Journal of Speech and Hearing Disorders* 39:169–77.

SERMAS, C. E., & N. D. COX (1982). The stutterer and stuttering: Personality correlates. *Journal of Fluency Disorders* 7:141–58.

SHAMES, G. H. (1986). Disorders of fluency. In G. H. Shames and E. H. Wiig (eds.), *Human Communication Disorders: An Introduction.* 2nd ed. Columbus, Ohio: Charles E. Merrill.

SHAMES, G. H. (1981). Relapse in stuttering. In E. Boberg (ed.), *Proceedings of the Banff Conference on the Maintenance of Fluency.* New York: Elsevier.

SHAMES, G. H. (1978). Operant conditioning and therapy for stuttering. In *Conditioning in Stuttering Therapy.* Memphis: Speech Foundation of America, no. 7.

SHAMES, G. H. (1975). Operant conditioning and stuttering. In J. Eisenson (ed.), *Stuttering: A Second Symposium.* New York: Harper & Row.

SHAMES, G. H., & D. B. EGOLF (1976). *Operant Conditioning and the Management of Stuttering.* Englewood Cliffs, N.J.: Prentice Hall.

SHAMES, G. H., D. B. EGOLF & R. C. RHODES (1969). Experimental programs in stuttering therapy. *Journal of Speech and Hearing Disorders* 34:30–47.

SHAMES, G. H., & C. L. FLORANCE (1982). Disorders of fluency. In G. H. Shames & E. H. Wiig (eds.), *Human Communication Disorders.* Columbus, Ohio: Charles E. Merrill.

SHAMES, G. H., & C. L. FLORANCE (1980). *Stutter-Free Speech: A Goal for Therapy.* Columbus, Ohio: Charles E. Merrill.

SHAMES, G. H., & H. RUBIN (1986). Concluding remarks. In G. H. Shames & H. Rubin (eds.), *Stuttering Then and Now.* Columbus, Ohio: Charles E. Merrill.

SHAMES, G. H., & C. E. SHERRICK (1963). A discussion of nonfluency and stuttering as operant behavior. *Journal of Speech and Hearing Disorders* 28:3–18.

SHANE, M. L. S. (1955). Effect on stuttering of alteration in auditory feedback. In W. Johnson (ed.), *Stuttering in Children and Adults.* Minneapolis: University of Minnesota Press.

SHEEHAN, J. G. (1980). Problems in the evaluation of progress and outcome. In W. H. Perkins (ed.), *Strategies in Stuttering Therapy.* Seminars in Speech, Language, and Hearing. New York: Theime-Stratton.

SHEEHAN, J. G. (1979). Level of aspiration in female stutterers: Changing times. *Journal of Speech and Hearing Disorders* 44:479–86.

SHEEHAN, J. G. (1978). Stuttering and recovery. In H. H. Gregory (ed.), *Controversies about Stuttering Therapy.* Baltimore: University Park Press.

SHEEHAN, J. G. (1975). Conflict theory and avoidance-reduction therapy. In J. Eisenson (ed.), *Stuttering: A Second Symposium.* New York: Harper & Row.

SHEEHAN, J. G. (1970). *Stuttering Research and Therapy.* New York: Harper & Row.

SHEEHAN, J. G. (1968). Reflections on the behavioral modification of stuttering. In *Conditioning in Stuttering Therapy.* Memphis: Speech Foundation of America, no. 7.

SHEEHAN, J. G. (1958). Conflict theory of stuttering. In J. Eisenson (ed.), *Stuttering: A Symposium.* New York: Harper & Row.

SHEEHAN, J. G. (1953). Theory and treatment of stuttering as an approach-avoidance conflict. *Journal of Psychology* 36:27–49.

SHEEHAN, J. G. (1951). The modification of stuttering through nonreinforcement. *Journal of Abnormal and Social Psychology* 46:51–63.

SHEEHAN, J. G. Relapse and recovery. In *Stuttering Transfer and Maintenance.* Memphis: Speech Foundation of America, no. 19.

SHEEHAN, J. G., R. G. HADLEY & E. GOULD (1967). Impact of authority on stuttering. *Journal of Abnormal Psychology* 72:290–93.

SHEEHAN, V. (1986). Approach-avoidance and anxiety reduction. In G. H. Shames & H. Rubin (eds.), *Stuttering Then and Now.* Columbus, Ohio: Charles E. Merrill.

SHERRARD, C. A. (1975). Stuttering as "false alarm" responding. *British Journal of Disorders of Communication* 10:83–91.

SHINE, R. E. (1980a). Direct management of the beginning stutterer. In W. H. Perkins (ed.), *Strategies in Stuttering Therapy.* Seminars in Speech, Language, and Hearing. New York: Thieme-Stratton.

SHINE, R. E. (1980b). *Systematic Fluency Training for Young Children: A Fluency Training Kit.* Tigard, Ore.: C. C. Publications.

SHIRKEY, E. A. (1987). Forensic verification of stuttering. *Journal of Fluency Disorders* 12:197–204.

SHULMAN, E. (1955). Factors influencing the variability of stuttering. In W. Johnson (ed.), *Stuttering in Children and Adults.* Minneapolis: University of Minnesota Press.

SHUMAK, I. C. (1955). A speech rating situation sheet for stutterers, In W. Johnson (ed.), *Stuttering in Children and Adults, Thirty Years of Research at the University of Iowa.* Minneapolis: University of Minnesota Press.

SIEGEL, G. M. (1976). Experimental modification of speech dysfluency. In B. B. Gray and G. England, *Stuttering and the Conditioning Therapies.* Monterey, Calif: Monterey Institute for Speech and Hearing.

SIEGEL, G. M. (1970). Punishment, stuttering, and disfluency. *Journal of Speech and Hearing Research* 13:677–714.

SIEGEL, G. M., & D. HAUGEN (1964). Audience size and variations in stuttering behavior. *Journal of Speech and Hearing Research* 7:381–88.

SIEGEL, G. M., J. LENSKA & P. BROEN (1969). Suppression of normal speech disfluencies through response cost. *Journal of Applied Behavioral Analysis* 2:265–76.

SIEGEL, G. M., & R. R. MARTIN (1968). The effects of verbal stimuli on disfluencies during spontaneous speech. *Journal of Speech and Hearing Research* 11:358–64.

SIEGEL, G. M., & R. R. MARTIN (1967). Verbal punishment of disfluencies during spontaneous speech. *Language and Speech* 10:244–51.

SIEGEL, G. M., & R. R. MARTIN (1966). Punishment of dysfluencies in normal speakers. *Journal of Speech and Hearing Research* 9:208–18.

SIEGEL, G. M., & R. R. MARTIN (1965a). Experimental modification of disfluency in normal speakers. *Journal of Speech and Hearing Research* 8:235–44.

SIEGEL, G. M., & R. R. MARTIN (1965b). Verbal punishment of disfluencies in normal speakers. *Journal of Speech and Hearing Research* 8:245–52.

SILBER, S. (1973). Fairy tales and symbols in hypnotherapy of children with certain speech disorders. *International Journal of Clinical and Experimental Hypnosis* 21:272–83.

SILVERMAN, E-M. (1980). Communication attitudes of women who stutter. *Journal of Speech and Hearing Disorders* 45:533–39.

SILVERMAN, E-M. (1974). Word position and grammatical function in relation to preschoolers' speech disfluency. *Perceptual and Motor Skills* 39:267–72.

SILVERMAN, E-M. (1973a). The influence of preschoolers' speech usage on their disfluency frequency. *Journal of Speech and Hearing Research* 16:474–81.

SILVERMAN, E-M. (1973b). Clustering: A characteristic of preschoolers' speech disfluency. *Journal of Speech and Hearing Research* 16:578–83.

SILVERMAN, E-M., & D. E. WILLIAMS (1967). A comparison of stuttering and nonstuttering children in terms of five measures of oral language development. *Journal of Communication Disorders* 1:305–9.

SILVERMAN, E-M., & C. H. ZIMMER (1982). Demographic characteristics and treatment experiences of women and men who stutter. *Journal of Fluency Disorders* 7:273–85.

SILVERMAN, F. H. (1980). The stuttering problem profile: A task that assists both client and clinician in defining therapy goals. *Journal of Speech and Hearing Disorders* 45:119–23.

SILVERMAN, F. H. (1976). Do elementary school stutterers talk less than their peers. *Language, Speech, and Hearing Services in Schools* 7:90–92.

SILVERMAN, F. H. (1975). How "typical" is a stutterer's stuttering in a clinical environment? *Perceptual and Motor Skills* 40:458.

SILVERMAN, F. H. (1974). Disfluency behavior of elementary school stutterers and nonstutterers. *Language, Speech, and Hearing Services in Schools* 5:32–37.

SILVERMAN, F. H. (1972a). An approach to defining goals for stuttering therapy. *Perceptual and Motor Skills* 34:414.

SILVERMAN, F. H. (1972b). Disfluency and word length. *Journal of Speech and Hearing Research* 15:788–91.

SILVERMAN, F. H. (1971a). The effect of rhythmic auditory stimulation on the disfluency of nonstutterers. *Journal of Speech and Hearing Research* 14:350–55.

SILVERMAN, F. H. (1971b). A rationale for the use of the hearing-aid metronome in a program of therapy for stuttering. *Perceptual and Motor Skills* 32:34.

SILVERMAN, F. H., H. KLINGER, L. LUSTBADER, J. FARRELL & A. D. MARTIN (1972). The effects of subliminal drive stimulation on the speech of stutterers. *Journal of Nervous and Mental Disorders* 155:14–21.

SILVERMAN, F. H., E. M. SILVERMAN & M. MEAGHER (1979). Bibliography of literature pertaining to the onset, development, and treatment of stuttering during the preschool years. *Journal of Fluency Disorders* 4:171–203.

SILVERMAN, F. H., & W. D. TROTTER (1973). Impact of pacing speech with a miniature electronic metronome upon the manner in which a stutterer is perceived. *Behavior Therapies* 4:414–19.

SILVERMAN, F. H., & D. E. WILLIAMS (1972). Obtaining self-ratings of amount of stuttering in specific situations from elementary school children. *Language, Speech, and Hearing Services in Schools* 3:36–37.

SILVERMAN, F. H., & D. E. WILLIAMS (1968). A proportional measure of stuttering adaptation. *Journal of Speech and Hearing Research* 11:444–46.

SKINNER, B. F. (1958). *Verbal Behavior.* New York: Appleton-Century-Crofts.

SKINNER, B. F. (1938). *The Behavior of Organisms.* New York: Appleton-Century-Crofts.

SLOCUM, Y. S. (1987). A survey of expectations about group therapy among clinical and non-clinical populations. *International Journal of Group Psychotherapy* 37:39–54.

SLORACH, N. (1971). Twenty years of stuttering therapy. *Journal of the Australian College of Speech Therapists* 21:19–23.

SODERBERG, G. A. (1971). Relations of word information and word length to stuttering disfluencies. *Journal of Communication* 4:9–14.

SODERBERG, G. A. (1967). Linguistic factors in stuttering. *Journal of Speech and Hearing Research* 10:801–10.

SOMMERS, R. K., K. BOBKOFF-LEVENTHAL, J. A. APPLEGATE & P. A. SQUARE (1979). A critical review of a recent decade of stuttering reserch. *Journal of Fluency Disorders* 4:223–37.

SOMMERS, R. K., W. A. BRADY & W. H. MOORE (1975). Dichotic ear preferences of stuttering children and adults. *Perceptual and Motor Skills* 41:931–38.

SOMMERS, R. K., & M. E. HATTON (1985). Establishing the therapy program: Case finding, case selection, and case load. In R. J. van Hattum (ed.), *Organization of Speech-Language Services in Schools: A Manual.* San Diego: College-Hill Press.

SPEECH FOUNDATION OF AMERICA (SFA). Memphis.
    (1987) *Do You Stutter? A Guide for Teens.* no. 21.
    Stuttering Therapy: Prevention and Intervention with Children. no. 20.
    Stuttering Therapy: Transfer and Maintenance. no. 19.
    Counseling Stutterers. no. 18.
    Stuttering, an Integration of Contemporary Therapies. no. 16.
    Self-Therapy for the Stutterer. 3d ed., no. 12.
    (1981) *If Your Child Stutters—A Guide for Parents.* no. 11.
    (1974) *Therapy for Stutterers.* no. 10.
    To the Stutterer. no. 9.
    (1971) *Stuttering: An Account of Intensive Desensitization.* Demonstration Therapy. no. 8.
    (1970) *Conditioning in Stuttering Therapy.* no. 7.
    Stuttering: Successes and Failures in Therapy. no. 6.
    (1962) *Stuttering: Its Prevention.* no. 3.
    (1960) *Stuttering: Training the Therapist.* no. 5.
    Stuttering Words. no. 2.

SPIELBERGER, C. D. (1966). Theory and research on anxiety. In C. D. Spielberger (ed.), *Anxiety and Behavior.* New York: Academic Press.

SPILKA, B. (1954). Some vocal effects of different reading passages and time delays in speech feedback. *Journal of Speech and Hearing Disorders* 19:37–47.

SPUEHLER, H. E. (1962). Delayed sidetone and auditory flutter. *Journal of Speech and Hearing Research* 5:124–32.

STAMPFL, T. G., & D. J. LEVIS (1967). Essentials of implosive therapy: A learning-theory based psychodynamic behavioral therapy. *Journal of Abnormal Psychology* 72:496–503.

STARBUCK, H. B., & M. D. STEER (1954). Adaptation effect and its relation to thoracic breathing in stutterers and non-stutterers. *Journal of Speech and Hearing Disorders* 19:440–49.

STARKWEATHER, C. W. (1987). *Fluency and Stuttering.* Englewood Cliffs, N.J.: Prentice Hall.

STARKWEATHER, C. W. (1987). Talking with parents of young stutterers. In *Counseling Stutterers*. Memphis: Speech Foundation of America, no. 18.

STARKWEATHER, C. W. (1986). The development of fluency in normal children. In H. H. Gregory (ed.), *Stuttering Therapy: Prevention and Intervention with Children*. Memphis: Speech Foundation of America, no. 20.

STARKWEATHER, C. W. (1982a). Stuttering and laryngeal behavior: A review. *ASHA Monographs* no. 21. Rockville, Md.: American Speech, Language and Hearing Association.

STARKWEATHER, C. W. (1982b). Stuttering in children: An overview. *Journal of Child Communication Disorders* 6:5–14.

STARKWEATHER, C. W. (1981). Speech fluency and its development in normal children. In N. J. Lass (ed.), *Speech and Language: Advances in Basic Research and Practice*. New York: Academic Press.

STARKWEATHER, C. W. (1980). A multiprocess behavioral approach to stuttering therapy. In W. H. Perkins (ed.), *Strategies in Stuttering Therapy*. Seminars in Speech, Language, and Hearing. New York: Thieme-Stratton.

STARKWEATHER, C. W. (1973). A behavioral analysis of Van Riperian therapy for stutterers. *Journal of Communication Disorders* 6:273–91.

STEIN, J. (ed. chief) (1967). *The Random House Dictionary of the English Language*. New York: Random House.

ST. LOUIS, K. O. (ed.) (1986). *The Atypical Stutterer*. New York: Academic Press.

ST. LOUIS, K. O. (1979). Linguistic and motor aspects of stuttering. In N. J. Lass (ed.), *Speech and Language: Advances in Basic Research and Practice*. New York: Academic Press.

ST. LOUIS, K. O., P. L. CLAUSELL, J. N. THOMPSON & C. C. RIFE (1982). Preliminary investigation of EMG biofeedback induced relaxation with a preschool aged stutterer. *Perceptual and Motor Skills* 55:195–99.

ST. LOUIS, K. O., & A. R. HINZMAN (1986). Studies of cluttering: Perceptions of cluttering by speech-language pathologists and educators. *Journal of Fluency Disorders* 11:131–49.

ST. LOUIS, K. O., A. R. HINZMAN & F. M. HULL (1985). Studies of cluttering: Disfluency and language measures in young possible clutterers and stutterers. *Journal of Fluency Disorders* 10:151–72.

STOCKER, B. (1980). *The Stocker Probe Technique: For Diagnosis and Treatment of Stuttering in Young Children*. Tulsa: Modern Educational Corporation.

STOCKER, B., & L. J. GERSTMAN (1983). A comparison of the probe technique and conventional therapy for young stutterers. *Journal of Fluency Disorders* 8:331–39.

STOCKER, B., & E. PARKER (1977). The relationship between auditory recall and dysfluency in young stutterers. *Journal of Fluency Disorders* 2:177–87.

STRANG, H. R., & S. C. MEYERS (1987a). Training effective stuttering skills through the use of a microcomputer. *Journal of the American Voice I/O Society* 4:20–29.

STRANG, H. R., & S. C. MEYERS (1987b). A microcomputer simulation to evaluate and train effective intervention techniques in listening partners of preschool stutterers. *Journal of Fluency Disorders* 12:205–16.

STROMSTA, C. (1986). *Elements of Stuttering*. Oshtemo, Mich.: Atsmorts Publishing.

STROMSTA, C. (1965). A procedure using group consensus in adult stuttering therapy. *Journal of Speech and Hearing Disorders* 30:277–79.

STROMSTA, C. (1964). EEG power spectra of stutterers and nonstutterers. *Journal of the American Speech and Hearing Association* 6:418–19.

TATCHELL, R. H., S. VAN DEN BERG & J. W. LERMAN (1983). Fluency and eye contact as factors influencing observers' perception of stutterers. *Journal of Fluency Disorders* 8:221–31.

TATE, M. W., & W. L. CULLINAN (1962). Measurement of consistency of stuttering. *Journal of Speech and Hearing Research* 5:272–83.

TATE, M. W., W. L. CULLINAN & A. AHLSTRAND (1961). Measurement of adaptation in stuttering. *Journal of Speech and Hearing Research* 4:321–39.

TAYLOR, I. K. (1966). What words are stuttered? *Psychological Bulletin* 65:233–42.

THOMPSON, J. (1984). Update: School-aged stutterers. *Journal of Fluency Disorders* 9:199–206.

TIFFANY, W. R. (1963). Slurvian translation as a speech research tool. *Speech Monographs* 30:23–30.

TIFFANY, W. R., & C. N. HANLEY (1956). Adaptation to delayed auditory sidetone. *Journal of Speech and Hearing Disorders* 2:164–72.

TIFFANY, W. R., & HANLEY, C. N. (1954). An investigation into the use of electromechanically delayed side tone in auditory training. *Journal of Speech and Hearing Disorders* 19:367–73.

TORNICK, G. B., & O. BLOODSTEIN (1976). Stuttering and sentence length. *Journal of Speech and Hearing Research* 19:651–54.

TRAVIS, L. E. (1978). The cerebral dominance theory of stuttering, 1931–78. *Journal of Speech and Hearing Disorders* 43:278–81.

TRAVIS, L. E. (1971). The unspeakable feelings of people with special reference to stuttering. In L. E. Travis (ed.), *Handbook of Speech Pathology*. Englewood Cliffs, N.J.: Prentice Hall.

TRAVIS, L. E. (1931). *Speech Pathology*. New York: Prentice Hall.

TROTTER, W. D. (1960). The speech of young stutterers in the presence of their mother. *Central States Speech Journal* 12:51–54.

TROTTER, W. D. (1956). Relationship between the severity of stuttering and word conspicuousness. *Journal of Speech and Hearing Disorders* 21:198–201.

TROTTER, W. D., & M. F. BERGMANN (1957). Stutterers' and nonstutterers' reactions to speech situations. *Journal of Speech and Hearing Disorders* 22:40–45.

TROTTER, W. D., & M. M. LESCH (1967). Personal experiences with a stutter-aid. *Journal of Speech and Hearing Disorders* 32:270–72.

TROTTER, W. D., & F. H. SILVERMAN (1974). Does the effect of pacing speech with a miniature metronome on stuttering wear off? *Perceptual and Motor Skills* 39:429–30.

TROTTER, W. D., & F. H. SILVERMAN (1973). Experiments with the stutter-aid. *Perceptual and Motor Skills* 36:1124–30.

TURNBAUGH, K. R. (1983). Personal correspondence.

TURNBAUGH, K. R., & B. E. GUITAR (1981). Short-term intensive stuttering treatment in a public school setting. *Language, Speech, and Hearing Services in Schools* 12:100–106.

TURNBAUGH, K. R., B. E. GUITAR & P. R. HOFFMAN (1981). The attribution of personality traits: The stutterers and nonstutterers. *Journal of Speech and Hearing Research* 24:288–91.

TURNBAUGH, K. R., B. E. GUITAR & P. R. HOFFMAN (1979). Speech clinicians' attribution of personality traits as a function of stuttering severity. *Journal of Speech and Hearing Research* 22:37–45.

TYRE, T. E., S. A. MAISTO & P. J. COMPANIK (1973). The use of systematic desensitization in the treatment of chronic stuttering behavior. *Journal of Speech and Hearing Disorders* 38:514–19.

ULLIANA, L., & R. J. INGHAM (1984). Behavioral and nonbehavioral variables in the measurement of stutterers' communication attitudes. *Journal of Speech and Hearing Disorders* 49:83–93.

VAN DANTZIG, M. (1940). Syllable-tapping: A new method for the help of stammerers. *Journal of Speech Disorders* 5:127–32.

VAN RIPER, C. (1982). *The Nature of Stuttering*. Englewood Cliffs, N.J.: Prentice Hall.

VAN RIPER, C. (1979). To Banff—with love. *Western Michigan Journal of Speech, Language, and Hearing* 15:1–3.

VAN RIPER, C. (1978). *Speech Correction Principles and Methods*. Englewood Cliffs, N.J.: Prentice Hall.

VAN RIPER, C. (1975). The stutterer's clinic. In J. Eisenson (ed.), *Stuttering: A Second Symposium*. New York: Harper & Row.

VAN RIPER, C. (1973). *The Treatment of Stuttering*. Englewood Cliffs, N.J.: Prentice Hall.

VAN RIPER, C. (1972). Stuttering therapy in 2050 A.D., In L. I. Emerick & C. E. Hamre (eds.), *An Analysis of Stuttering*. Danville, Ill.: The Interstate.

VAN RIPER, C. (1971a). Symptomatic therapy for stuttering. In L. E. Travis (ed.), *Handbook of Speech Pathology and Audiology*. New York: Appleton-Century-Crofts.

VAN RIPER, C. (1971b). The rhythm method. *California Journal of Communication Disorders* 2:3–6.

VAN RIPER, C. (1965). Clinical use of intermittent masking noise in stuttering therapy. *Journal of the American Speech and Hearing Association* 7:381.

VAN RIPER, C. (1959). Binaural speech therapy. *Journal of Speech and Hearing Disorders* 24:62–63.

VAN RIPER, C. (1958a). Experiments in stuttering therapy. In J. Eisenson (ed.), *Stuttering: A Symposium*. New York: Harper & Row.

VAN RIPER, C. (1958b). The effect of punishment upon frequency of stuttering spasms (1937). In C. F. Diehl (ed.). *A Compendium of Research and Theory on Stuttering.* Springfield, Ill.: Charles C. Thomas.

VAN RIPER, C. (1937). Effect of devices for minimizing stuttering on the creation of symptoms. *Journal of Abnormal and Social Psychology* 32:185–92.

VAN RIPER, C., & L. EMERICK (1984). *Speech Correction Principles and Methods.* Englewood Cliffs, N.J.: Prentice Hall.

VAUGHN, J. E., C. K. HENRICKSON & J. A. GRIESHABER (1974). A quantitative study of synapses on motor dendritic growth cones in the developing mouse spinal cord. *Journal of Cellular Biology* 60:664–72.

VENKATAGIRI, H. S. (1982). Reaction time for /s/ and /z/ in stutterers and nonstutterers: A test of discoordination hypothesis. *Journal of Communication Disorders* 15:55–62.

VENKATAGIRI, H. S. (1980a). The core disruption under DAF: Evidence from adaptation studies. *Journal of Communication Disorders* 13:365–71.

VENKATAGIRI, H. S. (1980b). The relevance of DAF-induced speech disruption to the understanding of stuttering. *Journal of Fluency Disorders* 5:87–98.

WAKABA, Y. Y. (1983). Group play therapy for Japanese children who stutter. *Journal of Fluency Disorders* 8:93–118.

WALL, M. J. (1980). A comparison of syntax in young stutterers and non-stutterers. *Journal of Fluency Disorders* 5:345–52.

WALL, M. J., & F. L. MEYERS (1984). *Clinical Management of Childhood Stuttering.* Baltimore: University Park Press.

WALL, M. J., & F. L. MEYERS (1982). A review of linguistic factors associated with early childhood stuttering. *Journal of Communication Disorders* 15:441–49.

WALL, M. J., C. W. STARKWEATHER & H. CAIRNS (1981). Syntactic influences on stuttering in young child stutterers. *Journal of Fluency Disorders* 6:283–98.

WALTON, D., & M. D. MATHER (1963). The relevance of generalization techniques to the treatment of stammering and phobia symptoms. *Behavior Research and Therapy* 1:121–25.

WATTS, F. (1973). Mechanisms of fluency control in stutterers. *British Journal of Disorders of Communication* 8:131–38.

WATTS, F. (1971). The treatment of stammering by the intensive practice of fluent speech. *British Journal of Communication Disorders* 6:144–47.

WEBSTER, L. M. (1970). A clinical report on the measured effectiveness of certain desensitization techniques with stutterers. *Journal of Speech and Hearing Disorders* 35:369–76.

WEBSTER, R. L. (1979). Empirical considerations regarding stuttering therapy. In H. H. Gregory (ed.), *Controversies about Stuttering Therapy.* Baltimore: University Park Press.

WEBSTER, R. L. (1974). Behavioral analysis of stuttering: Treatment and theory. In M. Calhoun (ed.), *Innovative Treatment Methods in Psychopathology.* New York: John Wiley.

WEBSTER, R. L., & B. B. LUBKER (1968). Interrelationships among fluency producing variables in stuttered speech. *Journal of Speech and Hearing Research* 11:754–66.

WEINER, A. E. (1984a). Patterns of vocal fold movement during stuttering. *Journal of Fluency Disorders* 9:31–49.

WEINER, A. E. (1984b). Stuttering and syllable stress. *Journal of Fluency Disorders* 9:301–5.

WEINER, A. E. (1978). Vocal control therapy for stutterers: A trial program. *Journal of Fluency Disorders* 3:115–26.

WEISS, D. A. (1967). Similarities and differences between cluttering and stuttering. *Folia Phoniatrica* 19:98–104.

WEISS, D. A. (1964). *Cluttering.* Englewood Cliffs, N.J.: Prentice Hall.

WEISS, D. A. (1960). Therapy of cluttering. *Folia Phoniatrica* 12:216–28.

WELLER, H. C. (1941). Vegetative rhythm determinative of speech patterns. *Journal of Speech Disorders* 6:161–71.

WELLS, G. B. (1987). *Stuttering Treatment: A Comprehensive Clinical Guide.* Englewood Cliffs, N.J.: Prentice Hall.

WELLS, P. G., & M. T. MALCOLM (1971). Controlled trial of the treatment of 36 stutterers. *British Journal of Psychiatry* 119:603–5.

WEPMAN, J. M. (1939). Familial incidence in stammering. *Journal of Speech Disorders* 4:199–204.

WEST, R. (1942). The pathology of stuttering. *The Nervous Child* 2:96–106.

WESTLEY, C. E. (1979). Language performance of stuttering and nonstuttering children. *Journal of Communication Disorders* 12:133–45.

WEUFFEN, V. M. (1961). An investigation of the word-finding of normal and stuttering school age children from 8 to 16 years. *Folia Phoniatrica* 13:255–68.

WEXLER, K. B., & E. D. MYSAK (1982). Disfluency characteristics of 2, 4, and 6-year-old males. *Journal of Fluency Disorders* 7:37–46.

WHITE, P. A., & S. R. C. COLLINS (1984). Stereotype formation by inference: A possible explanation for the "stutterer" stereotype. *Journal of Speech and Hearing Research* 27:567–70.

WIENER, N. (1948). Cybernetics. *Scientific American* 179:14–19.

WILKINS, C., R. L. WEBSTER & B. T. MORGAN (1984). Cerebral localization of visual stimulus recognition in stutterers and fluent speakers. *Journal of Fluency Disorders* 9:131–41.

WILLIAMS, A. M., & C. J. MARKS (1972). A comparative analysis of ITPA and PPVT performance of young stutterers. *Journal of Speech and Hearing Research* 15:323–29.

WILLIAMS, D. E. (1986). Emotional and environmental problems in stuttering. In H. H. Gregory (ed.), *Stuttering Therapy: Prevention and Intervention with Children*. Memphis: Speech Foundation of America, no. 20.

WILLIAMS, D. E. (1957). A point of view about stuttering. *Journal of Speech and Hearing Disorders* 22:390–97.

WILLIAMS, D. E. Working with children in the school environment. In *Stuttering Therapy: Transfer and Maintenance*. Memphis: Speech Foundation of America, no. 19.

WILLIAMS, D. E. Talking with children who stutter. In *Counseling Stutterers*. Memphis: Speech Foundation of America, no. 18.

WILLIAMS, D. E., F. H. SILVERMAN & J. A. KOOLS (1969a). Disfluency behavior of elementary-school stutterers and nonstutterers: The consistency effect. *Journal of Speech and Hearing Research* 12:301–7.

WILLIAMS, D. E., F. H. SILVERMAN & J. A. KOOLS (1969b). Disfluency behavior of elementary school stutterers and nonstutterers: Loci of instances of disfluency. *Journal of Speech and Hearing Research* 12:308–18.

WILLIAMS, D. E., F. H. SILVERMAN & J. KOOLS (1968). Disfluency behaviors of elementary school stutterers and nonstutterers: The adaptation effect. *Journal of Speech and Hearing Research* 11:622–30.

WILLIAMS, J. (1983). Using a computer to control stuttering. *Rehabilitative Literature* 44:74–75.

WILLIAMS, J. D. (1984). Comments on the use of the "Edinburgh Masker" device. DeKalb, Ill.: Northern Illinois University, undated, received 1984.

WILLIAMS, J. D., & R. B. MARTIN (1974). Immediate versus delayed consequences of stuttering responses. *Journal of Speech and Hearing Research* 17:569–75.

WINGATE, M. E. (1988). *The Structure of Stuttering, a Psycholinguistic Analysis*. New York: Springer-Verlag.

WINGATE, M. E. (1986a). Physiological and genetic factors. In G. H. Shames & H. Rubin (eds.), *Stuttering Then and Now*. Columbus, Ohio: Charles E. Merrill.

WINGATE, M. E. (1986b). Adaptation, consistency and beyond: II. An integral account integral account. *Journal of Fluency Disorders* 11:37–53.

WINGATE, M. E. (1986c). Adaptation, consistency and beyond: I. Limitations and contradictions. *Journal of Fluency Disorders* 11:1–36.

WINGATE, M. E. (1984a). Definition is the problem. *Journal of Speech and Hearing Disorders* 49:429–31.

WINGATE, M. E. (1984b). Fluency, disfluency, dysfluency, and stuttering. *Journal of Fluency Disorders* 9:163–68.

WINGATE, M. E. (1984c). Stutter events and linguistic stress. *Journal of Fluency Disorders* 9:295–300.

WINGATE, M. E. (1984d). A rational management of stuttering. In M. Peins (ed.), *Contemporary Approaches to Stuttering Therapy*. Boston: Little, Brown.

WINGATE, M. E. (1984e). The recurrence ratio. *Journal of Fluency Disorders* 9:21–29.

WINGATE, M. E. (1984f). Pause loci in stuttered normal speech. *Journal of Fluency Disorders* 9:227–35.

WINGATE, M. E. (1983). Speaking unassisted: Comments on a paper by Andrews et al. *Journal of Speech and Hearing Disorders* 48:255–63.

WINGATE, M. E. (1980). On the hedge—Daly and Kimbarrow exchange. *Journal of Speech and Hearing Research* 23:217–18.

WINGATE, M. E. (1979a). The first three words. *Journal of Speech and Hearing Research* 22:604–12.

WINGATE, M. E. (1979b). The loci of stuttering: Grammar or prosody? *Journal of Communication Disorders* 12:283–90.

WINGATE, M. E. (1977a). The immediate source of stuttering: An integration of evidence. *Journal of Communication Disorders* 10:45–51.

WINGATE, M. E. (1977b). Criteria for stuttering. *Journal of Speech and Hearing Research* 20:596–607.

WINGATE, M. E. (1976). *Stuttering Theory and Treatment.* New York: John Wiley.

WINGATE, M. E. (1971a). Phonetic ability in stuttering. *Journal of Speech and Hearing Research* 14:189–94.

WINGATE, M. E. (1971b). The fear of stuttering. *Journal of the American Speech and Hearing Association* 13:3–5.

WINGATE, M. E. (1969a). Sound mindedness as a factor in stuttering. *Proceedings of the 77th Annual Convention of the American Psychological Association.* 4:581–82.

WINGATE, M. E. (1969b). Sound and pattern in "artificial" fluency. *Journal of Speech and Hearing Research* 12:677–86.

WINGATE, M. E. (1967a). Stuttering and word length. *Journal of Speech and Hearing Research* 10:146–52.

WINGATE, M. E. (1967b). Slurvian skill of stutterers. *Journal of Speech and Hearing Research* 10:844–48.

WINGATE, M. E. (1966a). Stuttering adaptation and learning: I. The relevance of adaptation studies to stuttering as "learned behavior." *Journal of Speech and Hearing Disorders* 31:148–56.

WINGATE, M. E. (1966b). Stuttering adaptation and learning: II. The relevance of adaptation studies to stuttering as "learned behavior." *Journal of Speech and Hearing Disorders* 31:148–56.

WINGATE, M. E. (1966c). Prosody in stuttering adaptation. *Journal of Speech and Hearing Research* 9:550–56.

WINGATE, M. E. (1966d). Behavioral rigidity in stutterers. *Journal of Speech and Hearing Research* 9:626–30.

WINGATE, M. E. (1964a). A standard definition of stuttering. *Journal of Speech and Hearing Disorders* 29:484–89.

WINGATE, M. E. (1964b). Recovery from stuttering. *Journal of Speech and Hearing Disorders* 29:312–21.

WINGATE, M. E. (1962a). Evaluation and stuttering: I. Speech characteristics of young children. *Journal of Speech and Hearing Disorders* 27:106–15.

WINGATE, M. E. (1962b). Evaluation and stuttering: II. Environmental stress and critical appraisal of speech. *Journal of Speech and Hearing Disorders* 27:244–57.

WINGATE, M. E. (1962c). Evaluation and stuttering: III. Identification of stuttering and the use of a label. *Journal of Speech and Hearing Disorders* 27:368–77.

WISCHNER, G. J. (1952). Anxiety reduction as reinforced in maladaptive behavior: Evidence in stutterer's representations of the moment of difficulty. *Journal of Abnormal Social Psychology* 47:566–71.

WISCHNER, G. J. (1950). Stuttering behavior and learning: A preliminary theoretical formulation. *Journal of Speech and Hearing Disorders* 15:324–35.

WOHL, M. T. (1970). The treatment of non-fluent utterance—a behavioral approach. *British Journal of Disorders of Communication* 5:66–76.

WOHL, M. T. (1968). The electronic metronome—an evaluative study. *British Journal of Disorders of Communication* 3:89–98.

WOHL, M. T. (1966). Reciprocal inhibition—a process of continuous diagnosis. In *Speech Pathology Diagnosis: Theory and Practice.* Report of the National Conference of the College of Speech Therapists. Edinburgh: E. & S. Livingstone.

WOLK, L. (1986). Cluttering: A diagnostic case report. *British Journal of Disorders of Communication* 21:199–207.

WOLPE, A. (1957). Play therapy, psychodrama, and stuttering. In L. E. Travis (ed.), *Handbook of Speech Pathology.* New York: Appleton-Century-Crofts.

WOLPE, J. (1973). *The Practice of Behavior Therapy.* New York: Pergamon Press.

WOLPE, J. (1958). *Psychotherapy by Reciprocal Inhibition.* Stanford, Calif.: Stanford University Press.

Woods, C. L. (1977). Dimensions of the stutterer stereotype. *Australian Journal of Human Communication Disorders* 5:119–25.

Woods, C. L. (1976). Stigma of a disorder. *Australian Journal of Human Communication Disorders* 4:133–39.

Woods, C. L. (1974). Social position and speaking competence of stuttering and normally fluent boys. *Journal of Speech and Hearing Research* 17:740–47.

Woods, C. L., & D. E. Williams (1976). Traits attributed to stuttering and normally fluent males. *Journal of Speech and Hearing Research* 19:267–78.

Woods, C. L, & D. E. Williams (1971). Speech clinicians' conception of boys and men who stutter. *Journal of Speech and Hearing Disorders* 36:225–34.

Work, R. S. (1985). The therapy program. In R. J. van Hattum (ed.), *Organization of Speech-Language Services in Schools: A Manual.* San Diego: College-Hill Press.

Yairi, E. (1983). The onset of stuttering in two- and three-year-old children: A preliminary report. *Journal of Speech and Hearing Disorders* 48:171–77.

Yairi, E. (1982). Longitudinal studies of disfluencies in two-year-old children. *Journal of Speech and Hearing Research* 25:155–60.

Yairi, E. (1973). Item analysis for parental behaviors rated by stutterers and nonstutterers. *Perceptual and Motor Skills* 36:351–52.

Yairi, E. (1972). Disfluency rate and patterns of stutterers and nonstutterers. *Journal of Communication Disorders* 5:225–31.

Yairi, E., & B. Lewis (1984). Disfluencies at the onset of stuttering. *Journal of Speech and Hearing Research* 27:154–59.

Yairi, E., & D. E. Williams (1971). Reports of parental attitudes by stuttering and by non-stuttering children. *Journal of Speech and Hearing Research* 14:596–604.

Yairi, E., & D. E. Williams (1970). Speech clinicians' stereotypes of elementary-school boys who stutter. *Journal of Communication Disorders* 3:161–70.

Yates, A. J. (1963). Delayed auditory feedback. *Psychological Bulletin* 60:212–32.

Yates, A. J. (1963). Recent empirical and theoretical approaches to the experimental manipulation of speech in normal subjects and in stammerers. *Behavioral Research Therapy* 1:95–119.

Yonovitz, A., W. F. Sheperd & S. Garrett (1977). Hierarchical stimulation: Two cases of stuttering modification using systematic desensitization. *Journal of Fluency Disorders* 2:21–28.

Young, E. H. (1965). The motokinesthetic approach to the prevention of speech defects including stuttering. *Journal of Speech and Hearing Disorders* 30:269–73.

Young, M. A. (1975a). Onset, prevalence, and recovery from stuttering. *Journal of Speech and Hearing Disorders* 40:49–58.

Young, M. A. (1975b). Comment on "Stuttering frequency and the onset of phonation." *Journal of Speech and Hearing Research* 18:600–602.

Young, M. A. (1975c). Observer agreement for marking moments of stuttering. *Journal of Speech and Hearing Research* 18:33–40.

Young, M. A. (1965). Audience size, perceived situational difficulty, and stuttering frequency. *Journal of Speech and Hearing Research* 8:401–7.

Young, M. A. (1961). Predicting ratings of severity of stuttering. *Journal of Speech and Hearing Disorders* 7:31–54.

Zalosh, S., & L. F. Salzman (1965). Aftereffects of delayed auditory feedback. *Perceptual and Motor Skills* 20:817–23.

Zemlin, W. R. (1980). *Speech and Hearing Science, Anatomy and Physiology.* Englewood Cliffs, N.J.: Prentice Hall.

Zimmerman, G. (1980a). Articulatory dynamics of fluent utterances of stutterers and non-stutterers. *Journal of Speech and Hearing Research* 23:95–107.

Zimmerman, G. (1980b). Articulatory behaviors associated with stuttering: A cinefluoro-graphic analysis. *Journal of Speech and Hearing Research* 23:108–21.

Zimmerman, G. (1980c). Stuttering: A disorder of movement. *Journal of Speech and Hearing Research* 23:122–36.

INDEX